The RN First Assistant

An Expanded Perioperative Nursing Role

Second Edition

The RN First Assistant

An Expanded Perioperative Nursing Role

Second Edition

Jane C. Rothrock, RN, DNSc, CNOR
Professor, Perioperative Nursing
Delaware County Community College
Media, Pennsylvania

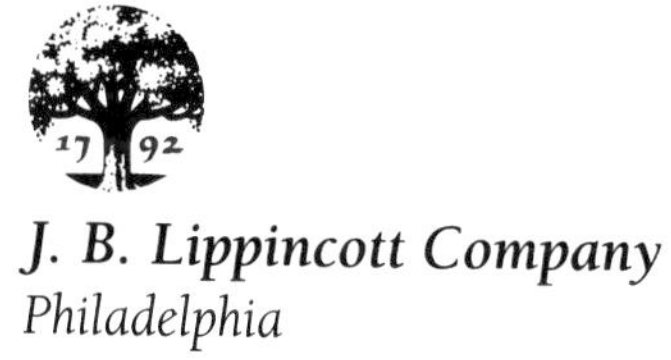

J. B. Lippincott Company
Philadelphia

Sponsoring Editor: David P. Carroll
Coordinating Editorial Assistant: Patty L. Shear
Interior Designer: Ellen Dawson
Cover Designer: Linda Baris
Production Manager: Janet Greenwood
Production: Tapsco, Inc.
Compositor: Tapsco, Inc.
Printer/Binder: R. R. Donnelley & Sons

Second Edition

 Printed in the United States of America. For information write J. B. Lippincott Company, 227 East Washington Square, Philadelphia, Pennsylvania 19106.

6 5 4 3 2

Library of Congress Cataloging in Publications Data

The RN first assistant : an expanded perioperative nursing role /
[edited by] Jane C. Rothrock. — 2nd ed.
p. cm.
Includes bibliographical references and index.
ISBN 0-397-55014-6 (hardcover)
1. Operating room nursing. 2. Surgical nursing. I. Rothrock, Jane C., 1948– .
[DNLM: 1. Operating Room Nursing—methods. 2. Surgical Nursing—methods.
WY 162 R627]
RD32.3.R6 1993
610.73'677—dc20
DNLM/DLC
for Library of Congress

92-48997
CIP

Any procedure or practice described in this book should be applied by the healthcare practitioner under appropriate supervision in accordance with professional standards of care used with regard to the unique circumstances that apply in each practice situation. Care has been taken to confirm the accuracy of information presented and to describe generally accepted practices. However, the authors, editors, and publisher cannot accept any responsibility for errors or omissions or for any consequences from application of the information in this book and make no warranty express or implied, with respect to the contents of the book.

Every effort has been made to ensure drug selections and dosages are in accordance with current recommendations and practice. Because of ongoing research, changes in government regulations and the constant flow of information on drug therapy, reactions and interactions, the reader is cautioned to check the package insert for each drug for indications, dosages, warnings and precautions, particularly if the drug is new or infrequently used.

This book is dedicated to
my partner in life,
Joseph Trimble Rothrock III

CONTRIBUTORS

Arthur S. Brown, MD
Professor and Head
Division of Plastic and Reconstructive Surgery
Robert Wood Johnson Medical School at Camden
Camden, New Jersey

Rudolph C. Camishion, MD
Professor of Surgery and Head
Division of General Surgery
University of Medicine and Dentistry of New Jersey
Robert Wood Johnson Medical School at Camden
Camden, New Jersey

Jacqueline Daly, RN, MSN, CNOR, RNFA
Assistant Director, Perioperative Education
Nursing Operating Room Services
Cedars-Sinai Medical Center
Los Angeles, California

Nancy B. Davis, RN, NP, CNOR
Nurse Practitioner
Cardiovascular and Chest Surgical Associates
Boise, Idaho

Christine C. Espersen, RN, CNOR, RNFA
Cardiac Surgery
Buffalo General Hospital
Buffalo, New York

Denise Jackson, RN, BSN, CNOR, RNFA
RN First Assistant
Shannon Medical Center
San Angelo, Texas

Sergius Pechin, MD, FACS
Faculty, RN First Assistant Program
Delaware County Community College
Media, Pennsylvania

Jane C. Rothrock, RN, DNSc, CNOR
Professor, Perioperative Nursing
Delaware County Community College
Media, Pennsylvania

Robert H. Sculthorpe, DO
Associate Professor and Chairman
Department of Anesthesiology
College of Osteopathic Medicine
Southeastern University of the Health Sciences
Miami, Florida

Patricia C. Seifert, RN, MSN, CNOR, RNFA
OR Coordinator, Cardiac Surgery
Arlington Hospital
Arlington, Virginia

Chester R. Smialowicz, MD
Specialist in Infectious Diseases
Cherry Hill, New Jersey

Richard K. Spence, MD
Professor of Surgery and Head
Section of Vascular Surgery
Robert Wood Johnson Medical School at Camden
Camden, New Jersey

LIST OF REVIEWERS

Althea Dunscombe, RN, CNOR, RNFA
RN First Assistant
Professional Assistants, PRN
Venice, FL

Lynn Martin Carter, RN, BSN, CNOR, RNFA
Project Director, Surgical Services
Wilkes-Barre General Hospital
Wilkes-Barre, PA

Sheila L. Fruehauf, RN, BS, CNOR, RNFA
RN First Assistant
Millard Fillmore Hospitals
Buffalo, NY

Marlene Craden, RN, CNOR, RNFA
RN First Assistant
Millard Fillmore Hospitals
Buffalo, NY

Susan Renee Tatum, RN, MN, CNOR, CNAA
OR Consultant
Baxter Healthcare Corporation
Lake Bluff, IL

Kathleen T. Flynn, RN, MS, CNS
Visiting Faculty, University of Massachusetts
School of Nursing
Amherst, MA

Jane Hershey Johnson, RN, MSN, CNOR, RNFA
Perioperative Nursing Faculty
Delaware County Community College
Media, PA

Jody L. Evans, RN, BSN, CNOR, RNFA
RN First Assistant
Seattle, WA

Dale A. Smith, RN, CNOR, RNFA
RN First Assistant
Brighton Medical Center
Portland, ME

Vicki J. Fox, RN, MSN, CNS, CNOR
Specialty Nursing Services, PC
Tyler, TX

M. Betsy Martino, RN, CNOR, RNFA
RN First Assistant
Medical Center of Delaware
Christianna, DE

PREFACE

In her *Notes on Nursing,* Florence Nightingale suggested the very essence of what perioperative nurses and RN first assistants are doing in the 1990s to meet the challenges of the 21st century:

> No system can endure that does not march. Are we walking to the future or to the past? Are we progressing or are we stereotyping? We remember that we have scarcely crossed the threshold of uncivilized civilization in nursing; there is still so much to do. Don't let us stereotype mediocrity. We are still on the threshold of nursing.

This second edition of *The RN First Assistant—An Expanded Perioperative Nursing Role* is intended to march to the future with the hundreds of RN first assistants who are determined to design that future and cross its threshold. They impel me to march with them; their eagerness, enthusiasm, vibrancy, and commitment enriches my being and my writing. They want to know "why," and I am compelled to want to find an answer with them. They want to know "how," and I am compelled to work with them to discover "how." They would never accept mediocrity in themselves and never expect it from me. The revision of this book is intended to keep us on the threshold.

All of the chapters in this edition have undergone revision, some major and some not so major. The need for only minor revison to many chapters is due in part to the fine work of the contributors to the first edition, whose names you will find in a footnote on the first page of each chapter. There are some new chapters, and I am beyond delighted that some of my former students have contributed their talents and knowledge to walk us forward in our quest to seek better ways and become the best at providing assistance at surgery.

There is no doubt in my mind that we have not written the last word on the RN first assistant. No one who reads these pages will doubt that we still have many unresolved issues and that nursing is changing constantly. Much of what happens in our future will depend on us and our endurance, stamina, courage, and fortitude. The future for the RN first assistant is bright, because that future rests with the nurses who are providing the service. My confidence and belief in them gives me great hope and enormous pride. Many of them (over 750) have been in one of my classes. They are my legacy, and they are the ones who will open a better way in the future. They will choose the road that is best for RN first assistants, and I will be there walking and marching with them.

Jane C. Rothrock

ACKNOWLEDGEMENTS

Perhaps one of the most difficult of the many tasks of editing a book is the concern that your attempt to acknowledge and thank all of the people who saw the project to fruition will fall short on recognizing all those who should be recognized. I am, at the outset, indebted to all of my students who learn with their minds and speak with their hearts. They generously give me courage, motivation, and inspiration. I am also grateful to all of the contributors and reviewers, whose intimate knowledge of the art and science of first assisting enabled them to grasp the significance of the book's content. To the people at J. B. Lippincott, particularly David Carroll and Patty Shear, I thank you for steering me in the right direction with your perceptive editing and expert guidance. To my colleagues at Delaware County Community College, thank you for sharing my passion about the RN first assistant. Finally, I need to name the people who always give me love and understanding when I am working on a book; they excuse me for being so busy, call me back when I'm taking a break, ask how it's going when I have to miss their company, and patiently wait for our quality time together. Thanks, Joe, Dad and Sally, Jan, Harold, Rachael, Brittany, Rick, Sue and Sean. You always care about my causes and share my hopes and dreams, with unfailing faith and constancy.

CONTENTS

The RN First Assistant

An Expanded Perioperative Nursing Role

Second Edition

1 History of the RN First Assistant Role

*Jane C. Rothrock**

> Each regiment in this civilian army had brought its own physician. Medical and surgical treatment by these men—known as regimental surgeons—seemed even less likely of success than that of their military brothers. They were hometown doctors of varied ability, and needed only the approval of the regimental commander and a rubber stamp from the colonial legislature before receiving their commissions.[1]

The origins of the nurse's role as assistant during surgery are evidenced throughout history. For centuries, nurses have assisted physicians during surgical procedures in the home and the hospital. The evolution of medicine and surgery is paralleled by the development of professional nursing and the place of the nurse in the operating room.[2] In particular, wounds inflicted during war and the new technology needed to repair these wounds created the opportunity and the need for the nurse to act as a surgical assistant.

In the 18th century there was little formal education available for nurses or surgeons. In 1775, during the Revolutionary War, less than 300 of the 3,500 regimental surgeons had received a medical degree. Most physicians in colonial times were apprentice trained. The primary qualification for these apprentice "doctor's boys" was the ability to stand the sight of blood.[3] Apprenticeships lasted from 3 to 6 years, after which the fledgling new physician was ready to do bloodletting, tooth-pulling, wound dressing, and minor surgery. Advanced skills were learned on the battlefield, where wounds,

---

* *The authors of this chapter in the first edition were Rena Lawrence and Sally A. Lawrence.*

burns, and fractures were treated and amputations and trepanning skull fractures were undertaken. The surgeon was attended by a "surgeon's mate"; nurses, who were females, were kept from the battlefield and waited to attend the soldiers as they were removed to a hospital.

In this era, assumption of the role of "nurse" was even less standardized than the apprenticeship system for surgeons. Throughout the colonial era, caring for friends and relatives was an important societal role for women. Nursing was often taught from mother to daughter or learned by a domestic servant as part of her job. Ministering to the sick was expected of all women in the family. Nursing was a woman's duty, and as the economy began to expand, older widows and spinsters from the working class "professed" themselves as nurses. Also known as "natural-born" nurses, these women often came to their profession when other forms of employment were closed to them; nursing then became their obvious choice for work.[4] Working either in the home or hospital, many of these nurses were devoted women who demonstrated caring and concern in their duties. However, the quality of their efforts and their skills were more disparate than similar; some blundered badly beyond their capabilities or knowledge.[5]

Advances in science, the work of Florence Nightingale, and the introduction of formal training for nurses furthered the development of the role of nurse as first assistant.[6] Nightingale defined nursing as "putting the patient in the best condition for nature to act upon him."[7] She emphasized cleanliness, quiet, and environmental control, all of which are important to both the caring and the curing roles of nursing and vital to effective surgical intervention.

IMPACT OF WARTIME

CRIMEAN WAR

During the Crimean War, from 1854 to 1856, Florence Nightingale and her staff of 125 nurses provided nursing services at the Barrack Hospital in Turkey. The hospital, with 4,000 patients in a facility designed to care for 1,700, was infested with maggots, lice, rats, and other vermin.[8] There were no clean dressings, clothing, or bedding. Food and water were extremely limited; there was no soap or water for cleaning either the patients or the hospital. Physicians were in drastically short supply, nurses were essentially nonexistent, and patients cared for one another.

Emphasizing cleanliness and environmental control, Nightingale instituted sanitation measures and obtained needed food, water, and supplies. She stressed the importance of the nurse's role in managing and supervising patient units and the operating room. Her care, combined with her vigilance, her identification of the role of cleanliness in infection control, and her insistence on environmental sanitation, became basic principles for managing a hospital as well as critical elements in nursing interventions in the operating room. She cautioned the surgical nurse to "be ever on the watch, ever on guard, against want of cleanliness, foul air, want of light, and of warmth."[9]

The role of nurse as first assistant was initially conceived during Nightingale's tenure. At the physician's side, the nurse prepared wounds for surgery and assisted during the surgical procedure. Meticulous care of the surgical site and prevention of infection were of paramount importance. The perioperative role, beginning on the patient ward with sanitation and care of the sick, accompanying the patient to the operating room and acting as a nurse participant, and resuming care activities of the postoperative patient and wound, became the basis for role evolution.

AMERICAN CIVIL WAR

During the Civil War, 1861 to 1865, conditions in hospitals and operating rooms were similar to those found in the Crimea. Dorothea Dix, Florence Nightingale's American counterpart, and a nursing force of 10,000 provided care to thousands of wounded soldiers. Cleanliness and infection control were the primary nursing directives. Dix adopted and practiced many of the principles established by Nightingale, and this war again saw the nurse assuming responsibilities of the first assistant in surgery. Amputation was the predominant surgical procedure.[10] Abdominal surgery was extremely high risk; hemorrhage and infection were grave complications. Postoperative infection and bleeding were of such magnitude that nurses continuously concerned themselves with tying off bleeders and cauterizing blood vessels with heat. The primary disinfectant used by the nurse was alcohol, although in 1865 Lister began to use carbolic acid to soak dressings, slowly reducing the 45.7% surgical mortality rate associated with limb amputation.[11]

Nurses of the Civil War era left important legacies as they worked to improve patient welfare and influence wartime health policies. Nursing care in the United States was revolutionized during this war, and nurses were influential in creating the impetus for change. With its incredible demands for the care of hospitalized soldiers, the Civil War triggered the beginning of respectable, well-educated women extending their knowledge of nursing care outside their own circle of family and friends. Social barriers were breached as more women knowledgeable in the principles of nursing care began to practice nursing in hospitals. This was not accomplished without overcoming the prejudices of head surgeons in the hospitals, however. Woolsey related these prejudices in her diary:

> Hardly a surgeon of whom I can think received or treated them (women nurses) with even common courtesy. Government had decided that women should be employed, and the army surgeons—unable, therefore, to close the hospitals against them—determined to make their lives unbearable that they should be forced in self-defense to leave . . . Some of the bravest women I have ever known were among the first company of army nurses. They saw at once the position of affairs, the attitude assumed by the surgeons, and the wall against which they were expected to break and scatter; and they set themselves to undermine the whole thing.[12]

The nurses of the Civil War won the grudging respect of surgeons and were often idolized by their patients. Despite the fact that army surgeons initially wished to bar them from hospitals, these nurses went on to become regional and national heroes. Using perseverance, plain talk, and political power, they radically transformed the care of hospitalized soldiers.[13]

SPANISH-AMERICAN WAR

The Spanish-American War, in 1898, had one major land battle that resulted in 968 casualties and 5,438 deaths from disease due to poor sanitation and yellow fever.[14] An all-graduate nurse staff replaced medical corpsmen in caring for the war victims. Although surgery was limited, advances were made in preventing transfer of disease and infection. These epidemiologic discoveries helped to both advance surgical recovery and expand the role of the nurse first assistant. After the war, government investigations led to the founding of the Army and Navy Nurse Corps. These corps helped stabilize the role of the nurse as first assistant and led to advanced specialization in operating room nursing.

WORLD WAR I

During World War I, 8,587 American nurses cared for 184,000 wounded and sick soldiers on the European front.[15] This war also saw a large volume of amputations for which the nurse acted as first assistant. The nature of the wounds mandated the need to remove much dead and devitalized tissue. Frequently, stretchers were placed directly on the operating table. With clothing quickly cut away, one nurse would begin to administer chloroform and ether while another nurse, functioning as first assistant, cleaned the wound with gasoline, then iodine, and began the procedure of wound debridement.[16]

The use of gas warfare created new problems. The gas destroyed lung tissue and caused massive burns; in particular, the eyes, face, and hands were severely affected by first-degree burns.[17] Again in a first assistant role, the nurse assumed primary responsibility for burn dressing, wound debridement, and pinch grafting. The nursing emphasis on infection prevention continued to direct care activities.

The nursing literature of the era generated ideas regarding the changing focus of nursing roles. Themes that emerged related to, in part, the nature of nursing education. The need for educational preparation that developed the individual, allowed for the acquisition of general knowledge, educated the nurse for citizenship and social reform, and developed patterns of critical thinking would eventually have a strong influence on the nursing profession and on the education of its practitioners.[18]

WORLD WAR II

During World War II, more and more nurses functioned as first assistants in both civilian and military facilities. On the civilian front, 23% of the available patient beds and operating rooms were not used because nursing personnel were scarce. Student nurses represented 80% of the work force in the 1,300 hospitals with schools of nursing or affiliated with schools of nursing. By 1944, casualties numbered as high as 1,750 per day.[19] "Give us nurses; 10,000 needed overnight" became the national call.[20] By June 1945, 29% of all graduate nurses were on duty with the armed forces.[21]

The combination of personnel shortages and high casualty rates gave impetus to the continued need for the RN to act as first assistant. In this role, nurses opened and closed wounds; the surgeon performed the internal interventions. Tying and clamping of bleeders was a routine nursing function. Nursing experience with abdominal and chest surgery was increasing, and nurses sometimes performed procedures such as tracheostomy and chest tube insertion. New sorting and treatment possibilities—such as triage, antibiotic therapy, transfusions, and rehabilitation—led both nursing and medicine into the fledgling technological era of health care. At no other time in American history were nurses in greater demand. Nursing roles expanded in response to this demand, and the RN first assistant filled a patient care need with efficiency and acumen.

World War II also brought important changes in American society that affected nurses. The changing roles of women, increasing levels of education among the general population, advances in medical science, and altered economic conditions contributed to changing patterns of nursing practice. Nursing in the home increasingly shifted to clinics and hospitals as a result of the public health movement. Nursing curricula began to accommodate advances in science, especially medical science, to prepare nurses not only with knowledge but also with an understanding of both the "what" and "why" of changes in nursing practice. This upgrading of nursing's educational standards was opposed by many physicians and hospital administrators, who were concerned about possible reductions in nursing school enrollments, the possibility of nurses becoming more independent in their actions and less obedient to the demands of physicians, the threat of competition by highly educated nurses taking over aspects of the physician's role, and the possibility of such educated nurses passing judgment on physicians' work.[22] Despite such opposition, however, the need for a strong science background and critical thinking and judgment abilities would continue to make itself felt in the educational preparation of the RN first assistant. Unquestioning obedience was no longer compatible with standards of nursing behavior or with the practice of nurses who met the rigorous demands of perioperative patient care during the war.

KOREAN WAR

The Korean War, 1950 to 1953, witnessed the expansion of the nurse's role as first assistant in Mobile Army Surgical Hospitals. These MASH units were each staffed with 16 skilled nurses who perfected the role of first assistant. Skill and knowledge were essential; nurses worked long hours assisting in complex procedures under adverse conditions. Triage became a nursing responsibility during this war. Nurses assessed patient injury, prioritized casualties for surgery, provided initial emergency intervention, and administered emergency medical services. Eventually, the role of the medical corpsman evolved as a part of wartime medicine, but this did not deter some nurses from holding onto the role and responsibility that had evolved for the RN first assistant. This role continued to be important to the military forces in both Vietnam and the Middle East during "Desert Storm."

THE STUDENT NURSE AS FIRST ASSISTANT

From 1873 until the early 1930s, hospital nursing staffs often consisted of a superintendent of nurses (who was a graduate nurse) and nursing students. As late as 1926, 549 nursing schools had no full-time graduate teachers; the remaining 894 schools had from one to six graduate teaching faculty.[23] In 1927, as many as 73% of the hospitals with nursing schools had no graduate nurses employed for general duty. Hospitals without schools were staffed by attendants.[24] Graduate nurse staffs increased slightly during the 1930s but decreased again in the 1940s. Even from 1944 to 1945, student nurses provided nearly 80% of the nursing services in hospitals affiliated with schools.[25] Consequently, hospital operating room nurses were often students.

Various early nursing texts referred to the nursing role in the operating room, describing the perioperative nurse as a provider of indirect and direct nursing care and as a first assistant. Weeks, in 1890, stated that two nurses were in attendance at the operating table, emphasizing the participant nature of their roles: "You are present not as a spectator, but as an assistant."[26] In 1901 Luce described the role of the operating room nurse: "The operating room nurse assists the surgeon with sponges, ligatures, and sutures; she keeps the instruments clean and ready for use, and is sometimes required to hold retractors or specula."[27]

Usually four nurses participated in a surgical procedure; these nurses were sometimes referred to as a permanent operating room nurse, a senior operating room nurse, and two junior operating room nurses.[28] The nurse in charge of the room, called the circulating nurse in later years, prepped and draped the patient in the etherizing room while the surgeon completed another patient procedure. Two nurses were in attendance with the surgeon at the operating table. One of these two nurses was to retract viscera, assist during the surgery, and attend to the routine of closure.[29, 30, 31, 32] The other nurse was often referred to as the "sponge" nurse. Senn described the practice of sponging: "If asked to do the sponging, she (nurse) does not wipe but merely compresses the bleeding parts, allowing the sponge to absorb what it will."[33] The fourth nurse administered anesthesia.[34, 35, 36]

Over the years, the vital nature of anesthesia administration and of the role of first assistant became recognized, and students were not permitted to fill these roles. By the 1930s, anesthesia was administered only by graduate nurses. By the 1960s, only graduate nurses were permitted to act as first assistants.

THE PRIVATE DUTY NURSE AS FIRST ASSISTANT

From 1873 to the late 1920s, private duty nursing was the primary area of employment for the graduate nurse. A limited amount of this private duty was performed by students, who were sent into private homes by proprietary hospital schools to render nursing service. During this time, and even until the late 1920s, many surgical procedures were performed in the home. Wound morbidity and mortality were lower for persons receiving surgery in the home than for those receiving surgery in the hospital.

Early nursing literature described processes used to prepare the home for surgery. Descriptions included precise suggestions for creating suitable conditions for operating. Instructions were offered for converting the kitchen and stove into a good operating room and sterilizer.[37] DeLee provided a detailed description of how to prepare the home for obstetric procedures, including vaginal forceps delivery, craniotomy, decapitation, and abdominal caesarean section.[38] DeLee advised that " . . . a kitchen or library table makes an excellent operating table; a sewing table does well for the instruments and basins; a euchre table gives additional space. Two kitchen chairs with a table board on them makes an excellent side table."[39]

Weeks described in detail the practice of cauterizing vessels with nitrate of silver and tying off bleeders. This was an essential part of the nurse first assistant role. According to Weeks, "the artery is picked up by a pair of forceps, and a ligature tucked firmly about it. A ligature should be about eighteen inches long . . . Test its strength well, so as to leave no chance of its breaking when strained; and if you have to tie, be sure and make it a firm knot."[40] She went on to detail how to make the surgeon's reef knot, the surgeon's knot, and the cat's paw, complete with diagrams and the dictate that nurses practice these knots.

EDUCATION OF THE NURSE FOR THE OPERATING ROOM

Formal schools of nursing in the United States originated in 1873 and were modeled on the Nightingale schools in England. In the early years of nursing education, the theory component included the use of surgical instruments, hemostasis, and preparation of the patient for surgery. Perhaps no better metaphor of the importance of the nurse in surgery during this time period exists than Thomas Eakin's painting *The Agnew Clinic*. This famous painting reflects Eakin's fascination with the new hospitals in the 19th century. Lynaugh suggested that by asking Mary Clymer, a student at the new school of nursing at the Hospital of the University of Pennsylvania, to pose for the scene in the surgical amphitheatre, Eakins "sought to convey a new ideal of professional training and competence set against disease, pain, and death. In his portrait, she [Mary Clymer] stands in the shaft of light that is counterpoint to the figure of Agnew, the famous surgeon memorialized in the painting. She is there as Eakin's symbol of a vibrant age, full of optimism and promise."[41]

The contributions of the nurse in the surgical amphitheatre and then the operating room were widely acknowledged as vital to the success of the operation and to the surgical patient's welfare. The number of hours in theory instruction gradually increased, and the National League for Nursing Education began publishing curriculum guides for schools. The 1937 edition of this publication recommended that operating room theory and practice be covered in the second year of 3-year diploma programs and that students be prepared to assist in operations and emergencies.[42]

In 1933 the Committee on the Grading of Nursing Schools reported that nursing schools placed a high priority on operating room nursing and that most schools included the recommended 6- to 8-week clinical rotation for this specialty. Objectives for the curricular undertaking in operating room nursing included an understanding of the relationship between the procedure and the patient's safety, an improvement in skill in nursing patients in the operating room, and an understanding of operating room techniques and their scientific basis.[43] In 1942 the National League for Nursing Education, in an attempt to alleviate the nursing shortage and prepare practitioners in a shorter time, proposed three different plans to reduce the 36-month diploma program. Consistently, the high priority given to operating room nursing resulted in the recommendation that this experience be increased from 6 weeks to 8 weeks.[44] Beginning in 1945, nursing education made earnest and valid efforts to transform the role of the student as nonpaid hospital employee to that of academic participant. Essential to this transformation was the use of full-time, qualified nurse faculty to guide academic development. These changes had a negative impact on operating room nursing. The expense of the small ratio of faculty to students in the operating room was not cost-effective, and students' clinical experience in the operating room began to decrease in schools.

Compounding this problem was the emergence of specialization by surgeons and by operating room nursing staffs. As early as 1961, a surgical nursing textbook stated that "in these days of specialization, it is essential that knowledge be built on a foundation of sound basic science, for then it does not matter whether work is done in a plastic, thoracic, or general surgery unit."[45] The rapid development of new surgical treatments and new knowledge required operating room nurses to become versatile members of the surgical team. The role of circulating nurse became increasingly complex; this nurse simultaneously became instructor, supervisor, and patient care manager in the assigned operating room. The scrub nurse of the 1970s needed "above all else, experience. This must be intelligent experience, based on a thorough understanding of each proposed surgical procedure and a careful observation and anticipation of each step in the operation."[46] To help students fully appreciate the importance of these nursing roles, authors specified various assignments and purposes for the student nurse's first, second, third, and fourth operating room experiences.[47] Based on the view that only highly trained and experienced personnel could fulfill the complicated and highly responsible functions of operating room nurse, it was believed that student nurses should be advanced slowly and progressively during their surgical experiences. Nursing curricula, on the other hand, could ill afford the time required for this slow progression. "Scrubbing up to assist the surgeon" was a duty that a ward nurse should be familiar with, but that was performed by nurses who specialized in the operating room.[48] Soon, the goals of student rotations also became more oriented toward familiarization with the role than toward skill or competency in it.

Despite the efforts of the Association of Operating Room Nurses (AORN), with its well-designed and patient-focused learning modules for nursing educators who oversaw curricular content for nursing in the operating room, by the 1980s experience for students in the perioperative nursing role had all but disappeared from basic nursing curricula. The long-term impact of this change and its influence on not only perioperative nursing but all of nursing have yet to be determined.

FACTORS INFLUENCING THE FIRST ASSISTANT ROLE, 1945 TO 1992

The period following World War II was marked by major increases in hospital construction, increases in elective surgery procedures, and a continued severe nursing shortage. The preferred solution to the health care personnel emergency was to free the nurse to nurse, a solution proposing that specific tasks and nonnursing duties could be performed by less-skilled personnel. Brown was the primary originator and long-term advocate of this concept. Writing in 1948, she stated that "the graduate staff nurse should be freed, or should free herself, to the maximum degree from those relatively unimportant duties still performed by her in order that she may concentrate her whole attention, within the voluntary hospital, upon the acutely ill and those in greatest need of total care."[49]

Brown also emphasized that no institution should pay for nursing services that could be performed as effectively by a person with shorter preparation than the RN. The Brown Report called for increasing use of practical nurses, licensing of practical nurses, use of paid aides to take the place of volunteers who had been used during the war years, and use of a new group of nonnursing personnel classified as technicians.[50] The Brown Report was readily accepted by hospital administrators, third-party payers, and unemployed military corpsmen. The practical nurse entered the operating room and was rapidly followed by the operating room technician. Both of these workers quickly began to replace the RN at the operating table, as scrub nurse and as first assistant.

By 1965 the use of operating room technicians had become an accepted practice. The mid-1960s also brought the return of large numbers of independent duty corpsmen. These persons had received the equivalent of practical nurse training in their military programs. They were also proficient in the execution of emergency medical measures. Increasing numbers of these corpsmen entered the civilian job market each year. Coupled with a physician shortage, these events abetted the emergence of yet another health care worker who entered the operating room. These workers have become the physician's assistant in today's market. By 1970, the physician's assistant was functioning as first assistant during surgery. With the advent of the technician and the physician's assistant, the roles of the professional nurse in the operating room, as scrub person and first assistant, were seriously threatened.

The 1970s and 1980s were marked by articulate debate and concerted attempts to clarify the role of the professional nurse in the operating room. The philosophical premise on which the operating room nurse has explored role ambiguity and role clarification is the concern with providing safe, economical patient care. It is this concern with the patient that has driven and continues to drive the activity surrounding research on the perioperative role, scope of practice for RN first assistants, and third-party reimbursement.

By 1980 the American College of Surgeons (ACS) had defined the duties of the first assistant. In this definition the role of the RN as provider of first assistant services was affirmed. However, the ACS emphasized that when the RN functions in this capacity, those assigned duties must fall within the scope of the nurse's State Nurse Practice Act.

In 1980 AORN developed guidelines for the RN functioning as first assistant. These guidelines also emphasized that when the RN serves as first assistant, the first assistant functions must fall within the scope of the pertinent Nurse Practice Act.[51]

By 1983 the RN was permitted to function in the role of first assistant in 17 states. However, only the state of Washington clearly stated that the RN could function as a first assistant and still function within the scope of the Nurse Practice Act. The majority of states considered first assistant practice to be a delegated medical function or a function regulated by hospital policy. Twelve states firmly stated that the RN could not function as a first assistant because this function was not clearly identified within the scope of their Nurse Practice Acts. Many other states continued to study the question.[52]

In 1983 AORN appointed a task force to study and clarify the role responsibilities and qualifications of the RN first assistant. The task force issued its report and presented its findings as guidelines for position assumption; the AORN House of Delegates approved these in that same year. Thus a landmark movement to return nurses to their rightful role as first assistant took shape in this country. Committed to and energized by the issue, perioperative nurses became politically active patient advocates.

An event in Pennsylvania portrayed what was occurring across the nation. On June 19, 1980, the Pennsylvania State Board of Nurse Examiners ruled that RNs could not function as first assistants and further stated that any nurse who did function as a first assistant would be liable for malpractice. As the RN first assistant movement swept the country, Pennsylvania nurses began taking steps to reverse the Board's position. AORN members contacted

Board members and set up a process of dialogue and debate. These nurses extensively interviewed and surveyed practicing operating room nurses and clearly identified for the State Board what nonnurses were doing as first assistants and the inherent danger of such practice for the consumer. A detailed plan of action was developed. Information relative to the AORN goal was disseminated to other nursing organizations in an attempt to gain and solidify professional nursing support. In November 1984, representatives of the Pennsylvania Council of Operating Room Nurses met with the State Board of Nurse Examiners to discuss proposed changes in the interpretation of the Nurse Practice Act.

During the November meeting of the Pennsylvania State Board of Nurse Examiners, the previous ruling concerning first assistant practice was withdrawn. The State Board ruled that first assisting did fall within the scope of nursing practice under the Professional Nurse Act. This decision was made possible because the Board stated that according to the Pennsylvania Professional Nurses Law's definition of nursing, nursing practice is allowed if it provides for "provision of care supportive to or restorative of life and well being and executing medical regimens as prescribed by a licensed physician or dentist."[53] In addition, provision for allowing the RN to function as a first assistant was covered under rules and regulations relating to the responsibilities of the RN in Section 21.11, General Functions, specifically:

> Carries out nursing care actions which promote, maintain, and restore the well being of individuals.
>
> The Board recognizes standards of practices and professional codes of behavior as developed by appropriate nursing organizations as the criteria for assuring safe and effective practice.[54]

Since 1985 there have been rapid, persistent, and promising efforts and events that have clearly confirmed the importance of the role of the RN first assistant. As first assistant educational courses began to flourish, the ranks of perioperative nurses prepared to assist at surgery swelled. Legislative efforts were initiated, seeking third party reimbursement from both private and federal payers. The *Core Curriculum For The RN First Assistant* was published in 1990, and activities were undertaken to develop a certification examination for RN first assistants in 1992. Repeated surveys of Boards of Nursing indicated that by 1992 no states ruled that assisting at surgery by the RN was outside the scope of nursing practice. Instead, all states had either rendered an opinion that the RN could first assist or had declined to render an opinion.

In testimony of AORN on reimbursement for nonphysician providers before the Physician Payment Review Commission, it was noted that:

> The RN first assistant is a very versatile professional whose contribution to the patient is not limited to intraoperative "assisting" the surgeon. Preoperatively, the RN first assistant is involved in taking the patient history and doing the physical examination. They also teach the patient, order routine laboratory tests, check the x-rays, evaluate the patient's emotional status, and check

> on last-minute details of the surgery schedule. Immediately before the surgery, the RN who will later assist the surgeon assists the anesthesiologist with insertion of intraoperative monitoring lines and preliminary procedures. Intraoperatively, the RN first assistant assists the surgeon with the surgical procedure itself. Specific tasks are directly related to the specialty, training, and education of the RN first assistant. Virtually every surgical specialty uses RN first assistants. More than 40% work in general surgery, with 24% evenly split between orthopedic and cardiovascular specialties. Plastic surgery, gynecology, and ophthalmology are also popular specialties who utilize the services of a RN first assistant. RN first assistants are experts in their area of practice. For example, those who are employed by cardiovascular surgeons may in fact harvest veins for cardiac bypass surgery. The specific procedures for which an RN first assistant is credentialed would be determined by the individual hospital credentialing procedure. All RN first assistants do not do the same procedures, but they do share common skills such as retraction, tying sutures, clamping bleeding vessels, and closing incisions. Postoperatively, the RN first assistant makes rounds to evaluate the patient's condition and remove sutures, chest tubes, central monitoring lines, and in some cases intra-aortic balloons. Many RN first assistants also see patients in the physician's office postdischarge, at which time they do a great deal of patient teaching.[55]

The window of opportunity for RN first assistants is wide open in the 1990s. The nursing literature has provided cumulative evidence that nurses deliver cost-effective care that can be substituted for a physician's care in many instances. Studies have been done linking surgical volume with lower inpatient mortality and indicating that hospitals with a larger proportion of RNs provide better care as measured by lower mortality rates. The problem with many of these studies, however, is that they do not isolate or measure the specific nursing contributions to improvements in patient care. The clarion call for the 1990s must be the development of a body of research that validates the contributions of the RN first assistant. Such research should focus on operating room productivity, quality and outcomes of care, intraoperative contributions, practice settings, roles and responsibilities, effects of collaboration, nurse-generated innovations, cost-effectiveness, utilization, and reimbursement patterns. As RN first assistants develop this body of knowledge, what is now only intuitively and experientially known will become visible and evident to all who seek to confirm the value of the RN first assistant to the efficient and effective care of perioperative patients.

CONCLUSION

The role of first assistant has always been an integral part of perioperative nursing. Although specific aspects of role dimension have been modified throughout history, the vital nature of the knowledge base and the skill level possessed by the perioperative nurse have always pointed to this person as the best prepared nursing team member to provide care to the surgical patient. For a time this role, as well as the quality of health care provided to the consumer, was at risk. By 1985 the role of the RN as first assistant had made a full historical circle and repeated itself. The future will determine the full impact of the importance of the RN first assistant role as well as its impact on nursing itself, nursing in the perioperative arena, and quality perioperative patient care.

REVIEW QUESTIONS

Please select the best response to the following questions. Answers are provided at the conclusion of the review question section.

1. During colonial development in the United States
   a) nursing service had a distinctive role
   b) nursing of the sick was done by women in the home
   c) colonial medicine was in the hands of educated physicians
   d) boards of health instituted important sanitation measures
2. In the early part of the 18th century, hospitals became so crowded that cleaning was impossible in a hospital ward. This furthered the belief that
   a) respectable people considered it a disgrace to send a relative to the hospital
   b) educated women and women of the upper class should participate in hospital nursing
   c) it was a woman's social responsibility to change these deplorable conditions
   d) nurses should be paid higher wages, considering their working conditions
3. The service of nursing began its slow climb up the ladder of respectability when Florence Nightingale sailed for Scutari in the Crimea in 1854. The results of her efforts are well known and proved the value of
   a) accepting female nurses in a military hospital
   b) nursing collaboration with medical staff
   c) having social contacts to purchase resources for care of the ill
   d) using prepared individuals (her 38 nurses) in the care of the ill
4. In her *Notes on Nursing*, Nightingale depicted nursing as
   a) performance of household and laundering chores
   b) the proper use of fresh air, light, warmth, and cleanliness
   c) unfailing loyalty and obedience to the physician
   d) the duty of devoted women, despite their subordinate position
5. At the beginning of the Civil War, there were no organized nursing groups, no ambulances, and no field hospital service. The woman appointed Superintendent of the Female Army of Nurses was
   a) Mary Ann Bickerdyke
   b) Louise Schuyler
   c) Dorothea Dix
   d) Louisa May Alcott
6. The goals of nursing leaders of the late 19th century focused on
   a) subverting medical opposition to female doctors
   b) developing schools of nursing in Universities
   c) trying to contain hospital costs for nursing service
   d) improving nursing service and widening opportunities for women

7. During World War I
   a) Clara Barton became Superintendent of the Army Nurse Corps
   b) some nurses served with surgical teams close to the front lines
   c) nursing care continued to consist of routine care and comfort
   d) nurses were forbidden assignment in camp, evacuation, or mobile hospitals
8. The nursing profession emerged from World War I with
   a) a deep sense of pride in its accomplishments
   b) little eagerness for a more independent status for nurses
   c) a sad lack of increased prestige in the eyes of the public
   d) a renewed zeal for private duty nursing
9. In the first third of the 20th century, nursing began to think of protecting those needing nursing service. Nurses realized that one way to do this was by
   a) organizing labor unions to improve working conditions
   b) using students, rather than graduates, to keep costs down
   c) changing the 24-hour work day to a 12-hour work day
   d) advocating nurse registration
10. There were 1,619 nurses serving in World War II who received medals for their service. For perioperative nursing and RN first assistants, one of the most important outcomes of this war was their
    a) replacement in operating rooms on the home front by practical nurses
    b) demonstrated ability in front-line aid stations and field hospitals
    c) development of psychosocial skills to keep up the morale of the wounded
    d) assignment to bedside nursing in war zones, which added a preoperative role dimension to their practice
11. At the close of the 1970s, nurses were finding themselves in conflict with demands from physicians to take on tasks once done only by physicians. For the RN first assistant, an example of such task conflict was
    a) performing blood pressure measurement
    b) expanding into labor and delivery to assist at complicated births
    c) tying surgical knots and suturing wounds
    d) administering intravenous conscious sedation
12. A study of nursing education with many implications for the contemporary nurse was *Nursing for the Future* by Esther Lucille Brown, published in 1948. Brown recommended that
    a) educational programs for practical nursing be improved but that practical nurses not be licensed
    b) the hospital environment foster the nurse's professional growth and free her to "nurse"
    c) specialty hospitals be expanded and educational programs for nurse specialists be developed
    d) education for nurses remain hospital-based to provide the requisite clinical skills demanded by medical advances
13. The 1984 AORN Official Statement on the RN First Assistant acknowledged the importance of this nursing practice area in achieving optimal results for the patient. To provide this type of assistant-at-surgery, AORN recommended that the RN first assistant

a) not concurrently function as a scrub nurse
b) obtain advanced preparation in a master's program
c) have CNOR as a minimal certification
d) be hired by a surgeon and be directly responsible to that surgeon

14. The term *perioperative* encompasses
    a) scrub nurses
    b) circulating nurses
    c) RN first assistants
    d) all of the above

15. In the 1990s, the role of the RN first assistant
    a) is primarily intraoperative
    b) is important in small hospitals without residents
    c) has expanded beyond the confines of the surgical suite
    d) is threatened by lack of nursing support

Answer Key

1. b	6. d	11. c
2. a	7. b	12. b
3. d	8. a	13. a
4. b	9. d	14. d
5. c	10. b	15. c

REFERENCES

1. Wilbur CK: Revolutionary Medicine. Chester, Globe Pequot Press, 1980
2. Colp R, Keller MW: Textbook of Surgical Nursing. New York, Macmillan, 1927
3. Wilbur, p 1
4. Reverby S: A caring dilemma: Womanhood and nursing in historical perspective. Nursing Research 36:5–11, 1987
5. Ibid, p 6
6. Atkinson DT: Magic, Myth, and Medicine. New York, World Publishing, 1956
7. Nightingale F: Notes on Nursing. New York, Dover Publications (Original work published 1859), 1969
8. Kalisch PA, Kalisch BJ: The Advance of American Nursing. Boston, Little, Brown & Co, 1978
9. Nightingale, p 71
10. Kalisch and Kalisch, pp 49–66.
11. Sigerist HE: The Great Doctors. New York, WW Norton & Co, 1933
12. Dannett SGL: Nobel Women of the North. New York, Thomas Yoseloff, 1959
13. Ragge MM: Nursing and politics: A forgotten legacy. Nursing Research 36:26–30, 1986
14. Kalisch and Kalisch, pp 216–220
15. Ibid, p 315
16. Quandt E: Active service on the western front. Am J Nurs 18:454–455, 1918
17. Interviews with nurses and patients who served during World War I. Lebanon Veterans Hospital, 1955–1957
18. Hanson KS: An analysis of the historical context of liberal education in nursing education from 1924–1939. J Prof Nurs 7:341–350, 1991
19. Kalisch and Kalisch, pp 471–478
20. Ibid, p 478

21. Ibid, p 483
22. Hanson, p 344
23. Some problems in grading our schools of nursing. Trained Nurse and Hospital Review 77, November, p 509, 1926
24. Kalisch and Kalisch, p 363
25. Ibid, p 478
26. Weeks CS: Textbook of Nursing, 2nd ed. New York, Appleton, 1897
27. Luce M: The duties of an operating room nurse. Am J Nurs 1:404–406, 471–473, 1901
28. Fowler RS: The Operating Room and the Patient. Philadelphia, WB Saunders, 1918
29. VanSyckel J: The operating room technique at St Luke's Hospital, New York. Am J Nurs 10:635–638, 1910
30. Colp and Keller, p 291
31. Bertella M: Operating room routine: The training of students. Am J Nurs 24:377–380, 1924
32. Colp and Keller, p 14
33. Senn N: A Nurse's Guide for the Operating Room. Chicago, WT Keene, 1902
34. Weeks, p 199
35. Senn, p 13
36. Kalisch and Kalisch, p 183
37. Woodbury LC: Surgical nursing. Am J Nurs 13:688–693, 1903
38. DeLee JB: Obstetrics for Nurses, 3rd ed. Philadelphia, WB Saunders, 1909
39. Ibid, p 181
40. Weeks, p 245
41. Lynaugh, J: Diary of a nurse. Nursing Research 40:254–255, 1991
42. Committee on Curriculum of the National League for Nursing Education: Nursing Schools of Today and Tomorrow, Final Report of the Committee on the Grading of Nursing Schools. New York, Committee on Grading of Nursing Schools, 1937
43. Stewart I: The Education of Nurses. New York, Macmillan, 1943
44. National League for Nursing Education: Nursing Education in Wartime (Complete Series of Fourteen Bulletins). New York, National League for Nursing Education, 1945
45. Taylor S, Worrall O: Principles of Surgery and Surgical Nursing. London, The English Universities Press Ltd, 1961
46. LeMaitre G, Finnegan J: The Patient in Surgery, Philadelphia, WB Saunders Co, 1970
47. Ibid, pp 87–120
48. Moroney J: Surgery for Nurses. London, Churchill Livingstone, 1971
49. Brown EL: Nursing for the Future. New York, Russell Sage Foundation, 1948
50. Ibid, pp 57–72
51. Task force defines first assisting. AORN J 39:502–503, 1984
52. Survey shows state board position on first assistant. AORN J 37:428–436, 1984
53. Professional Nursing Law, Commonwealth of Pennsylvania. Act 151, 1974
54. Rules and Regulations of the State Board of Nurse Examiners for Registered Nurses, Commonwealth of PA, 1983
55. Testimony of the Association of Operating Room Nurses on Reimbursement for Nonphysician Providers before the Physician Payment Review Commission, September 13, 1990

2 The Nurse Practice Act and Expanded Roles

Jane C. Rothrock*

The practice of nursing for both registered nurses (RNs) and licensed practical nurses (LPNs) or licensed vocational nurses (LVNs) is regulated by the law of each state. The law is set forth in a nurse practice act, which must be approved by the state senate and house and signed by the governor. In addition to the act, rules and regulations promulgated by the state board of nursing have the weight of law and clarify the implementation of the act. For example, the act requires that the RN have a current license to practice, and the rules and regulations spell out procedures and requirements for obtaining the license, including items such as required educational background and fees. Each nurse should have a current copy of his or her state nurse practice act. It is in reference to "the act" that first attempts are made to determine "what is nursing?"

PURPOSE OF THE PRACTICE ACT

The purpose of the law is to protect the consumer. By issuing licenses it is possible to control who practices nursing and to ensure that the practice meets approved standards. Also, by limiting the practice of nursing to licensees and restricting impostors, substandard care is avoided and nurses are protected from less qualified persons who may try to displace them.

Many health and other professions and occupations are regulated by the law in each state, and it is necessary to have a valid license to practice. A trend among other health care personnel is to press for the rights of licensure

---

* *The author of this chapter in the first edition was Janette L. Packer.*

so that their practice will be recognized, defined, and protected. It is necessary that nurses monitor this movement so that nursing practice is restricted to qualified personnel. In this period of growth in the health professions, various health-related groups want to carve niches within the health care industry. Professional nurses have a responsibility to make sure that patients receive the best possible care, which involves more than performing tasks. It also includes assessment, diagnosing, planning, implementing, evaluating outcomes of care, and teaching, which must take into account the total family and the various resources available.

EARLY LICENSURE EFFORTS

The idea of licensing nurses began in 1867 in England, where Dr. Henry Wentworth Ackland, a physician, made unsuccessful efforts to protect the public by recognizing qualified nurses. The banner was taken up by a nurse, Ethel Gordon Bedford Fenwick, but as early as the 1890s nurses were divided in their support of nursing licensure. Florence Nightingale was a strong opponent of licensure, because she was concerned that qualifications established for licensure would not give sufficient weight to moral characteristics. Knowing how hard Nightingale fought to raise nursing to a respected profession rather than merely the work of servants and prostitutes, it is understandable that she would be protective. But this divisiveness in nursing resulted in the delay of licensing in England until 1919, long after the first nurse practice act was passed in New Zealand in 1901.

In the United States, North Carolina passed its nurse practice act in 1903, followed shortly thereafter by New Jersey, New York, and Virginia. These acts included the major rights and requirements of nursing practice that remain relevant today. They specified the right to the title RN, required that graduates pass an examination, and provided a grandfather clause allowing those practicing to be licensed by waiver. The most impressive aspect of this success is that nurses managed to guide these acts through the legislative process at a time when women did not have the right to vote. This demonstrates what can be accomplished when nurses work together. The cooperative, dedicated work of these early nurse leaders should be an example to all nurses.

Chaska[1] divided the development of nursing legislation into three phases. In the first phase, from 1903 to 1938, the focus was primarily on registration. From 1938 to 1971, as the profession developed, the emphasis was on defining the scope of practice. We are now in the third phase, struggling with the concepts of advanced practice and the expanded role of the nurse, which will be discussed in more detail.

BOARDS OF NURSING

Each state or jurisdiction has its own board or boards; some have one board for RNs and another for LPNs. Boards are administered according to the statutes of the jurisdiction. Some nurse boards are under the jurisdiction of the education department; others are responsible to the commissioner of a bureau of professional regulation or licensure. The administrative organization has implications for the autonomy and independence of the board.

BOARD COMPOSITION

Appointment to the board varies in each state but usually requires senate approval; the appointment is made by the governor, commonly for a period of 4 to 6 years. In some states board members are elected. Most boards govern both RNs and LPNs and typically consist of RNs, LPNs, and consumers. In some states physicians serve on the nurse board. It is helpful to have a balanced board with members representing both practice and education as well as different regions of the state. All nurse members should be well prepared and active in professional nursing. The reasons for this will become apparent in the discussion of board functions.

NATIONAL COUNCIL OF STATE BOARDS OF NURSING

At the 1978 convention of the American Nurses Association (ANA), the delegates voted to form the National Council of State Boards of Nursing (NCSBN), comprised of the member boards. At the NCSBN annual meeting, two delegates from each member board vote on issues in the house of delegates meetings. The President and Board of Directors are elected and committees are elected or appointed as specified by the bylaws, mindful of the differing needs in each jurisdiction.

The purpose of the NCSBN, as stated in the preamble to the bylaws, is to provide an organization through which boards of nursing act and counsel together on matters of common interest and concern affecting public health, safety, and welfare, including the development of licensing examinations in nursing. Decisions and recommendations are made by the delegate assembly and the Board of Directors. Member boards are grouped into four geographic areas to meet to discuss local issues, review the effects of national-level proposals on the region, and share ideas and prepare presentations to the delegate assembly that have national impact.

Licensing Examinations

One of the most important services that the NCSBN provides for its member boards is preparing and delivering the National Council Licensing Examination for RNs (NCLEX-RN) and for LPNs (NCLEX-PN). The Board of Directors solicits from each jurisdiction the names of nurses knowledgeable in specialty fields representing both nursing service and education. From these names the examination writers are selected. A professional testing service constructs the examination based on the test plan. Each examination includes a few trial items that are analyzed for reliability and difficulty level. As all states have the same required score for passing the examination, endorsement of licensure from one state to another is facilitated. Provisions to protect the integrity of the examinations are supervised by the Administration of Examination Committee.

PURPOSE AND FUNCTIONS OF STATE BOARDS

The purpose of state boards is to protect the public by supervising the implementation of the practice act(s). "The power of each state legislature to regulate practice through licensure laws is a result of the federal Constitution's delegation of the police power to the individual states under the 'state rights' provision of Article X of the U.S. Constitution."[2] The function of each board is based on the contents of the practice act. As was discussed earlier, the acts have developed as the nursing profession has evolved and have arrived in their present form through negotiation with interest groups and the influence of legislators.

Nurse Practice Acts

In 1980 the ANA updated its 1955 statement and published a document entitled "The Nursing Practice Act: Suggested State Legislation."[3] Later, in 1982, the NCSBN published "The Model Nursing Practice Act."[4] Both of these publications were based on extensive preparation, including the findings of committees and suggestions and comments from members. The NCSBN used the results of a research project to formulate its model act, which was approved by the House of Delegates. Models provide guidelines for states rewriting their acts and provide a degree of consistency that facilitates interaction between states and reduces confusion for licensees.

Although the practice acts are similar in outline from state to state, they vary in detail, content, specificity, and length. All practice acts include a definition of nursing (which involves the scope of practice), and most include the organization of the state board, approval of nursing education programs, and conditions of licensure, including definition of violations and disciplinary actions. Other sections included by some states are definitions of advanced practice, expanded role, and entry level.

The first task of the act is to define the practice of nursing. Most states have a flexible definition that allows nurses to practice in the many varied situations in which nurses are placed—from critical care to preventive health care. Although necessary, this broad definition can be frustrating for the practicing nurse who wants specific answers to questions of scope of practice. Some of these answers may be found in the rules and regulations or in specific statements made by the state board.

Both the ANA and NCSBN model acts include definitions of RN and LPN practice (see Chart 2-1). In the drafts of the NCSBN definition of RN and LPN practice, comments and rationales were given for the recommended statements. It was explained that the definition of nursing purposely excluded educational preparation and responsibilities common to all health professions so that

CHART 2-1

Comparison of ANA and NCSBN Suggested Definitions of Nursing

Practice of Nursing (ANA)

The practice of nursing means the performance for compensation of professional services requiring substantial specialized knowledge of the biological, physical, behavioral, psychological, and sociological sciences and of nursing theory as the basis for assessment, diagnosis, planning, intervention, and evaluation in the promotion and maintenance of health; the case finding and management of illness, injury, or infirmity; the restoration of optimum function; or the achievement of a dignified death. Nursing practice includes but is not limited to administration, teaching, counseling, supervision, delegation, and evaluation of practice and execution of the medical regimen, including the administration of medications and treatments prescribed by any person authorized by state law to prescribe. Each registered nurse is directly accountable and responsible to the consumer for the quality of nursing care rendered.

The practice of practical nursing means the performance for compensation of technical services requiring basic knowledge of the biological, physical, behavioral, psychological, and sociological sciences and of nursing procedures. These services are performed under the supervision of a registered nurse and utilize standardized procedures leading to predictable outcomes in the observation and care of the ill, injured, and infirm; in the maintenance of health, in action to safeguard life and health; and in the administration of medications and treatments prescribed by any person authorized by state law to prescribe.

(From American Nurses' Association: The Nursing Practice Act: Suggested State Legislation, p 6. Kansas City, American Nurses' Association, 1980. Reprinted with permission.)

Practice of Nursing (NCSBN)

The "practice of nursing" means assisting individuals or groups to maintain or attain optimal health throughout the life process by assessing their health status, establishing a diagnosis, planning and implementing a strategy of care to accomplish defined goals, and evaluating responses to care and treatment. Registered Nurse. "Registered nurse" means a person who practices professional nursing by:

- assessing the health status of individuals and groups
- establishing a nursing diagnosis
- establishing goals to meet identified health care needs
- planning a strategy of care
- prescribing nursing interventions to implement the strategy of care
- implementing the strategy of care
- authorizing nursing interventions that may be performed by others and that do not conflict with this act
- maintaining safe and effective nursing care rendered directly or indirectly
- evaluating responses to interventions
- teaching the theory and practice of nursing
- managing the practice of nursing
- collaborating with other health professionals in the management of health care.

(continued)

CHART 2-1. ***Comparison of ANA and NCSBN Suggested Definitions of Nursing*** *(continued)*

Licensed Practical Nurse. "Licensed practical nurse" means a person who practices nursing by:

- contributing to the assessment of health status of individuals and groups
- participating in the development and modification of the strategy of care
- implementing the appropriate aspects of the strategy of care as defined by the board
- maintaining safe and effective nursing care rendered directly or indirectly
- participating in the evaluation of responses to interventions
- delegating nursing interventions that may be performed by others and that do not conflict with this act.

The licensed practical nurse functions at the direction of the registered nurse, licensed physician, or licensed dentist in the performance of activities delegated by the health care professional.

(From National Council of State Boards of Nursing: The Model Nursing Practice Act, 1982. Reprinted with permission.)

the definition clearly specifies what is the province of nurses. Most state definitions for RNs include the steps of the nursing process from assessment through evaluation, teaching, supervision, and also reference to professional judgment and accountability. Many include reference to nursing diagnosis; the definition often contains language similar to the following: "Nursing is the diagnosis and treatment of human responses to actual or potential health problems."

Scope of practice decisions may be in the form of rules and regulations, statements of policy, or informed opinions. Rules and regulations must be promulgated, which entails publication in the official state bulletin, usually allowing a period during which the public has an opportunity to respond. If there is very limited opposition or no opposition, the decision bears the weight of statutory law; if violated, legal action can be taken against the licensee. A statement of policy or an informed opinion may be used in case law. The only difference between the two is that the statement of policy is published in the state bulletin. However, depending on the statute, a waiting period for public comment is not always required. A licensee may perform an act defined as outside the scope of practice without legal repercussions, but if that nurse's practice is questioned, the licensee is subject to court hearing, where the opinion of the state board may be used by the prosecuting attorney.

Boards are frequently pressured by nurses and administrators to issue scope of practice decisions; this is one of the most perplexing areas of board function. When making such a decision, the board must consider many factors, such as the difference between practice in large urban medical centers and in small rural hospitals, implications for quality improvement and risk management, and educational opportunities and levels of preparation and competence of nurses.

Licensees should keep in mind that they should not undertake a task unless they believe that they can complete it safely—which presupposes knowledge of procedures necessary to deal with complications that may occur. This holds true in all situations except emergencies when life-saving measures are instituted. Because nursing is a profession, it carries with it certain responsibilities, including accountability and use of sound judgment.

Organization of the board includes such considerations as membership and meetings. Three types of meetings are possible: open meetings where decisions are made, which are open to the public; work sessions where the preliminary work is done in preparation for meetings; and executive sessions, which are closed to the public and during which private concerns such as personnel matters are discussed.

The extent of the board's responsibility for educational matters is defined in the practice act. Some laws require supervision only of programs leading to licensure, which would include baccalaureate and associate degree programs as well as diploma programs. Other state boards are authorized to monitor the RN/BSN completion programs and those programs offering a master's degree. The rules and regulations set forth standards for curriculum, faculty and administrators' qualifications, and student health and welfare policies. Educational institutions are visited on a regular basis.

Licensure

The board's last major function is concerned with issuing and taking action against licensees. The board in each state contracts with the NCSBN to administer the licensing examinations, issues licenses to the successful candidates, and endorses licenses from nurses in other jurisdictions.

Laws directly affecting licensure vary among jurisdictions. One of the most basic differences is whether licensure is permissive or mandatory. All of the early nurse practice acts were permissive. The first mandatory act was passed in New York in 1938, although it did not become effective until 1947. Under mandatory acts the nurse must obtain a valid license before practicing. Permissive laws regulate the use of titles, which means that individuals may perform nursing acts but may not use the title "nurse" or "registered nurse." By the mid-1980s, most states had adopted mandatory licensure.

A license is a property right and cannot be taken without due process, which entitles the licensee to a hearing. The most frequent basis for action against a licensee is substance abuse. Many states have agreements that allow action against a license to be taken in one state based on action taken in another state. The NCSBN maintains a national disciplinary data bank so that action taken in each state is reported nationwide; however, not all jurisdictions avail themselves of this service.

Actions taken are revocation or suspension of license, with or without probation. Revocation is for an unlimited period and suspension is for a specified period, but in both cases the licensee must surrender her or his license and cease practicing.

Laws are being passed that facilitate action against licensees. Mandatory reporting laws require that if one licensee knows or strongly suspects that another licensee is breaking the law (for example, diverting controlled substances), then the first licensee must report the second licensee's behavior within a specified time or else face punishment by law. Another provision of law is that the state board may automatically suspend a license for a limited period pending formal action if it is deemed dangerous for the licensee to continue to practice. Mandatory reporting and automatic suspension laws usually include a clause that protects a person taking action in good faith.

Probation is sometimes used in conjunction with suspension; that is, the suspension is stayed for probation. The terms of probation for substance abuse may include drug screens, reports from treatment programs, and work evaluations. The advantage to probation is that should the licensee break the terms of probation, then the license can be suspended immediately without the need for a second hearing. The advantage to the licensee is that she or he may continue to practice in a safe and supervised manner, thus encouraging rehabilitation.

Depending on state law, other situations may incur disciplinary action. Having been found guilty of a felony or being negligent or incompetent in the practice of nursing is usually grounds for action. Besides action against the licensee, fines also may be levied.

A suspended or revoked license may be reinstated. As mentioned before, suspensions frequently carry time limits; at the completion of this term, the licensee is usually requested to fulfill specific requirements to end the suspension. In cases of revocation, the plaintiff may at any time request reinstatement by board action. This frequently requires a formal hearing as the minimal condition for a decision.

MONITORING OF BOARDS OF NURSING

Most state professional and occupational boards are monitored by the state's "sunset law." The purpose of this law is to ensure that only viable boards are continued, which is a reasonable requirement as some boards do not even meet and some can rarely assemble a quorum to take action. Among boards, the nurse board usually has the highest number of licensees and many monitoring functions, so it conducts a large quantity of business.

Sunset Audit

The sunset audit involves investigation by an appointed group, usually supervised by a specified senate or house committee. The committee reviews all aspects of function including budget, number of cases investigated and completed, the consistency of minutes with actions, and the keeping of records. In addition to the internal audit, external professional groups and other licensees are invited to respond to questions regarding the operations of the board. Ideally, when the audit report is complete it is made available to the board for comment before being presented to the designated legislative committee at an open hearing. Testimony is heard and, based on all the findings, the practice act is revised as necessary. In revising the practice act, the responsible senate or house committee makes a recommendation that must be approved by both the senate and the house. If there is a difference of opinion, then a joint subcommittee is formed to negotiate agreement, and a date is set for final signature by the governor.

If the act is not acted on positively, then the board is disbanded. Many states include in their sunset laws a clause that creates a grace period for recreating or disbanding the board in an orderly way. This safeguard is the result of boards being disbanded because of a technical problem such as the legislature's not acting because of a heavy work schedule and then recessing. If the nurse board stopped functioning it would seriously affect licensees and the public. Among other things, no licenses could be issued or endorsed, no examinations could be given, and there would be no way to take action against licensees or to control practice.

Since the first sunset law was passed in Colorado in 1976, many states have accepted this procedure. As part of the process the acts are opened, thus creating an opportunity for special interest groups to submit recommendations for change. These recommendations must be carefully monitored so that the public is protected and the board can operate efficiently.

BEYOND THE GENERALIST

Movement toward advanced preparation or specialization in nursing, as in any other discipline, is initiated by three forces: new knowledge pertinent to the field, technologic advances, and response to public need or demand.[5] Since the 1900s, consistent with rapid advances in technology and evolving professional and social demands, the practice of nursing has become more complex. The changes have resulted in new patterns of nursing, each with their own roles and titles. Specialization in nursing practice has been a major advance in nursing over the last few decades. This can certainly be construed as healthy growth within the profession; the great need and demand for nursing specialties and nurse specialists is a vibrant source of nursing's strength.

One danger of such growth in specialties, however, is the confusion that this can create in the public's perception of the system. Other dangers lie in the lack of agreement about what constitutes each role, who should define the roles, and lack of clarity and consistency about who sets and implements standards. If state boards do become involved in credentialing advanced specialty practice, then they should be prudent. First, it is necessary to satisfy the "rational relationship" test by demonstrating that by recognizing these specialized groups the public welfare and safety will be protected. Related to this, there must be provision for taking action against the credential with a clear process for providing the licensees with due process to protect their rights. Second, there may be antitrust implications if there is a question of limiting access to the profession and thus restraining trade.

One requirement of a profession is that it be self-regulating. Nursing achieves this through the legislative authority vested in the nurse boards and through the definition of practice, ethical standards, certification of specialists, and criteria for accreditation developed by nursing organizations. In defining the general practice of nursing, the ANA and the NCSBN both have issued clear statements that are not in conflict and that are reflected to some degree in the majority of the acts. The situation becomes more complex when considering standards for advanced practice in the developing specialties. These standards may be implemented by government-supported agencies, such as state boards, or professional organizations such as the ANA or, for perioperative nurses, the Association of Operating Room Nurses (AORN).

Nursing specialties originate and are recognized in many ways. Some of these include recognition by educational programs, state or national certification programs, specialty organizations, and councils such as those of the ANA. New specialties and the bodies that recognize them continue to change and proliferate. Styles, in an attempt to review, summarize, and analyze specialties in nursing, identified the following characteristics as indices of the "maturity" of a specialty:

practice: The practitioner is defined as a professional nurse; differentiation is recognized (though not necessarily through certification) between a generalist in a specialty area and a master's-prepared clinical nurse specialist or practitioner; definitions of functions and areas of responsibility exist; standards of practice are defined.

education: A baccalaureate degree in nursing is the prerequisite for entry into a specialty education program (or there is an intent to implement this standard); graduate level and continuing education in the specialty are available (or emerging); the specialty organization is accredited as a provider of continuing education.

research and development: Visible support and resources exist; the knowledge base for the specialty is identified, empirically based, and identifiable as advanced nursing knowledge; research symposia are conducted regularly.

credentialing: A rigorous program of certification in the specialty is available; a procedure (or plan) for recertification exists.

organization: Concerns and interests of the specialty are represented by an organized body; standards for practice are established; interests of the specialty are represented to nursing-at-large and to other groups as appropriate.

publications: Refereed journals are published; other mechanisms for regular communication are available.

relationship with other professions and disciplines: The specialty recognizes and undertakes joint ventures with the ANA (as the official organization-at-large); communication links and cooperative efforts with other specialty organizations are maintained.[6]

Pressure on state boards to credential nurses in specialties is increasing, because recognition is needed for third-party reimbursement. Legitimacy for a specialty emanates in part from governmental or other third-party payers at the federal and state levels agreeing to reimburse certain "specialists." Reimbursement initiatives are occurring at the state level by amending state insurance laws to authorize payments for RNs with varied educational backgrounds, specializations, and certifications. At the federal level, however, most of the initiatives target advanced practitioners—usually specified as certified nurse practitioners, clinical nurse specialists, certified nurse midwives, and nurse anesthetists. These advanced practice nurse categories often emanate from definitions of "nonphysician providers" of Medicare services.

A significant change in the financing of health care services was the introduction of Medicare's prospective payment system. This major financing innovation has numerous evolving implications for nursing payment systems in terms of cost of nursing services, efficient use of nursing resources, and possible support for expanded nursing roles. With a primary objective of minimizing costs, evolving payment systems may underscore the desirability of using midlevel practitioners whenever feasible; access to this level of provider has significant cost-saving implications. As the groundwork for future health care reform is laid, nurses will need to identify the value of their services, identify the nursing component of certain "physician services," and seriously consider the relationship of relative value scales for nursing services. As the delivery of health care in this country is being restructured, provider payment reform—and not simply physician payment reform—is likely to become an important part of the restructuring process.[7,8,9]

Thus, definitions of advanced practice and their relationship to reimbursement for nursing services will be a major issue for the nursing profession for the remainder of this century. It will not be an easy debate; definitions, decisions, and regulation of such practice need to be refined. In 1985, the ANA clearly stated its opposition to including definitions of advanced practice in the practice acts, citing three main reasons: (1) the professional organization should define nursing practice, (2) other professions become involved with preparing the enabling rules, and (3) regulations may constrict practice.[10] In 1992, however, the multiple economic, legislative, and policy changes affecting health care are requiring new analyses of definitions and implications of advanced nursing practice.

ADVANCED PRACTICE ROLES

Definitions of advanced nursing practice should first be sought in a state's nurse practice act. As part of their accountability for protecting public health, welfare, and safety, boards of nursing are authorized to regulate nursing practice. Many boards have, through statutes and administrative rules, recognized some level of advanced nursing practice. For example, nurse practitioners (NPs) are specifically regulated in 36 states. In 6 states, they function under a broad scope of practice with no specific title protection. In other states, both Boards of Nursing and Medicine regulate NPs.[11] Thus, throughout the states, concepts and definitions of advanced nursing practice vary in interpretation and regulation.

In 1980, the ANA published "Nursing: A Social Policy Statement." Part of this policy statement addressed the nature and scope of nursing practice and described important characteristics of specialization. An integral philosophic thrust of the policy statement originated in the belief that nursing, and the authority to practice as a nurse, is based on a social contract between society and the professions. Society grants the professions authority over their functions and autonomy in the conduct of their affairs. In return, the professions must uphold this public trust by acting responsibly and regulating themselves to assure quality in performance of the profession.

As the nursing profession has matured, so have its body of knowledge and the needs and demands placed on it by the public. As complexity in required patient care services has grown, so has specialization in nursing. As early as 1957, an educational program for clinical nurse specialists was introduced, at Rutgers University. Shortly thereafter, other programs were developed, with many adding the functional role of teacher or administrator to the clinician role. The Master of Science in Nursing (MSN), or a similarly titled degree, is awarded for successful completion of the program. The course content includes core courses (for example, research and theory) along with advanced pathophysiology and nursing science. Clinical nurse specialists function in hospitals and other health care agencies in line and staff positions in the roles of consultants, teachers, researchers, and supervisors, and they accept responsibility for patients requiring complex nursing care.

Some literature and demonstration projects in the early 1960s described the change in role and functions of the nurse as "extender" functions. More commonly referred to as "physician extenders," early role responsibilities focused on illness-oriented care and the assumption of patient care activities that formerly had been part of medical management. Although this was a natural evolution of nursing practice, nurse practitioner programs soon developed that incorporated a health focus. By the late 1960s and early 1970s, the term "nurse practitioner" was being used to designate a nurse who had completed a course of study, either institutional- or program-based, that prepared the nurse for expanded practice. But as nursing began to recognize the need to move these educational programs into the mainstream of education, recommendations were initiated to reserve the title "nurse practitioner" for nurses prepared at the master's level, in recognition of the specialized knowledge and skills required for autonomous practice.

By 1985, the NCSBN had adopted a position paper on advanced clinical nursing practice. Like the ANA, the NCSBN defined the educational preparation as at least a master's degree and recommended that boards of nursing regulate this advanced nursing practice through designation/recognition. Of all the approaches for regulating advanced nurse practice that the NCSBN could have suggested, designation/recognition was the least restrictive. This approach has allowed boards of nursing to establish state-recognized credentials and authorize permission for a nurse to represent herself or himself with those credentials. Unfortunately, however, the resulting variability of titles, education, and scope of practice among jurisdictions has created problems in credentialing, practice parameters, and geographic mobility for designated/recognized nurses in advanced practice.

In 1992 the NCSBN issued a draft position paper that recommends licensure of advanced nursing practice roles in the categories of nurse anesthetist, nurse midwife, nurse practitioner, and clinical nurse specialist. Advanced practice of nursing by these four categories is "based on knowledge and skills acquired in basic nursing education; licensure as a registered nurse; graduate degree and experience in the designated area of practice, which includes advanced nursing theory, substantial knowledge of physical and psychosocial assessment, appropriate interventions, and management of health care status."[12] The NCSBN further elaborated the essential skills and abilities for advanced nursing within the designated area of practice as:

> assessing clients, synthesizing and analyzing data, and understanding and applying nursing principles at an advanced level
> providing expert guidance and teaching
> working effectively with clients, families, and other members of the health care team
> managing clients' physical and psychosocial health-illness status
> utilizing research skills
> analyzing multiple sources of data, identifying alternative possibilities as to the nature of a health care problem and selecting of appropriate treatment
> making independent decisions in solving complex client care problems
> performing acts of diagnosis and prescribing therapeutic measures consistent with the area of practice
> recognizing the limits of knowledge and experience, planning for situations beyond expertise, and consulting with or referring clients to other health care providers as appropriate.

The NCSBN position paper, if adopted, will facilitate direct reimbursement for advanced nurse practitioners. (Federal requirements for Medicare and Medicaid have focused on state authorizations and definitions.) It will also provide title protection to the roles and promote a high level of public protection.

THE RN FIRST ASSISTANT

Definitions and categories of advanced nursing practice do not include the specific title of "RN first assistant." While some RN first assistants have credentials as nurse practitioners or clinical nurse specialists, most do not. At one time, many states would not allow nurses to act as first assistants. In 1984, AORN issued an official statement confirming that in the absence of a qualified physician, RNs with appropriate knowledge and skills are the best-qualified nonphysician personnel to act as first assistant. This position statement (presented in Appendix I) also described the definition, scope of practice, qualifications, preparation, and establishment of practice privileges.[13]

Evolution of this role, and the increasing demand for it by both perioperative nurses and surgeons who value this patient care service, may be reviewed by examining the positions of the states and their boards of nursing. The February 1983 *AORN Journal* report of a first assistant survey listed each state's ruling on whether the RN may perform as first assistant: 17 states allowed RNs to act as first assistants, 14 did not, and 20 did not directly address the issue. In the January 1985 *AORN Journal*, the survey was updated, with 30 states allowing the RN to first assist, 9 clearly not allowing it, and 23 not giving a ruling interpretation. By 1990, only three states still did not permit the RN to first assist. By 1992, no state boards of nursing ruled that first assisting was outside the scope of nursing practice. There remain states where the board has chosen not to rule, however, and there is still active movement toward getting these states to issue opinions.

Many medical boards have a "right to delegate" clause under which the nurse has a broader scope of practice yet remains dependent on the physician. In nurse practice acts that are silent on the issue of first assisting, the inclusion in the act of some authority in accepting delegated medical acts or an "other acts" clause has been the basis for interpreting the act to permit first assisting because nothing in the act forbids it.[14] Most legal definitions of nursing are broad enough to permit a wide scope of practice. However, all RNs are clearly accountable for their actions and, therefore, are both legally and morally responsible for them.

INSTITUTIONAL LICENSURE AND EXPANDED PRACTICE

Institutional licensure, a process by which a state government regulates health institutions, has existed for many years. The focus has been on ensuring that health facilities have adequate standards to protect the consumer. For example, there must be sufficient footage around each patient's bed. A question raised repeatedly is whether institutional licensure should be extended to include personnel.

This terminology is somewhat confusing, because licensure is usually defined as a process by which permission is granted by a governmental agency, whereas credentialing is a more inclusive term including accreditation, licensure, and certification. Where institutional licensure exists, it refers to a situation whereby the institution sets practice within the state government regulations.

Nathan Hershey has long been a proponent of institutional personnel licensure over individual licensure. He clearly states how nurses would be given job descriptions and classifications by the institution, but believes that physicians should be excluded.[15]

If job classification is part of institutional licensure, a major drawback could be that systems may be developed by nonnurses who may interpret nursing care of patients in limited terms. Attention may be given only to physical tasks without understanding the nursing assessment, diagnosis, planning, and evaluation processes. The teaching and advocacy roles that nurses perceive as vital components in the nursing care of patients and families also may be omitted.

The first study of institutional licensure failed to show that the consumer was protected or that career mobility would not be inhibited. If the federal government tries to examine this option again, it probably will be through reimbursement control rather than through confrontation with the states.[16]

When the state board of nursing gives an opinion expanding the role of practice, it is incumbent on institutions employing nurses to decide whether that specific function is acceptable given their circumstances. This decision making usually includes the practice or standards and quality improvement committees, as well as the opinion of the risk manager or legal counsel. The AORN's "Quality Improvement Standards for Perioperative Nursing," Standard II, addresses institutional responsibility: "Delineate the scope of patient care activities or services."[17] This standard suggests that who is served, what services are provided, and who provides the service should be determined as part of the scope of patient care services. Clinical care activities such as circulating, first assisting, scrubbing, and educating patients should then be determined as part of the criteria for an institution meeting the standard.

Difficulties in decision making occur when functions are not clearly delineated. One reason for the lack of clarity is that levels of functions depend on many factors, such as educational preparation, available continuing education and staff development programs, availability to interns and residents, and the fact that nurses tend to be perceived as more capable at night and on weekends.

Another problem associated with expansion of nursing practice is that although nurses may be well prepared, capable of advanced practice, and permitted to perform specified tasks in one institution, these functions may not be approved in another institution. This situation may result in limited job mobility, with the nurse staying in one place and possibly receiving a relatively low salary.

There is no simple solution to this dilemma. Part of the answer lies with the institutions, which need to provide safe care for patients both for humane reasons and for self-protection in a litigious society. Another part of the answer lies with individual nurses, who must accept the increased responsibility and accountability associated with being a professional. Yet another part lies with the professional organizations and the state nurse boards, which need to work together to define nursing for the protection of the public. Underlying these suggestions is the need for nurses to work together to support each other and their administrators.

NURSING INITIATIVES TO INFLUENCE PRACTICE

Nurses have the potential to affect not only nursing, but the total health care delivery system through legislative action. This brings with it the need to act responsibly and in concert. Perhaps the most difficult part is setting up an information network. An immediate resource is the vice president for nursing, who should have copies of the nurse practice act and rules and regulations. The health care facility probably subscribes to the official state bulletin, which provides regular reports on the activities of the boards of nursing, medicine, health, welfare, and education. Nursing organizations, such as ANA, the National League for Nursing (NLN), and AORN, have publications that include legislative information; the RN first assistant must belong to the organizations to receive their mailings. In 1992, AORN supported the formation of speciality assemblies; the Specialty Assembly for RN First Assistants is an important resource when establishing an information network. Some state councils of operating room nurses have task forces or other subcommittees that monitor and respond to issues affecting the practice of RN first assistants. A newsletter for RN first assistants, "First Hand," is another information resource.[18]

State boards operate under the sunshine act, and meetings are open to the public. RN first assistants should set up a roster to send representatives to meetings. Another source of information is related to the professional nurse role as consumer advocate. Contacting local health agencies allows the RN first assistant to determine health care needs in specific geographic areas. Patients are another excellent source of information about needed services.

Once an information and resource base has been identified, the RN first assistant should start working with state representatives and senators in both the work district and area of residence. Useful strategies include building a working relationship with them before it becomes necessary to solicit their legislative support; becoming familiar with how they have voted on health issues; offering to assist with elections by making phone calls or campaigning in some other way; and, if there is pertinent legislation in the state house or senate, informing legislators of how it would affect health care. The RN first assistant also should know the legislative aides who are often available and frequently brief legislators on pending legislation.

It is easy to complain about the "system," but in a democracy the individuals are the system, which makes complaining rather futile. The RN first assistant should be a productive professional by knowing the issues, developing ways to be heard, and then acting in an effective way to improve the health care delivery system and nursing.

CONCLUSION

Nurse practice acts are statutes passed by state legislatures. They define what constitutes nursing. The state nurse practice acts also make provisions for creating state boards of nursing. State legislatures delegate "rule-making authority" to the board of nursing. It is this board that handles specific concerns regarding nursing practice and makes rules to more specifically implement and enforce the nurse practice act. All states have similar statutes that define the practice of medicine. RN first assistants should review both the medical practice act and their nurse practice act, as well as all relevant guidelines, qualifications, or other documents the board may have developed regarding the RN first assistant. Regardless of how the role is defined by the board, the RN first assistant must have the proper education and technical expertise to perform the nursing behaviors required of first assistants.[19]

The AORN official statement on RN first assistants requires didactic and supervised practice and education in surgical assistant content areas before the nurse can assume that role. Many state boards of nursing have adopted the AORN position in their decision that RNs may first assist as part of the scope of nursing practice.[20] Once the RN first assistant is clear about the position and opinions of the board of nursing and has obtained the requisite education for role assumption, clear institutional policies and credentialing mechanisms must be put in place to ensure that the nurse who acts as first assistant is qualified to do so. That is the topic of the next chapter.

REVIEW QUESTIONS

Use the following list of terms to identify the definitions in questions 1-12:

a. Attorney general opinion
b. Constitutional law
c. Law
d. Legal
e. License and licensure
f. Personal liability
g. Policies
h. Rules and regulations
i. Scope of practice
j. Standard of care
k. Standards
l. Statutes

1. _______: criteria of measuring and conformity to established practice
2. _______: branch of law dealing with organization and function of government
3. _______: guidelines within which employees of an institution must operate
4. _______: opinion of the attorney general; opinion is not law, but is given credence should litigation arise on the issue discussed in an opinion
5. _______: legislative enactments; acts of legislature declaring, commanding, or prohibiting something
6. _______: the sum total of man-made rules and regulations by which society is governed in a formally and legally binding manner
7. _______: permission granted by the state to conduct a certain activity that the state board regulates and controls
8. _______: clear and concise statements mandating or prohibiting certain activities
9. _______: each person is responsible for his or her own acts
10. _______: that area of practice legally considered to fall withn the expertise of the registered nurse
11. _______: permitted or authorized by law
12. _______: the professional is expected to exercise that degree of care that other reasonably prudent professionals would exercise under similar situations

Select the best response to the following questions.

13. Nurses may look to several sources of law to determine their scope of practice. These include
    a. the state nurse practice act
    b. rules and regulations
    c. attorney general opinions
    d. all of the above
14. The state's power and authority to regulate through licensure are primarily directed towards
    a. allowing for disciplinary action of licensees
    b. establishing a testing process to determine licensee competence
    c. protecting the public's health, welfare, and safety
    d. preventing encroachment on nursing practice
15. The organization that has as its purpose to provide an organization through which boards of nursing act and counsel together is the
    a. National League for Nursing
    b. National Council of State Boards of Nursing
    c. American Nurses' Association
    d. Association of Nurse Attorneys
16. Many nurse practice acts include a definition of nursing similar to which of the following?
    a. Nursing is the responsibility for knowing the law, practicing within legal boundaries, being accountable for judgments, and maintaining competency in its art and science.
    b. Nursing is the performance of selected acts requiring additional education and preparation.
    c. Nursing is an independent practice that does not require the supervision of a physician.
    d. Nursing is the diagnosis and treatment of human responses to actual or potential health problems.
17. When a state board of nursing gives an opinion regarding a practice issue (such as determining that the RN first assistant may harvest veins), then
    a. all RN first assistants may engage in the practice
    b. institutions must include this in their job descriptions for RN first assistants
    c. institutions may decide whether the function is acceptable as part of the job description
    d. the RN first assistant may legitimately bill the patient for the service

Consider the following situation and then mark "True" or "False" for the questions posed.

Rachael Hutting is a perioperative nurse with 4 years of experience in an operating room. She has her CNOR and is going to a nearby university to obtain her BSN. Rachael has a friend, Brittany, who is an RN first assistant. Brittany attended a college course that required 340 hours of study and supervised clinical practice in first assisting. Rachael also wants to first assist. She believes that her 4 years of experience and her CNOR have prepared her to take on this function. In determining whether Rachael is within the scope of nursing practice to first assist at surgery, the following are proper courses of action:

18. _______ Rachael sh... see whether other perioperative nurses in her AORN chapter are first assisting without having educational preparation.

19. _______ Rachael should write to AORN and request a resource packet on the RN first assistant.

20. _______ Rachael should write to the state board of nursing, requesting any guidelines, opinions, or rules or regulations about the RN first assistant.

21. _______ If the state board of nursing responds to Rachael that they have chosen not to address this issue, then Rachael cannot pursue her goal of first assisting at surgery.

22. _______ On reading her nurse practice act, Rachael notes a provision for "delegated medical acts." She correctly realizes that this might be a first avenue of further exploration.

23. _______ In reviewing the AORN official statement on RN first assistants, Rachael finds a definition stating that "the RN first assistant practices perioperative nursing and has acquired the knowledge, skills, and judgment necessary to assist the surgeon, through organized instruction and supervised practice."

24. _______ Rachael's state board of nursing has determined that first assisting at surgery is within the scope of nursing practice. Therefore, she no longer needs to concern herself with the AORN official statement.

25. _______ Rachael's state board of nursing has determined that first assisting at surgery is within the scope of nursing practice. Therefore, Rachael has the right to demand that her employing institution allow her to first assist, because it is law.

Answers

1. k
2. b
3. g
4. a
5. l
6. c
7. e
8. h
9. f
10. i
11. d
12. j
13. d
14. c
15. b
16. d
17. c
18. F (Although Rachael may be interested in this information, it does not obviate her responsibility for conforming to her state nurse practice act. That is the first source of authority. Rachael should also be guided by information from her specialty nursing association (AORN) and institutional guidelines. A nurse cannot assume that a practice is permissible simply because another nurse performs it.)
20. T

21. F (If the state board is silent on the issue, this does not mean that it is not permissible.)
22. T
23. T
24. F (Nursing practice acts of each state set bounds of practice for nurses licensed under those statutes and serve as a standard of practice. However, standards of practice from specialty nursing associations such as AORN can be used as guidelines for nursing practice. The AORN official position statement should not be ignored.)
25. F (Institutions have the right and responsibility to determine their own policies and procedures. An institution is not required to make provision for the role of RN first assistant simply because it has been determined by the board of nursing to be within the scope of nursing practice.)

REFERENCES

1. Chaska NL: The Nursing Profession: A Time to Speak, pp 613–614. New York, McGraw-Hill, 1983
2. Snyder M, LaBar C: Issues in Professional Nursing Practice. Nursing: Legal Authority for Practice, p 2. American Nurses' Association, 1984
3. American Nurses' Association: The Nursing Practice Act: Suggested State Legislation, p 6. Kansas City, American Nurses' Association, 1980
4. The Model Nursing Practice Act, pp 2–3. Chicago, National Council of State Boards of Nursing, 1982
5. Hoeffer B, Murphy, SA: Issues in Professional Nursing, 5th ed, p 337. New York, Macmillan, 1984
6. Styles MM: On Specialization In Nursing: Toward A New Empowerment. Kansas City, American Nurses' Foundation, 1989
7. Markus G: Considered approaches to physician payment in the '90s. Nurs Econ, 6:63–66, 98, 1988
8. Griffith H: Physician payment reform: Implications for nurses. Nurs Econ, 7:231–233, 1989
9. Jones KR: Evolution of the prospective payment system: Implications for nursing. Nurs Econ, 7:299–305, 1989
10. Piemonte RV: Credentialing: The Thread Between Licensure, Accreditation, and Certification, p 136. New York, National League for Nursing Pub. No. 15-1974, 1985
11. Pearson J: 1991-92 Update: How each state stands on legislative issues affecting advanced nursing practice. Nurse Practitioner, 17:15–23, 1992
12. National Council of State Boards of Nursing: Position Paper on the Licensure of Advanced Nursing Practice. Revised draft, August 13, 1992
13. AORN Official Statement on RN First Assistants, AORN J 39:403–506, 1984
14. Murphy EK: When is the RN first assistant practicing within the scope of nursing? AORN J, 40:256–260, 1984
15. Bullough B: The Law and the Expanding Nursing Role, 2nd ed, pp 111–112. New York, Appleton-Century-Crofts, 1980
16. Chaska NL: The Nursing Profession: A Time to Speak, p 329. New York, McGraw-Hill, 1983
17. Association of Operating Room Nurses: Standards and Recommended Practices for Perioperative Nursing. Denver, Association of Operating Room Nurses, 1992
18. First Hand, c/o QuestRN, Inc., P.O. Box 20, Wallingford, PA 19086
19. O'Neale M: Clinical issues. AORN J 48:520, 1988
20. Murphy EK: OR nursing law. AORN J 44:458, 1986

3 Institutional Credentialing of the RN First Assistant

Nancy B. Davis

In the 1990s there is little debate regarding the commonness of using RN first assistants or the effectiveness of such providers of patient care services. Through either rulings or opinions of boards of nursing, most states have determined that the practice of an RN as an assistant in surgery is either within the scope of nursing or permissible under a portion of the practice act that addresses delegated medical functions. Some states have gone so far as to publish sets of guidelines for RNs acting in this capacity. Nonetheless, most states would expect that such functions be performed only after practice privileges have been granted by a credentialing committee established by the institution. Clear definitions of the role of the RN first assistant must be established within institutional policy; policies should be explicit with regards to the knowledge and skills that an RN first assistant should possess. Institutional practice privileges can limit activities associated with practice as a RN first assistant, but they cannot expand the RN's practice beyond the legal parameters established by the state nurse practice act and the board's interpretation of the act.

CREDENTIALING AND PRACTICE PRIVILEGES

The Association of Operating Room Nurses (AORN) Official Statement on RN First Assistants (reprinted in Appendix I)[1] addresses the need to establish practice privileges in the institution where the nurse is practicing. The position of the American College of Surgeons (ACS) regarding qualifications of the first assistant in the operating room is that "practice privileges of those acting as first assistant should be based on verified credentials reviewed and approved by the hospital credentialing committee."[2] Such requirements are part of the institution's duty towards its patients—assuring that those persons who provide patient care services are qualified to do so. Practice privileges also meet the American Nurses' Association (ANA) requirement that the nursing profession provide methods of identifying and recognizing nurses with specialized skills and experience.[3]

The right to perform certain activities within an institution is a privilege granted through a "credentialing process." This process determines whether the individual is qualified to perform the activities for which the application is being made. This verification is essential for both employees and nonemployees of the institution, although it is possible that the institution's credentialing process will differ for employees and nonemployees. In both instances the credentialing process aims to ensure that established and accepted legal and professional standards for the nurse functioning in the role of first assistant are met. By verifying that the professional nurse is competent to function in the role of first assistant, the institution assures that patients will receive quality care and minimizes the liability exposure of itself and of its staff.[4]

It is important not to confuse the credentialing process with institutional licensure. The term "institutional licensure" has been discussed for several years without being widely accepted or implemented. This system would allow the institution to determine "who can do what" within the institution. Scope of practice would not be determined by professional standards or by legal action. Competency would be determined by standards set within each institution, and variations potentially could have a negative effect on the quality of patient care. Professional associations such as the ANA are opposed to the system of institutional licensure for obvious reasons.

HISTORY OF HOSPITAL CREDENTIALING

The hospital credentialing process was instituted for the purpose of granting hospital privileges to physicians. This process became necessary as increasing numbers of physicians began using hospitals. In the early 1900s there was a growing acceptance of hospitals as centers for treating patients with acute illnesses and for performing surgical interventions. More and more physicians wanted to use the hospital facility as a "workshop." Hospitals were eager for physicians to admit their patients, especially those patients able to pay the hospital for their care. Because physicians determined which patients were to be admitted, they were powerful in influencing how hospitals were managed and controlled.

Physicians who had obtained hospital privileges soon controlled the "credentialing process." Often, other physicians were not granted hospital privileges and were unable to use the hospital for their patients. In 1907 a survey of New York physicians in the Bronx and in Manhattan found that only 10% had hospital privileges. Those physicians who were excluded began establishing their own hospitals, and increasing competition forced hospitals to open their staff privileges to qualified physicians. By 1933, 75% of all physicians had some type of hospital privileges.[5]

Initially, the authority in hospitals passed from trustees to physicians because of financial reasons. In the 1930s and 1940s, however, hospital administrators began challenging physicians' authority over hospitals. Administrators assumed more authority, reflecting the increasing complexity of the hospital's internal organization and its relationship with outside agencies.

There are other reasons for increased control of hospitals by governing boards and administrators. Hospitals have a moral, ethical, and legal responsibility for overseeing the care that patients receive. Because they are legally responsible for physician competence, health care institutions cannot simply "rubber stamp" medical staff recommendations regarding staff privileges. Licenses convey the right to practice; hospital privileges provide the opportunity.

NONPHYSICIAN PROVIDERS

In recent years, nonphysician providers of patient care, such as nurse practitioners, physician assistants, and RN first assistants, have increased their efforts to obtain hospital practice privileges. Although economic independence is certainly a factor in this movement, a major force is the opportunity for professional autonomy. Opposition has come primarily from physicians concerned about the fragmentation of patient care and the competition for health care dollars. Antitrust actions have been initiated by nonphysicians who were denied hospital privileges. In 1982 Tennessee Federal Trade Commission testimony, it was asserted that "access to an essential facility—the hospital—by nonphysician providers in appropriate circumstances may lead to substantial consumer benefits. Both new consumer options and competitive pressures on practitioners already in the market (leading to lower cost and improvements in quality) have potentials for providing important improvements in consumer welfare in the health care field."[6]

THE JOINT COMMISSION ON ACCREDITATION OF HEALTH CARE ORGANIZATIONS

In 1918 the ACS established the Hospital Standardization Program, to standardize hospital care so that a minimum level of care could be ensured. In 1951 other organizations were asked to participate, and the Joint Commission on Accreditation of Hospitals (JCAH) was formed. Initially, the participating organizations were the American College of Physicians, the American Medical Association, the American Hospital Association, and the Canadian Medical Association. The Canadian Medical Association withdrew in 1959 to form its own organization. In 1979, the American Dental Association was granted

JCAH membership. As accreditation by JCAH extended to organizations other than hospitals, its name was changed to the Joint Commission on Accreditation of Health Care Organizations (JCAHO).

The Joint Commission accreditation process is voluntarily accepted by health care organizations. Currently, 8,400 healthcare organizations and programs are accredited by the Commission.[7] Reimbursement by third-party payers often requires Joint Commission approval of the institution. This economic determinant increases the use of the accrediting process. Additional benefits to the accredited institution include enhancement of community confidence in the facility; recruitment of medical staff; provision of educational tools to improve care, services, and programs; and partial or complete fulfillment of state/federal requirements for licensure/certification.[8]

To assist facilities seeking accreditation, Joint Commission publishes the *Accreditation Manual for Hospitals* (*AMH*), which identifies the standards to be met by the institution, specifies the characteristics of each standard, and describes the measures that the institution must implement to meet the standard. Credentialing procedures for RN first assistants who apply for practice privileges within the institution must comply with the Joint Commission requirements.

CREDENTIALING MECHANISMS

Institutions have credentialing mechanisms for granting or denying practice privileges. These mechanisms are based on standards that ensure the accountability and competence of the individual in performing activities within the institution.

In the 1992 *AMH*, Joint Commission standards address the need for the institution's governing body to approve the following:

- ☐ the medical staff
- ☐ the mechanism used to review credentials and to delineate individual clinical privileges
- ☐ recommendations of individuals for medical staff membership
- ☐ recommendations for delineated clinical privileges for each eligible individual
- ☐ the organization of the quality assessment and improvement activities of the medical staff as well as the mechanism used to conduct, evaluate, and revise such activities
- ☐ the mechanism by which membership on the medical staff may be terminated
- ☐ the mechanism for fair-hearing procedures.[9]

The governing body usually bases its approval on recommendations from the medical staff executive committee.

The Commission also posits that the medical staff is responsible for monitoring and evaluating the clinical performance of individuals with privileges. The Surgical and Anesthesia Services chapter of the *AMH* further emphasizes that there must be mechanisms to ensure that each practitioner provides only those services in which he or she has been determined to be competent.[10]

Clinical privileges are based on the individual's license, experience, competence, ability, and judgment. When an individual is being considered for reappointment to the medical staff, or when an individual's clinical privileges are being renewed or revised, information regarding the individual's professional performance, judgment, and clinical and technical skills must be assessed. The Commission fully expects that when an individual has performance problems that cannot be improved, modifications (or other appropriate action) in clinical privileges will be made.[11]

RN FIRST ASSISTANTS EMPLOYED BY THE INSTITUTION

Perioperative nursing in many institutions includes first assistant functions and nursing behaviors. Additional education and experience are necessary for nurses who act as first assistants. The AORN Official Statement on RN First Assistants clearly states that "the RN first assistant practices perioperative nursing and has acquired the knowledge, skills, and judgment necessary to assist the surgeon through organized instruction and supervised practice."[12] This education is often obtained by the perioperative nurse through matriculation in an educational program for RN first assistants. There are many of these programs available throughout the United States. Specific information regarding program prerequisites, length, and curricular content may be obtained from the *Specialty Course Directory* available from AORN.

Joint Commission standards state that "the governing body requires a process or processes designed to assure that all individuals who provide patient care services, but who are not subject to the medical staff privilege delineation process, are competent to provide such services."[13] Competence is the primary consideration in assigning responsibilities to nursing staff. Nursing care standards determine the scope of responsibility based on educational preparation, any applicable licensing laws or regulations, and assessment of current competence. Determination of competence includes an objective assessment of the nurse's performance in delivering patient care services. This process is defined by the institution in its policies and procedures.

Employee credentialing by the institution is a mechanism that can be used for meeting these requirements. This mechanism provides a method for ensuring that the nurse is competent to function in the first assistant role. Not only does this affect the quality of patient care, it also gives the nurse recognition for the skill and knowledge needed to function in this role.

The AORN perioperative nursing credentialing model describes a credentialing process that can be used by an institution.[14] This model is directed toward the credentialing of nurses practicing in the operating room. Specific criteria regarding the employee or new employee are verified by the institution. Files maintained on each employee, updated annually, should contain documentation of the following information:

- ☐ educational qualification (*i.e.*, diplomas, degrees, certificate of completion of RN first assistant program)

- ☐ licensure (verify original and copy for file)
- ☐ peer evaluation (references, letters of recommendation)
- ☐ certification (*i.e.*, CNOR, CRNFA)
- ☐ evidence of continuing education and inservice education
- ☐ verification of orientation
- ☐ job description and skill list
- ☐ performance appraisal and documentation of competence
- ☐ professional development activities (*i.e.*, professional association activity, research, publications) (see Figure 3-1).

Institutions in which first assisting is an expanded perioperative nursing role need to develop a job description specific to first assisting that identifies the qualifications, responsibilities, and functions for the position. The institution may wish to use the job description for the staff nurse position in the operating room that relates to the scrub position and develop a separate job description for first assisting as a supplement. Perioperative nursing staff may function in various roles, such as scrubbing, circulating, or first assisting. A sample job description is shown in Chart 3-1.

A skills list is used in conjunction with the job description. The list is based on the knowledge required to actualize the role and on the employee's ability to perform the specific tasks required. A skills list is maintained on each employee; often this will be the employee's responsibility. The skills may be incorporated in a checklist system or a gradation system, ranging from 1, "not performed," to 5, "able to teach." The skills list for the professional nurse acting as a first assistant must address behaviors specific to that role. The behaviors might be classified in terms of suturing, handling tissue, providing exposure, using instruments, and providing hemostasis. Documentation of the numbers and types of operative procedures in which the nurse has assisted is suggested. The skills list is useful for evaluating the nurse's performance and for providing evidence of continued competence. A sample skills checklist is shown in Chart 3-2.

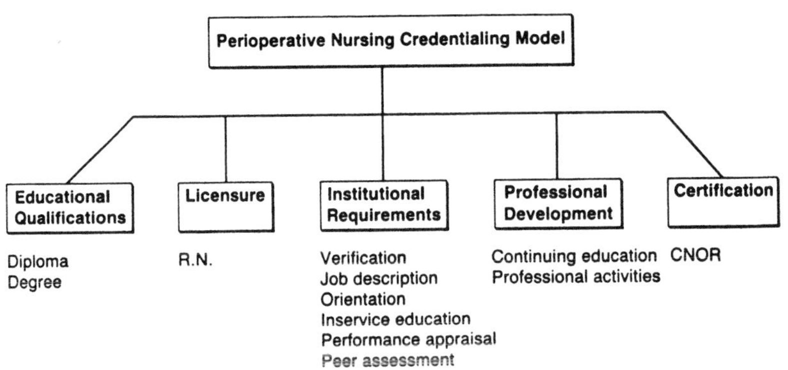

FIGURE 3-1
AORN's perioperative nursing credentialing model. *(Reprinted from AORN J 43(1), 1986. Copyright ©AORN, Inc., Denver, CO. All rights reserved)*

(text continues on page 47)

CHART 3-1

Millard Fillmore Hospitals Job Description

JOB TITLE: RN First Assistant **APPROVED BY:**
DEPARTMENT: Operating Room **DATE:**
REPORTS TO: (TITLE) Nursing Director
Surgical Services

MAIN FUNCTION: Under the direct supervision and direction of the operating surgeon functions during the assisting phase of the role until the conclusion of the operative procedure. Does not function concurrently as a scrub nurse.

DUTIES AND RESPONSIBILITIES:

1. Performs preoperative patient assessment and teaching.
2. Recognizes safety hazards and initiates appropriate corrective action.
3. Applies principles of asepsis and infection control skillfully.
4. Applies knowledge of surgical anatomy, physiology, and operative technique relative to operative procedures wherein the RN first assistant assists.
5. Performs positioning, prepping, and draping of the patient.
6. Provides hemostasis by clamping blood vessels, coagulating bleeding points, ligating vessels, and by other means as directed by the surgeon.
7. Provides exposure through appropriate use of instruments, retractors, suctioning, and sponging techniques.
8. Handles tissue as directed by the surgeon during the operative procedure.
9. Performs wound closure as directed by the surgeon; sutures the peritoneum, fascia, subcutaneous tissue, and skin.
10. Applies surgical dressings.
11. Assists with transfer of the patient from the operating room.
12. Performs postoperative patient evaluation and teaching.
13. Practices within limitations of preparation and experience.
14. Maintains continuing education relative to practice.

EDUCATION REQUIRED: (minimal formal education or its equivalent required to perform the job):

1. Graduate of approved school of nursing—RN
2. Completion of accredited course in RN first assisting

MINIMUM TIME TO LEARN JOB:
The minimum time required to learn job is 3–6 months; relative to opportunity for experience.

SPECIAL REQUIREMENTS: (registration, license, certification) OR OTHER HIRING SPECIFICATIONS (courses, studies, special skills needed or prior experience desired).

1. Licensed as a Registered Nurse in the State of New York
2. CPR Certification
3. CNOR Certification
4. Minimum 5 years diversified perioperative nursing experience; both scrubbing and circulating proficiency.

CHART 3-2

RN First Assistant Skills List

RN FIRST ASSISTANT NAME: ______________________

EVALUATOR: ______________________

DATE: ______________ YEARS PERIOPERATIVE EXPERIENCE: ______________

YEARS RN FIRST ASSISTANT: ______________

** Key	*1	2	3	4	5
A. 1. Identifies normal/abnormal anatomy.					
2. Participates in clinical decision making.					
3. Modifies techniques based on findings.					
4. Anticipates steps in surgical procedure.					
B. 1. Interviews patient and family preoperatively and assesses patient's needs.					
2. Implements and evaluates care plan.					
3. Implements revised care plan based on patient's outcomes.					
C. 1. Communicates relevant data to team members (physical findings, lab data, x-rays).					
2. Discusses radiological/surgical procedures to be implemented during surgery.					
3. Discusses unusual techniques/instruments required based on data collected.					
D. 1. Assists team members as needed.					
2. Collaborates with surgical team members to plan perioperative patient care plan.					
3. Analyzes critical situations and implements appropriate action.					
E. 1. Reports safety hazards and variances in aseptic technique.					
2. Relates changes in patient's condition.					
3. Demonstrates CPR technique.					
4. Reports concerns to appropriate members.					
5. Prioritizes calmly and efficiently in stressful or emergency situations.					
F. 1. Provides appropriate retraction.					
2. Demonstrates proper handling of tissue.					
3. Uses appropriate suctioning techniques.					
4. Demonstrates manual dexterity in the use of surgical instruments.					

CHART 3-2
RN First Assistant Skills List *(continued)*

** Key	*1	2	3	4	5
5. Provides hemostasis using:					
electrosurgery					
bipolar cautery					
clamps					
pressure/sponging					
collagens					
bone wax					
other (state)					
6. Demonstrates suturing skills:					
tying techniques					
ligating vessels					
wound closing					
approximation					
subcuticular closure					
skin closure					
staples					
securing drains					
7. Demonstrates appropriate use of instruments.					
G. 1. Reviews postoperative orders with surgeon and team members.					
2. Reports patient's status to PACU/OPU/ICU personnel.					
3. Participates in patient's and family's education and discharge planning.					

*As defined by Patricia Benner in "Novice to Expert," the Dreyfus Model, pages 21–32.

The Dreyfus Model (page 21) distinguishes between the level of skilled performance that can be achieved through principles and theory learned in the classroom and the context-dependent judgments and skills that can be acquired only in real situations.

STAGE 1. *NOVICE*

- □ has no experience of the situations in which he or she is expected to perform.
- □ is *given* context-free *rules* to guide actions to different *attributes.*
- □ is unfamiliar with goals and tools of patient care.

STAGE 2. *ADVANCED BEGINNER*

- □ *demonstrates* marginally acceptable performance and has coped with enough real situations to note the recurring "aspects of the situation."
- □ *formulates guidelines* (rather than rules) that dictate actions in terms of attributes and aspects.

(continued)

CHART 3-2
RN First Assistant Skills List *(continued)*

STAGE 3. *COMPETENT*

- □ begins to see his or her actions in terms of *long-range goals or plans* of which he or she is *consciously aware.*
- □ *establishes a prospective and a plan* based on considerable *conscious,* abstract, analytic contemplation of the problem and *helps to achieve efficiency and organization* (characteristic of this skill level).
- □ *begins to see* his or her actions in terms of long-range goals or plans of which she or he is consciously aware.
- □ *has a feeling of mastery* and has the *ability to cope with and manage the many contingencies* of clinical nursing.
- □ lacks speed and flexibility of the proficient nurse and does not base conclusions on salient points of the whole picture.

STAGE 4. *PROFICIENT*

- □ *perceives situations as a whole guided by maxims,* rather than in terms of aspects and attributes. Maxims reflect *nuances* of situations and provide directions as to what must be taken into consideration. *Perception is the key.* Practice is not "thought out" but "presents itself" based on experience and recent events.
- □ has a *holistic* undertaking of situations which improves decision making.

STAGE 5. *EXPERT*

- □ *possesses multifaceted knowledge with concrete referents* that cannot be put into abstract principles or explicit guidelines, but rather is based on an intuitive grasp of the situation. No longer relies on analytic principles (rules, guidelines, maxims) to connect his or her understanding of the situation, but zeroes in on the accurate region of the problem without wasteful consideration of a large range of unfruitful alternative diagnoses and solutions.
- □ *operates from a deep understanding of the total situation. The vision of "what is possible"* is one of the characteristics that separate competent from proficient and expert performance.
- □ *possesses an intuitive and holistic overview.*
- □ *implements rapid decision making.*

RN FIRST ASSISTANT NAME: ____________________

EVALUATOR: ____________________

DATE: ____________________

EXPLANATION OF CATEGORIES A, B, C, etc.

**** Key**	**Performance Evaluation**	**Criteria Met**
A.	Demonstrates knowledge base of procedures to which he or she is assigned.	________
B.	Assesses, plans, implements, and evaluates patients' needs and needs of the surgical team.	________
C.	Communicates relevant data to team members.	________
D.	Demonstrates qualities of a team member.	________
E.	Practices continuous surveillance as related to safety hazards, aseptic technique, and changes in patient's condition, and initiates appropriate action.	________
F.	Demonstrates assisting skills.	________
G.	Assists in planning the postoperative care and education of the patient and in the education of the family/others.	________

Florence T. Wilson, R.N., CNOR, RNFA
The Arlington Hospital
Arlington, Virginia

Division: Nursing Department of Surgery
Formulated: August, 1991
Revised: May, 1992

CHART 3-3

ANA Guidelines for Privileges

The ANA believes that nurses (external to organized nursing services) should have the opportunity, through the mechanism of nursing appointments, to gain access to the consumer in health care organizations for the purpose of providing continuity of care in an accountable systematic manner. The nurse appointment is a method of putting into operation the belief that all persons have the right to health care that is accessible, continuing, and comprehensive.

Because of the diversity of the various types of nursing practice, the nurse should apply for a specific type of appointment, one that is within the nurse's limits of competence and meets the consumer's and family's needs. The type(s) of appointment(s) requested may not encompass all the nurse's professional competencies but will reflect the desired area of practice of the nurse in the health care organization to which she applies.

Types of Appointments

The following are examples of types of appointments.

Type A. The appointee gives support to the consumer and family through the health care organization by:

1. providing data to nurses and other health care providers
2. participating in the planning for discharges with the health care team, including the consumer and family
3. maintaining contact with the consumer and family.

Type B. The appointee collaborates with physicians in implementing medical therapies in specified areas.

Type C. The appointee administers direct consumer nursing intervention by:

1. collecting data for nursing intervention, *e.g.*, health history, physical examination, limited laboratory work
2. identifying and providing a specific part of the nursing intervention.

Type D. The appointee provides consultation in a collaborative relationship that allows the appointee to be active in planning part or all of the nursing intervention (nursing order) in conjunction with the staff of the department of nursing services.

In general, there are two kinds of application for nursing services exclusively, as reflected in Types A, C, and D of the preceding examples; the other is for applicants interested in performing designated activities, as in Type B.

(Source: American Nurses' Association: Guidelines for Appointment of Nurses for Individual Practice Privileges in Health Care Organizations, pp 1–2. Kansas City, American Nurses' Association, 1978. Reprinted with permission.)

RN FIRST ASSISTANTS NOT EMPLOYED BY THE INSTITUTION

RNs not employed by an institution but who wish to function as first assistants within that institution must have practice privileges. Application for privileges is usually made through the medical staff, as an affiliate member. Nonphysicians are considered "limited" health care practitioners, in contrast to physicians. Practice privileges are based on the legal scope of the applicant's professional practice and on the need for the services that the individual desires to provide within the institution.

In some institutions, nurses are considered "dependent" practitioners. When functioning as a first assistant, the nurse is under the supervision of the surgeon and is, therefore, "dependent." The nurse's practice privileges usually require a professional association and collaboration with a specific surgeon or group of surgeons. According to the ANA's *Guidelines for Appointment of Nurses for Individual Practice Privileges in Health Care Organizations*, this is a Type B appointment: "The appointee collaborates with physicians in implementing medical therapies in specified areas."[15] (See Chart 3-3 for more details on the ANA guidelines.)

Although credentialing is done through the medical staff, the nursing department is also involved in the process. Standards for nursing care within the institution are the responsibility of the nursing department, and first assisting by RNs is considered a perioperative nursing role.

It is usually necessary for the applicant to provide the credentialing committee with information that might include a description of the role of the RN first assistant, the legal interpretation and constraints of the practice in the involved state, historical information, national trends, acceptance and support from professional associations (*i.e.,* AORN, ACS), as well as educational and certification credentials. This documentation should be gathered and submitted before applying for practice privileges; otherwise, the applicant may encounter resistance and negativism based on the institution's genuine concern for the quality of care when nurses assist in surgery. If negative attitudes exist within the institution, the nurse applying for privileges should remember that change occurs slowly and requires planning, patience, and persistence.

The application process begins with submission of the application form and requisite information to the appropriate committee; this will most likely be the operating room committee or surgical committee, if the medical staff is structured by services. From this committee, the application is usually sent to the executive committee of the medical staff and then to the governing body for the final decision.

Before applying for practice privileges, the nurse should review the institutional policies that apply to practicing within that health care setting. If the institution does not have a policy related to RN assistants or nonphysician assistants, such a policy should be developed and approved before the official application process can begin. Chart 3-4 lists the policy of a medical center in Boise, Idaho.

Institutional policies that govern the role of the RN first assistant should cover activities that may be performed by the nurse, qualifications required, and the mechanism for supervision by the surgeon. The nursing department, medical staff, and administration must be jointly involved in developing policies. AORN's Official Statement on RN First Assistants can provide general guidance to an institution in developing a policy that is specific to the institution.

CHART 3-4

Associated Health Care Professional Policy: Nonphysician First Assistant, St. Luke's Regional Medical Center

Purpose

The purpose of the nonphysician first assistant is to assist the surgeon/employer in those specific procedures that have been identified by the surgeon/employer, and that the nonphysician first assistant has demonstrated the knowledge, experience, and skill to perform as assistant for those procedures. The OR/Surgical Supervisory Committee grants privileges to the nonphysician first assistant.

Qualifications

A. Current Idaho registered nurse license or physician assistant registered with the Board of Medicine

B. Three years of experience as a registered nurse in the operating room with demonstrated knowledge and skill in those procedures for which requesting privileges as a first assistant or evidence of graduation from a physician assistant program with curriculum that includes courses in surgical procedures which have prepared the physician assistant to function in this role

C. Credentials approved by OR/Surgical Supervisory Committee through the following procedure:

1. Employing surgeon submits letter to the OR/Surgical Supervisory Committee requesting privileges for nonphysician first assistant and a copy of liability insurance coverage for nonphysician first assistant.
2. Applicant completes application for nonphysician first assistant privileges, including three current letters of references who can attest to the applicant's clinical skills and ability to perform procedures for which requesting privileges.
3. Submit completed application for nonphysician first assistant to the Medical Staff office, which will verify licensure or registration, insurance coverage, educational preparation, and references.
4. The Director of the Operating Room will orient the applicant to the operating room and complete a skills checklist of knowledge and skills requested by the applicant.
5. The OR/Surgical Supervisory Committee will review the application and recommendations. If all are satisfactory, the applicant will be appointed to Associate Health Care professional status for a 1-year period. Privileges are limited to the operating room.
6. Annual review of privileges will include recommendation by the Director of the Operating Room that the performance meets accepted standards. The Medical Staff office will verify continuation of insurance coverage, current licensure or certification, and continuing education.
7. Renewal of privileges will be granted by the OR/Surgical Supervisory Committee.

D. For privileges for the nonphysician first assistant to function outside the operating room, request must be made by the employing surgeon and reviewed by the OR/Surgical Supervisory Committee.

Date Reviewed: May 1990

(Source: Rules and Regulations, Article XVI, Associated Health Care Professional. Courtesy of St. Luke's Regional Medical Center, Boise, ID.)

When the nurse applies for institutional practice privileges, it is important to provide the information required by the Joint Commission. The 1992 AMH's Medical Staff section specifies that criteria for all applicants for medical staff privileges or delineated clinical privileges should include at least the following:

- ☐ evidence of current licensure
- ☐ relevant training and experience
- ☐ current competence (usually verified through references and peer recommendations)
- ☐ health status.[16]

Information regarding the applicant's licensure, specific training, experience, and current competence will be verified by the institution. Additional information, such as current professional liability insurance, likely will be requested. Medical staff bylaws or policies will also require provision of:

- ☐ information related to involvement in professional liability actions
- ☐ information related to any challenges (previously successful or currently pending) to licensure or registration or voluntary relinquishment of licensure or registration
- ☐ any limitation, reduction, or loss of privileges at another institution (voluntary or involuntary).

The institution is concerned with both legal constraints to practice and evidence of competence in relation to the activities or services that are to be provided by the applicant. Chart 3-5 provides a sample application for medical affiliate staff privileges.

AORN's Official Statement on RN First Assistants provides additional information regarding the credentialing process. It calls for a mechanism for the following:

- ☐ assessing individual qualifications for practice
- ☐ assessing continuing proficiency
- ☐ evaluating performance annually
- ☐ assessing compliance with relevant institutional and departmental policies
- ☐ defining lines of accountability
- ☐ retrieving documentation of participation as first assistant.[17]

The ACS's Qualifications of the First Assistant in the Operating Room address applying for practice privileges by surgeon assistants and physician assistants. The criteria outlined could be applied to professional nurses applying for practice privileges as first assistants. These criteria include the following:

- ☐ outline of qualifications and credentials
- ☐ request to "assist in a surgeon's practice including assisting at the operating table"
- ☐ identity of the surgeon responsible for the applicant's performance
- ☐ requirement that the qualifications be reviewed and approved by the hospital (institutional) board.[18]

CHART 3-5

Application for Medical Affiliate Staff Privileges

Name: ______________________________ Category:
First Middle Last
( ) Medical Student
( ) Resident
( ) CRNA
( ) 1st Assistant
( ) Psychologist
( ) Private Scrub
( ) Other (Specify) __________

Residence Address: ______________________________

Phone: __________ Date of Birth: __________

Employer: ______________________________

Address: ______________________________ Phone: __________

Position/Duties: ______________________________

____

EDUCATION:
College or University: ______________________________

Degree: ______________________________ Date: __________

College or University: ______________________________

Degree: ______________________________ Date: __________

EXPERIENCE:
Hospital: __________ From/to: __________ Position: __________

Hospital: __________ From/to: __________ Position: __________

Have your privileges at any hospital ever been denied, suspended, diminished, revoked, or not renewed? Yes _____ No _____ If Yes, please explain in detail on separate sheet.

Other qualifications and special training: ______________________________

____

____

Current Licensure/Certification:
STATE: _____ /______________ Expiration Date: __________

STATE: _____ /______________ Expiration Date: __________

Has your license or certificate to practice in any jurisdiction ever been suspended, revoked, or not renewed? Yes _____ No _____ If Yes, please explain in detail on separate sheet.

Membership in Professional Organizations:

____

____

(continued)

CHART 3-5
Application for Medical Affiliate Staff Privileges *(continued)*

Continuing Education:

____

____

HEALTH ASSESSMENT
Have you ever abused or been addicted to drugs and/or alcohol?
No _____ Yes _____
Have you ever been hospitalized for drug- and/or alcohol-related problems?
No _____ Yes _____
If you answered "Yes" to any of the above questions, please explain fully on the attached.

Please list three (3) medical references, able to attest to your current competence at performing the privileges you request (include address and phone).

____

____

____

List below the nature and scope of those privileges you are requesting as a staff affiliate: ____

____

____

____

____

____

____

In making application to affiliate status of the medical staff of St. Luke's Regional Medical Center, I agree to abide by the medical and dental staff bylaws, rules, and regulations, as well as the bylaws and policies of the hospital which pertain to me.

I attest that I am physically and mentally capable of accepting appointment to affiliate status and any privileges granted to me. I fully understand that any significant misstatement in or omissions from this application constitute cause for summary dismissal from the staff.

Signature of Applicant ________________________ Date ____________

PLEASE ATTACH CERTIFICATE OF LIABILITY INSURANCE

(Courtesy of St. Luke's Regional Medical Center, Boise, ID)

When an application for practice privileges is submitted, the institution usually requests specific information related to first assistant activities. The request may be for information in the form of a narrative description of the nurse's role, or for a checklist. The nurse may apply for privileges in all surgical specialties or apply for privileges in a specific surgical area or areas, such as cardiovascular, orthopedics, and so on. The privileges will be granted only in those specialty areas designated by the applicant. Examples of activities to include on the application are:

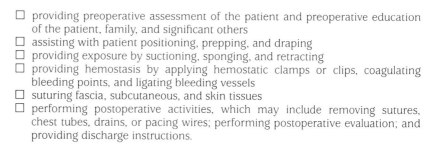

- ☐ providing preoperative assessment of the patient and preoperative education of the patient, family, and significant others
- ☐ assisting with patient positioning, prepping, and draping
- ☐ providing exposure by suctioning, sponging, and retracting
- ☐ providing hemostasis by applying hemostatic clamps or clips, coagulating bleeding points, and ligating bleeding vessels
- ☐ suturing fascia, subcutaneous, and skin tissues
- ☐ performing postoperative activities, which may include removing sutures, chest tubes, drains, or pacing wires; performing postoperative evaluation; and providing discharge instructions.

It may be necessary to identify specific operative procedures in which the nurse will be assisting as either first or second assistant. It is important to state that intraoperative activities will be performed under the supervision of the operating surgeon.

Privileges may be granted on a temporary basis, providing an opportunity to evaluate the nurse's competence as a first assistant. The provisional period required after the initial appointment to the medical staff can vary from 3 months to 2 years. At the end of this provisional period, the institution decides either to continue, expand, or curtail the nurse's practice privileges. All appointments and reappointments, as well as renewal or revision of clinical privileges, are made for a period not longer than 2 years.

Reappointment or renewal of practice privileges will be determined in relation to competence. Information concerning professional performance, judgment, and clinical or technical skills will be requested during the reappointment process. Peer recommendations are part of the basis for reappointment; these, as well as documentation of continuing education activities, should be prepared. Also required are recommendations from the department or major clinical service where the RN first assistant functions.

For applicants who are denied clinical privileges or receive adverse decisions, the Joint Commission requires that institutions offer a mechanism for appropriate action, including a fair hearing and an appeal process. Sex, race, creed, and national origin are not bases for decisions on granting or denying appointment or clinical privileges. The institution must abide by antitrust laws that prohibit restraint of trade or attempts to monopolize by excluding certain providers from access to the institution. The bylaws of the medical staff must define the criteria for admission to or denial of medical staff privileges within the institution. Decisions or recommendations cannot be made on the basis of competitive considerations.[19] The RN first assistant who is denied staff privileges may find it necessary to seek legal advice or counsel prior to appealing the institution's decision.

APPLYING FOR PRIVILEGES AS A RN FIRST ASSISTANT INTERN

The importance of educational preparation for assisting at surgery is well documented. In its Official Statement on RN First Assistants, AORN clearly states that "the RN first assistant practices perioperative nursing and has acquired the knowledge, skills, and judgment necessary to assist the surgeon through organized instruction and supervised practice."[20] The AORN's *Core Curriculum for the RN First Assistant* further emphasizes that "the RN first assistant, through organized instruction and supervised clinical practice, develops the cognitive, psychomotor, and affective behaviors necessary to function interdependently . . . using the nursing behaviors appropriate for, and unique to, the qualified perioperative nurse/RN first assistant."[21]

The 1990s have seen a significant interest in and institutional need for nurses to act as first assistants. Although it may seem expedient to assign a perioperative nurse who is available to assist, "expediency, however, does not make the practice advisable. If an injury occurs because a nurse who has not received adequate instruction and who is not acting pursuant to an institutional policy assumes the role of a first assistant, the consequences to that nurse and to that institution can be severe."[22]

Most educational programs for RN first assistants require a clinical internship, during which the nurse builds on a knowledge base acquired through classroom instruction. The internship is supervised by faculty or a surgeon and an experienced RN first assistant. These internships often require acquisition of a depth and breadth of clinical skills. For example, one collegiate program for RN first assistants requires an average of 240 hours of internship.[23] To engage in such internship activities, the RN first assistant may need to apply for privileges as an RN first assistant intern. The delineation of privileges may vary from institution to institution, and is often based on the clinical requirements of the educational program. A sample application for RN first assistant internship privileges is shown in Chart 3-6.

CONCLUSION

A credentialing process provides a system in the institution for identifying and recognizing the individual nurse's knowledge and skill. This is important as a quality assessment and improvement mechanism that validates the nurse's competence to function as a first assistant. With credentialing, the institution has a method for evaluating each nurse and assigning specific aspects of patient care based on the nurse's qualifications. Assigning the most qualified nurse to each patient care domain should result in increased productivity and efficiency.

CHART 3-6

Application For RNFA Internship Privileges

I ____,
request permission to practice as an RN First Assistant intern at Millard Fillmore Hospitals. The anticipated time frame for my clinical internship activities will be from:

____________________ to ____________________.

Attached you will find verification of:

1. Enrollment in an accredited RN first assistant course requiring a clinical internship experience
2. Goals and objectives for the internship
3. Clinical activities associated with the internship
4. CNOR status
5. RN Licensure
6. Malpractice insurance.

____
Signature of Applicant Date

Privileges Granted ______
Denied ______ Date ____________________

(Courtesy Millard Fillmore Hospitals, Buffalo, NY)

A credentialing system can be used for identifying the educational needs of individual staff members. A nurse's personal professional growth can be enhanced with such a system. Viewed in this framework, a credentialing system benefits the nurse, the institution, and the patient.

REVIEW QUESTIONS

1. A surgeon tells an RN first assistant to execute a medical order they both know is not part of the nurse's practice privileges. The patient is injured and sues the RN first assistant. In terms of the RN first assistant's liability,
   a. The surgeon's verbal assurance to the RN first assistant will provide adequate protection from legal liability to the patient.
   b. The nurse practice act addresses the function; therefore, no one can sue the RN first assistant.
   c. The hospital may hold the RN first assistant liable for performing a function for which she or he was not granted practice privileges.
   d. The borrowed servant law absolves the RN first assistant from responsibility.

2. Because most nurse practice acts either permit the nurse to function as assistant in surgery, or are silent on it,
   a. most hospitals must also permit it
   b. clear definitions of the role still need to be established in the institution
   c. surgeons may determine the role functions by the captain of the ship doctrine
   d. a nurse who functions as an RN first assistant could not be sued for wrongful conduct
3. While employed as an RN first assistant at a hospital with a job description for the role, and credentialed by the institution to perform the role, RN first assistant Hutt negligently injures a patient. Which of the following conclusions (if any) would apply?
   a. If the injured patient sues and collects damages from the hospital, RN first assistant Hutt cannot also be held liable.
   b. RN first assistant Hutt cannot be held liable under any circumstances, because the hospital, by virtue of the job description and credentialing mechanism, has agreed to assume all liability.
   c. Both RN first assistant Hutt and the hospital can be held liable for the negligence.
   d. None of the conclusions apply.
4. The law will absolve RN first assistants from liability
   a. if they are employed by a hospital with a credentialing mechanism for RN first assistants even if the nurse practice act is silent on scope of practice for RN first assistants
   b. if they can show they were carrying out a surgeon's orders
   c. in both of the above instances
   d. in neither of the above instances
5. A surgeon may safely assume that
   a. any perioperative nurse on staff is competent to carry out first assisting functions
   b. some surgical maneuvers cannot be delegated to a RN first assistant no matter what the circumstances
   c. a surgical technician can never carry out a function as well as a perioperative nurse
   d. as long as the RN first assistant has practice privileges, she or he is competent to carry out any assigned assisting duties
6. A perioperative patient care coordinator directs a RN first assistant intern to assist at major abdominal surgery even though the intern has only assisted at minor procedures in the past. As a result of the intern's lack of competence, the patient is injured. On what basis could the RN first assistant intern be held liable?
   a. for not discussing with the coordinator his or her limitations prior to assisting at the surgery
   b. for not carrying student liability insurance
   c. both of the above
   d. neither of the above
7. Credentialing processes
   a. place the burden of liability on the nurse
   b. attempt to decrease institutional liability

c. are required by the AORN and ANA
d. are part of the institution's duty towards patients

8. If using the perioperative credentialing model as a guideline, files maintained would contain annual documentation of

a. changes in the nurse practice act
b. a review by the risk manager of liability claims
c. performance appraisal and documentation of competence
d. current membership in the RN first assistant Specialty Assembly

9. When an institution develops a job description for the RN first assistant, it should

a. be separate from descriptions of staff nurse
b. not be part of nonphysician credentialing
c. require a master's degree (or evidence of a degree in progress)
d. be specific to assisting functions and responsibilities

10. Joint Commission standards require

a. a process that ensures that all individuals who provide patient care services are qualified to do so
b. that only medical staff appointments are subject to competence review and privilege granting/renewal
c. additional education and experience for nurses who request privileges as first assistants
d. advanced certification as an RN first assistant or physician assistant for any nonphysician provider of assistant at surgery services

Indicate whether each of the following statements is true (T) or false (F):

11. _______ The rights to perform certain activities within an institution are privileges granted through a credentialing process.

12. _______ Joint Commission requires that credentialing processes be the same for institutional employees and nonemployees.

13. _______ By verifying that an applicant is competent to function as a first assistant, the institution ensures that patients will receive quality care.

14. _______ Credentialing by an institution as an RN first assistant is the same as being given institutional licensure as an RN first assistant.

15. _______ Competence is the only requirement in determining assignment of an RN first assistant to a patient procedure.

16. _______ A skills list should be used in conjunction with a job description as evidence of the RN first assistant's continued competence.

17. _______ If an RN first assistant is granted "limited" privileges, it means that his or her competence is not yet at a level deserving "full" privileges.

18. _______ When applying for institutional practice privileges, the RN first assistant should be prepared to provide information on relevant training and/or experience.

19. _______ It is a violation of the RN first assistant's privacy to be queried regarding any professional liability actions.

20. _______ It is important that institutions have mechanisms for retrieving documentation of the RN first assistant's participation in surgical procedures as a first assistant.

ANSWER KEY

1. c
2. b
3. c
4. d
5. b
6. a
7. d
8. c
9. d
10. a
11. T
12. F (Credentialing processes are often different for employees and nonemployees.)
13. T
14. F (Institutional licensure would allow an institution to determine "who can do what" without regards to professional standards. Credentialing processes, on the other hand, rely on many professional standards to ensure competence and appropriate scope of practice delineations.)
15. F (Competence is important in assignment, but there must be an institutional position description that clearly identifies what is permissible.)
16. T
17. F ("Limited" privileges usually refer to the RN first assistant's nonphysician status, not to competence.)
18. T
19. F (This is permissible and relates to the institution's duty to provide quality care by competent professionals.)
20. T

REFERENCES

1. Association of Operating Room Nurses: AORN official statement on RN first assistants. AORN J 39:404–405, 1984
2. American College of Surgeons: Qualifications of the first assistant in the operating room. AORN J 32:1012, 1980
3. Nursing: A Social Policy Statement. Kansas City, American Nurses' Association, 1980
4. Jessee W: Delineating clinical privileges, QRB June 1987 13:209–213, 1987
5. Starr P: The Social Transformation of American Medicine, pp 162, 167. New York, Basic Books, 1982
6. The question of hospital privileges for allied health professionals. QRB January 1984 19:18, 1984
7. Joint Commission on Accreditation of Health Care Organizations: Handout, OR Manager's Conference, Boston. Chicago, Joint Commission on Accreditation of Health Care Organizations, 1991
8. Ibid
9. Joint Commission on Accreditation of Health Care Organizations: Accreditation Manual for Hospitals, p 62. Chicago, Joint Commission on Accreditation of Health Care Organizations, 1992
10. Ibid, p 165
11. Ibid, p 64

12. Association of Operating Room Nurses, p 404
13. Joint Commission on Accreditation of Health Care Organizations, p 28 1992
14. Association of Operating Room Nurses: Perioperative nursing credentialing model. AORN J 43:262–264, 1986
15. American Nurses' Association: Guidelines for Appointment of Nurses for Individual Practice Privileges in Health Care Organizations. Kansas City, American Nurses' Association, 1978
16. Joint Commission on Accreditation of Health Care Organizations, p 56
17. Association of Operating Room Nurses, p 405
18. American College of Surgeons, p 1012
19. Scott PE: Legal considerations. *In* Care Of The Surgical Patient, Vol. II Scientific American, Inc, 1991:X3-1–X3-12
20. Association of Operating Room Nurses, p 404
21. Vaiden R, Fox V, Rothrock JC: Core Curriculum for the RN First Assistant, p I-1. Denver, Association of Operating Room Nurses, 1991
22. Murphy EK: OR nursing law. AORN J 45:140–142, 1987
23. RN First Assistant Program, Delaware County Community College, Media, PA, 1991

BIBLIOGRAPHY

Apostoles F, Naschinski C: Instituting a clinical privileging process for nurses. JONA 17:33–38, 1987

Ball J: Credentialing versus performance: A new look at old problems, QRB December 1984, 10:397–401, 1984

Bradley D: Employee credentialing a quality assurance tool. J Qual Assur Spring 1984, pp 19–20, 1984

Durham J, Hardin S: Nurse psychotherapists' experiences in obtaining individual practice privileges. Nurse Pract 10:62–67, 1985

Gilbert B: Relating quality assurance to credentials and privileges. QRB May 1984, 10:130–135, 1984

Hesterly S: Nurse credentialing in an acute care setting. J Nurs Qual Assur 5: 18–26, 1991

Manley M: Clinical privileges for nonhospital-based nurses, Am J Nurs October 1981, 81:1822–1825, 1981

Murphy E: OR nursing law: When is the RN first assistant protected by institutional policy? AORN J 40:436–440, 1984

Pollard M, Schultheiss P: FTC and the professions: Continuing controversy, Nurs Econ 1:158–163, 1983

Quigley P, Hixon A, Janzen,S: Promoting autonomy and professional practice: A program of clinical privileging. J Nurs Qual Assur 5: 27–32, 1991

Richards G: Nonphysician practitioners make slow steady headway on staff privileges, Hospitals December 16, 1984, pp 82–86, 1984

Rose M: Laying siege to hospital privileges. Am J Nurs May 1984, 84:613–615, 1984

Rowland H, Rowland B: Hospital Administration Handbook, pp 717–718. Rockville, MD, Aspens Systems, 1984

Smith T: A structured process to credential nurses with advanced practice skills. J Nurs Qual Assur 5: 40–51, 1991

Trostoriff D: Medical staff privileging: How to avoid pitfalls in the administrative process. QRB, June 1987, 13:198–204, 1987

Wehrhagen R, McKiernan N: Credentialing and clinical privileges: Experiences at a tertiary care center. J Nurs Qual Assur 5: 33–39, 1991

Zimble J, Wendorf B: Credentialing within the quality assurance structure. QRB December 1984, 10:380–384, 1984

4 Microbiologic Basis of Asepsis

Chester R. Smialowicz

Combinations of socioeconomic factors, scientific discoveries, and public demand have resulted in significant changes in surgical technology and patient care practices. The well-known trend towards ambulatory surgery has altered traditional admission patterns, changed patient profiles, made tracking outpatient infection rates more difficult, and decreased average lengths of stay. Concomitantly, these changes have altered the demographics of inpatients, creating higher-risk pools within health care institutions. Surgical wound infections have remained a serious concern in the 1990s. Protecting patients through improving the quality of care is the clarion call for health care professionals. Although infection rates vary with the type of procedure, patient profiles, wound classification, and the appropriate use of antibiotics, the skill of surgical teams and the maintenance of aseptic technique continue to undergird efforts to protect patients.

NURSING DIAGNOSIS AND OUTCOME GOALS

It has been estimated that surgical wound infections account for 20% of all nosocomial infections; one-third of all excess hospital days have been attributed to managing these infections.[1] Superficial wound infections, which occur above the fascial plane, account for 60% to 80% of surgical wound infections.[2] Deep surgical wound infections, below the fascial plane, may affect bone, muscle, and internal organs.

The nursing diagnosis High Risk for Infection recognizes these particular problems. As the RN first assistant explores the microbiologic basis for this nursing diagnosis, it becomes evident that the high risk for wound infection is related, in part, to impaired skin integrity secondary to the surgical incision. Once the skin is violated, tissue is exposed to potential inoculation by endogenous and exogenous microorganisms. Having made this assessment, the RN first assistant establishes an outcome goal that the patient will have an integral wound that is free of infection, as evidenced by criteria such as the absence of redness, heat, tenderness, and drainage on postoperative wound evaluation. Intraoperatively, fundamental principles of aseptic technique will be implemented to facilitate goal achievement. Understanding the microbiologic basis for these actions promotes technique based on principled rationale rather than on ritualism.

THE HISTORY OF SURGICAL ASEPSIS

Even before man was able to see microorganisms, their presence and contagiousness were appreciated. In 1546, Girolamo Fracastoro described the significance of direct contact in the spread of infection. This was almost 100 years before Leeuwenhoek invented the microscope and saw the first microbe. In 1847, Ignacz Semmelweis demonstrated that puerperal fever was carried on the unclean hands of medical personnel. He came to this conclusion while investigating the death of a friend who sustained a small finger laceration while performing an autopsy on a patient who had died with puerperal sepsis. Determined to intervene in the chain of infection, Semmelweis advocated disinfection of hands between patient examinations (scrubbing the hands with soap and warm water and cleansing with a nail brush), isolation of infected patients, and nontraumatic examination of the uterus. Through these efforts, he was able to decrease infection rates from 18% in 1847 to 1% in 1848. Semmelweis went on to demonstrate that linens and instruments could also carry infection. His early efforts led to the recognition that the hands of members of the surgical team carry a significant patient risk if not properly decontaminated. Antiseptics that bind to the stratum corneum and have persistent action are the most appropriate for surgical scrubs; alcohol, chlorhexidine, and iodophors are currently recommended.

Florence Nightingale, in 1854, urged hospitals and surgeons to publish operative mortalities. Nightingale was convinced of the environment's role in the spread of infection. Her efforts in this respect are well documented and relevant even today. Her unrelenting belief that nurses could intervene in the epidemiology of infection continues to influence the nursing process and the nursing role in the infection control committee. RN first assistants have an important role to play in incorporating their nursing functions into indicator criteria and surveillance programs in an effort to identify predictive outcomes for surgical patients as part of institution-wide quality assessment and improvement activities.

Pasteur's work with fermentation in 1857 contributed dramatically to the recognition of the role of airborne contamination in infection and laid to rest the idea that pus was a "laudable" event in the wound healing process. Lister, in 1867, disinfected open wounds in compound fractures with carbolic acid and began using carbolic dressings to protect wounds. Although pouring antiseptic solutions into wounds goes back to ancient times and is even recorded by Luke in the Bible, Lister is remembered as the father of antisepsis. Early nursing textbooks recount the procedure by which nurses followed Dr. Lister's techniques, fumigating and soaking surgical supplies with carbolic acid.

Progress against surgical morbidity and mortality was rapid and continuous in the late 19th century. Bergmann was instrumental in designing the steam sterilizer in 1880; Neuber's surgical team donned caps and gowns in 1881; and gloves became part of the scrub team attire in 1894. By 1896 the surgical team began wearing masks, and the importance of barriers was confirmed. Alexander Fleming, working in a different theoretical framework, directed reconsideration of using antiseptic agents in surgical wounds. He posited that these agents did more harm to the tissues than they did to the bacteria themselves. In 1939 Fleming described the bactericidal properties of a *Penicillium* mold. Although his simple discovery opened the door to the complex world of antibiotics, it must be appreciated that, despite their effectiveness, antibiotics are not a substitute for aseptic surgical technique.

PATHOGENICITY OF MICROORGANISMS

Only a small fraction of the myriad microorganisms in our environment cause human disease; of these, only a few cause surgical wound infections. The human host has many barriers and defense mechanisms that prevent pathogens from causing infection. Even our own bacteria play a role in infection prevention. Humans have normal skin and mucosal flora that have been shown to be protective by virtue of competitive inhibition with pathogenic organisms.

Once pathogens attach to their host cell surface receptors, they demonstrate their virulence through a number of mechanisms. Toxin production was one of the first described methods of pathogenicity. Diphtheria, tetanus, and botulism are microorganisms that rely on toxin production. Protective outer coatings, called capsules, are used by other microorganisms, such as *Staphylococcus*, *Streptococcus*, *Neisseria*, and *Hemophilus*, to avoid being ingested by white blood cells. The capsule contributes to the organism's pathogenicity. The host relies on the normal humoral immune system of antibodies to coat the capsule and, after coating, to fix complement to this antibody-coated organism. Once the complement has been fixed, the organism is prepared for sequestration by the normal spleen. Any breech in this system, such as is seen in the antibody-deficient or asplenic patient, makes the patient vulnerable to the encapsulated organism.

Some organisms can live outside the host. They are able to survive phagocytic digestion and remain viable within legions of antibodies in complement. These intracellular organisms can live and multiply for years within the phagocyte, surfacing later to cause clinical disease, as witnessed by the tuberculosis bacillus and pathogenic fungi. These organisms tend to cause chronic illness with a more insidious onset. Other organisms, such as viruses, rickettsiae, and chlamydia, must live within the cell and use the host's metabolic machinery for growth and reproduction. These obligate cellular parasites can resurface repeatedly, causing recurrent clinical disease. The herpes family of viruses are such host parasites.

Although some organisms possess high degrees of innate virulence and have no difficulty overcoming the host defense mechanisms, other less virulent organisms—the ones usually responsible for postoperative infections—rely on a break in the host's defense systems. Burns, trauma, and surgery violate the most effective host barrier, the skin. With such a violation, even low-virulence organisms, such as *Staphylococcus epidermidis* and *Diphtheroides*, can enter and cause infection. Medications such as antibiotics destroy the patient's normal protective flora. Radiation and chemotherapy suppress the phagocytes and lymphocytes or damage the mucosal barriers of the bowel. Disease states that result in poor nutrition and organ dysfunction leave the host with little resistance. However, the event that allows for the invading organisms to penetrate into the vulnerable interior of the weakened human host is modern surgical technology. Many postoperative infections result from pathogens that the patient acquires during the hospital stay.

MICROBES OF SURGICAL IMPORTANCE

In the past 10 to 15 years, surgical wound surveillance has revealed that the most common organisms isolated from clean, clean-contaminated, and contaminated surgical wounds are *Staphylococcus aureus*, coagulase-negative staphylococcus, enterococcus, and *Pseudomonas*.[3] Since 1984, *Staphylococcus epidermidis* has often been implicated as a wound isolate. The type and virulence of an invading organism plays a pivotal role in the likelihood of infection.

STAPHYLOCOCCI

The staphylococci are morphologically gram-positive, non-spore-forming, nonmotile microbes that form in clumps and are pyogenic. *Staphylococcus aureus*, isolated from approximately 15% of infected surgical wounds, was once thought to be the only pathogenic form of the species, but *S. epidermidis* is frequently becoming resistant and causative in clean wound infections, especially with implant surgery. Staphylococci are ubiquitous in the environment, often carried in the nasopharynx. They cause infections commonly characterized by odorless, red, tender wounds with creamy exudate. Septicemia and deep organ involvement can also occur, usually after local involvement. The degree of infection depends on the specific extracellular enzymes and toxins produced by the causative organism. Staphylococcal organisms are resistant to destruction by heat and chemical disinfectants. This ability to survive in adverse conditions makes the role of barrier materials critical in infection control in the perioperative suite.

STREPTOCOCCI

Streptococci are morphologically gram-positive cocci in chains that are non-spore-forming and nonmotile. They are pyogenic and often classified in the laboratory according to their hemolytic properties. Surgical patients in all age groups may have mucous membranes colonized with group B streptococci; sites of colonization include the vaginal mucosa, the male urethral meatus, the throat, and the rectum.[4] These organisms are spread by hand-to-hand contact, as droplet contaminants, and as dust-borne bacteria. In their pathogenic form, they usually inhabit a wound in association with other organisms. They may be implicated in wound infection following caesarean birth or gynecologic procedures or in systemic infection, particularly in immunocompromised patients. They are commonly present in lower gastrointestinal surgery, in diffuse cellulitis, and in vascular stasis ulcers and gangrene in diabetic patients. Group A streptococci may cause cutaneous infections, while Group B streptococci can cause significant infections in neonates. They are easily destroyed by heat and chemical antisepsis.

ENTERIC BACILLI

The enteric bacilli are gram-negative, non-spore-forming, aerobic inhabitants of the gastrointestinal tract. Types include *Escherichia coli*, *Proteus mirabilis*, *Klebsiella*, and *Enterobacter*. When these microbes are implicated in wound infection, it is most often an autoinfection by the patient's endogenous flora. When they appear in wound infections, the wound is usually necrotic and purulent. They occur following bowel surgery where there has been no prep, with ruptured appendix, and with diverticulitis, presenting as a diffuse peritonitis. The enteric bacilli can also cause infection following instrumentation of the gastrointestinal tract and septicemia in the necrotic tissue of burn patients. These microbes are destroyed by heat and chemical disinfection.

PSEUDOMONAS

Small, slender, rod-shaped, gram-negative, and non-spore-forming, *Pseudomonas* is found environmentally in water and soil and decomposing organic matter. It is often a secondary invader in wound infections; its presence is detected by a characteristic bluish-green wound discharge with an acrid, musty odor. *Pseudomonas* will also cause pneumonia, often fatal for the patient on a respirator. Although it is susceptible to destruction with heat and antibiotics, it commonly occurs after prolonged use of broad-spectrum antibiotics.

CLOSTRIDIA

The *Clostridia* are anaerobic, gram-positive spore-formers, classified by typology as *C. tetani*, *C. wellchii*, *C. sordelli*, and so on. These microorganisms are found in the soil and in the colon, where the spores may remain viable for years. In their pathogenic form, they are the causative organisms in tetanus, forming a powerful neurotoxic exotoxin that causes spasms of voluntary muscle, and in gas gangrene. They occur in deep necrotic wounds associated with trauma. Because they are spore-forming, they are highly resistant to destruction.

Any of these microorganisms can cause contamination by direct contact with sterile and unsterile surfaces, as moisture droplets contaminating a sterile surface, by being airborne, or as hematogenous infectants carried by the patient's blood. Sources for these microbes include the patient's skin, the scrub team's skin, the bloodstream, the patient's respiratory tract, the team's respiratory tracts, the drapes, instruments, sutures, room air, the team's uncovered hair, and the patient's gastrointestinal tract. It is not surprising, then, that recommended practices for basic aseptic technique elaborate the perioperative team's responsibilities in minimizing wound contamination from identified microbial reservoirs present during surgery.

PROPHYLACTIC ANTIBIOTICS

Whenever consideration is given to the use of prophylactic antibiotics to prevent wound infection, it is important to remember that antibiotics are never a substitute for surgical asepsis. Prophylactic antibiotics are administered when bacterial contamination is expected; thus, they usually are not indicated in clean operations if the patient has no host risk factors. Host risk factors include abdominal surgery, an operation likely to last more than 2 hours, and patients with more than three concomitant diagnoses. However, if the surgery involves placement of a prosthetic device, open-heart procedures, or procedures involving the aorta or vessels in the groin, then antibiotic prophylaxis is usually indicated. Such prophylaxis is also indicated in clean-contaminated,

contaminated, and infected operations. The antibiotic selected should be effective against the most likely pathogen associated with the type of surgery being performed and should have a sufficiently long half-life to maintain tissue levels during the operation. Second doses are indicated when the surgery exceeds either 3 hours or the half-life of the antibiotic. Prolonged use of prophylaxis is not indicated; usually a single dose that is the same strength of a therapeutic dose, administered preoperatively, is adequate. The single dose is often administered intravenously by anesthesia.

TOPICAL ANTIMICROBIAL AGENTS

Topical antimicrobial agents, in the form of powders, sprays, ointments, or solutions, have been studied for years. Data indicate that no one agent has been shown to be clearly superior. Furthermore, when systemic antibiotics are administered, the contribution of additional topical agents seems unclear. Topical agents are also used intraperitoneally. Studies with agents such as kanamycin, used topically in an established peritonitis, indicate that the topical agent can decrease the rate of wound infection and other infectious complications. The question is whether the topical agents add anything when used in addition to systemic prophylaxis.

Recent studies indicate that they probably do not. The peritoneal lining will easily transport intravenously administered antibiotics to the peritoneal cavity more effectively than will instilling the antibiotic directly into the abdominal cavity.

ENTERAL PROPHYLAXIS

Studies on normal pharyngeal flora indicate that alpha hemolytic streptococci can inhibit the growth of *Staphyloccus aureus*, *Meningococcus*, and *Pneumonococcus* by more rapid use of growth metabolites in the surrounding environment. Normal flora also help by stimulating nonspecific protective antibodies to pathogenic strains that attempt to colonize the human host. Strains of *E. coli* have been shown to stimulate cross-reacting antibodies against *Hemophilus*; it is believed that these cross-reacting antibodies are more important in protecting children against *Hemophilus* infections than are subclinical infections with *Hemophilus* itself. A similar protective effort is provided by the anaerobes of the colon, which produce short-chain, organic fatty acids that inhibit strains of *Salmonella*, *Shigella*, *Pseudomonas*, and other pathogenic organisms from colonizing in the colon. This has been demonstrated clinically on oncology units, where extensive use of antibiotics often results in destruction of a patient's normal colonic flora followed by *Pseudomonas* colonization of the colon.

The same struggle for the balance of power in the battle of the colonic flora has resulted in the emergence of a new clinical syndrome: pseudomembranous colitis. Over the past two decades, epidemiologists have come to recognize that many persons carry a potentially dangerous organism—*Clostridium difficile*—in their colonic flora. It is generally held in check by the normal colonic flora; however, when a person carrying this organism is given antibiotics, especially broad-spectrum antibiotics that destroy the normal colonic flora, *C. difficile* begins to multiply because it no longer has competition. Should it reach significant numbers, it produces a toxin that inflames the colon and can cause potentially fatal diarrhea syndrome. The causative agent is resistant to all antibiotics except vancomycin and metronidazole.

Although mechanical cleansing of the colon in preparation for surgery reduces total fecal mass, it does not significantly reduce the number of bacteria in residual colonic material. Antimicrobials are required to obtain a significant reduction in the bacterial count. It is generally agreed that these drugs should be able to suppress both aerobes and anaerobes; the human colon and distal small intestine support a reservoir of these microbes. Numerous studies of poorly absorbable agents that attack the aerobic and anaerobic flora have been studied; erythromycin-neomycin oral programs are currently the most popular. Combined with mechanical cleansing, these oral agents, administered at 1:00 p.m., 2:00 p.m., and 11:00 p.m. on the day before surgery scheduled for about 8:00 a.m. the next day, provide both local (intraluminal) and systemic (serum) protection.[6] Many surgeons use both oral and parental antibiotics combined with mechanical cleansing. There is evidence that a single parental dose of a cephalosporin with aerobic and anaerobic activity, administered intravenously within 30 minutes of the incision, along with mechanical cleansing and oral antibiotics, may be particularly beneficial in operations lasting longer than 3 hours.[7]

SYSTEMIC ANTIBIOTIC PROPHYLAXIS

Systemic antibiotics are used following an assessment of the need for prophylaxis. Two initial determinations relate to consideration of wound-related factors and whether the patient is at risk for endocarditis. If the patient has a prosthetic heart valve or a history of either rheumatic fever or endocarditis, parental antibiotics (ampicillin and gentamicin) will be given; if the risk is relatively low, then oral amoxicillin or erythromycin may suffice. Wound-related factors take into consideration the categorization of the procedure as clean, clean-contaminated, contaminated (including nontraumatic abdominal procedures and trauma surgery), or infected. In clean surgery involving a catheter for dialysis or nutrition, a shunt, a pacemaker, or a prosthetic device (such a valve or a vascular or orthopedic implant), antibiotic prophylaxis will be implemented.

The choice of antibiotic depends on the sensitivity of the expected infecting organisms. New broad-spectrum and more expensive antibiotics claim usefulness, but they have yet to demonstrate superiority over the older, proven antibiotics such as cefazolin, which has been studied in well-controlled clinical trials. A first-generation cephalosporin, cefazolin is ideal for prophylaxis, has proven effective against both gram-positive and gram-negative bacteria, has a low rate of allergic response, is cost-effective and easy to administer. It is often the choice for clean or clean-contaminated prophylaxis unless the patient is allergic; in these cases, vancomycin may be substituted. Intravenous administration at the induction of anesthesia is probably sufficient; there is mounting evidence for single-dose prophylactic therapy. Prolonged administration of prophylactic antibiotics, whether before or after surgery, will only lead to stimulation and colonization of resistant hospital flora.

CLINICAL AND LABORATORY DIAGNOSIS OF INFECTION

In normally responsive patients (those who are not compromised), infection usually presents with the cardinal signs of inflammation: redness, heat, pain, and swelling. These signs represent the host response to infection. The clinical sign of fever, which is 38° centigrade (100.4° F) or higher, occurs after normal postoperative temperature elevation has resolved. The white blood cell (WBC) count is usually elevated, and the presence of infection is confirmed by laboratory assessment. Gram's stain for preliminary information on the characteristics of the microorganism facilitates early identification and treatment. Culture of the wound, sputum, urine, or drainage, under aerobic or anaerobic conditions, enables specific identification. Antibiotic sensitivities guide specific antimicrobial treatment. A WBC count and blood chemistries are also obtained. Chest x-ray, aspiration of potentially infected fluid, or ultrasonography or computed tomography (CT) scan of the operative site may also be required to make an appropriate diagnosis and guide appropriate therapy.

Infection in compromised patients who are elderly, have sustained major trauma, have a chronic disease or end-organ failure, or are undergoing chemotherapy may not be as clinically straightforward. These patients may have such clinical manifestations of infection as confusion, hypotension, fluid retention, ileus, delayed wound healing, or gastric bleeding. Creatinine clearance may be altered, with a subsequent elevation in serum creatinine and blood urea nitrogen (BUN) levels. Empirical antibiotic therapy in these patients may be instituted before laboratory confirmation. Septic shock may be manifested by tachycardia; hypotension; initially warm, then cold and dry extremities; generalized flushing; and a hypermetabolic state.

ANTIBIOTICS IN THE TREATMENT OF POSTOPERATIVE INFECTIONS

The spectrum of systemic antibiotics available to the clinician for the treatment of postoperative wound infections is vast. The RN first assistant will need to read drug literature and pharmacology texts to become familiar with specific treatment regimens. The RN first assistant must keep in mind that antibiotic therapy cannot replace wound drainage when an abscess or wound hematoma is present. Antibiotics cannot replace surgical debridement of devitalized or necrotic tissue, especially when anaerobic organisms are involved. Antibiotics usually fail when a prosthetic implant has become infected early in the postoperative course. Postoperative irrigation of infected wounds with antibiotic solution has not been shown to be more beneficial than simple mechanical cleansing. In fact, continuous antimicrobial irrigation systems have been shown to allow resistant hospital organisms to enter the wound. The systemic antibiotics generally penetrate adequately into the wound infection, obviating the need for antibiotic irrigations.

When a physician selects an antibiotic, consideration is given to factors such as the patient's antibiotic allergic history and renal and hepatic function (the modes of antibiotic clearance from the body). The antibiotic must be able to penetrate to the infected area. The physician must determine the causative organism through Gram's stain and culture and sensitivity, selecting an agent that will be efficacious, provide narrow-spectrum coverage to prevent damage to the patient's protective flora, and be the least toxic, all for the lowest price. It is these kinds of complex decisions that keep the consultative field of infectious disease a growing and viable subspecialty.

INFECTIONS THAT PATIENTS TRANSMIT TO THE SURGICAL TEAM

The perioperative environment should provide safety for the patient and the surgical team. The perioperative staff should be protected from environmental hazards, including infectious agents. The team itself, through meticulous and frequent handwashing and the use of protective asepsis, can initiate important activities that protect against contact with infectious hazards.

BACTERIAL AND FUNGAL INFECTIONS

Bacterial and fungal infections that a patient might have at the time of surgery generally do not carry a risk of contagiousness to the surgical team. Even when the patient is colonized with resistant organisms, team members rarely become colonized except for the transient colonization of the hands. Health care personnel with normal pharyngeal-tracheal membranes will not become colonized with hospital gram-negative rod flora, because organisms such as *Pseudomonas* cannot adhere to normal mucosal membranes. Even if colonization by the patient's bacterial or fungal flora occurs, team members do not become clinically infected because they lack the one thing the patient has been subjeced to—an invasive procedure.

Tuberculosis is probably the only common bacterial infection that the surgical patient can transmit to the surgical team. Even this would be unusual, since only the pulmonary source is felt to be the root of spread, and prolonged contact is usually required. Tuberculosis of nonpulmonary sites that might require surgery would not be contagious to the surgical team through surgical manipulation of the tubercular site during the operation. On rare occasions, an intraoperative stab wound of a member of a surgical team with an instrument contaminated with *Mycobacterium tuberculosis* might result in a cutaneous tubercular lesion.

RESPIRATORY INFECTIONS

Many viral infections can theoretically be transmitted by the respiratory route to susceptible perioperative personnel. In reality, this rarely occurs, because a patient generally is not sent to the operating room if he or she has a respiratory illness. Also, exposure to a patient carrying a contagious respiratory virus, even one as highly infectious as the influenza virus, is for only a short time. Masks worn by the surgical team, coupled with the anesthesia mask and closed breathing circuit of the anesthetized patient, act as effective barriers to droplet spread of respiratory viruses.

TYPE A HEPATITIS

Of all the potentially contagious infections to which the surgical team is exposed, the hepatitis viruses pose the greatest threat. Type A hepatitis, formerly known as "infectious" hepatitis, is transmitted only by the fecal-oral route. Even if a surgical patient harbored this virus during a colonic or hepatic procedure, the risk to a gloved and gowned surgical team member would be almost nonexistent. With the availability of serological tests to study the epidemiology of Type A hepatitis, study results indicate that the prevalence among hospital personnel and the general population is the same. Therefore, the hospital employee is at no greater occupational risk for this infection than is the general population. Although there currently is no vaccine to prevent Type A hepatitis, immune serum globulin (HBIG) in the dose listed in Table 4-1, given to an individual who has sustained direct contamination of a mucosal surface with potentially infectious material within 2 hours of exposure, will be 90% effective in preventing infection. It is also important to note that 50% of the adult population already has protective antibodies to Type A hepatitis from childhood exposure. This virus is now felt to be a common childhood viral illness that usually results in subclinical infection with no permanent liver damage, no chronic carrier state, and no associated mortality.

TYPE B HEPATITIS

Data on hepatitis B virus (HBV) infections are not as reassuring. HBV is clearly the most common and potentially dangerous infection to which the surgical team may be exposed. An estimated 5,900 to 7,400 health care workers contract it each year.[8] HBV is a double-stranded DNA virus spread by percutaneous inoculation or contamination of mucosal membranes with infected body fluids. Although all body fluids of infected patients contain the virus, only blood, blood products, saliva, and semen are documented as being able to transmit it. Generally, the incubation period ranges from 40 to 180 days, but occasionally, when the vehicle of spread is a blood transfusion or cutaneous inoculation, the incubation period can be as short as a few weeks. Therefore, it is important that HBIG be given as directed in Table 4-1 as soon after inoculation as possible, at least within the first week after exposure. It is estimated that 1 million persons are chronically infected with HBV, and approximately 1.5% of all hospital admissions have active HBV infection. Surgical patients at greatest risk of carrying HBV are those who have received multiple blood transfusions, dialysis patients, gay men, and intravenous drug users. Nurses at greatest risk are those working in the emergency department, in dialysis, and in perioperative care units. Approximately 25–30% of the members of the surgical team test positive for hepatitis B surface antibody (HBsAg), compared with a general population rate of 3–10%. Unlike hepatitis A virus infection, HBV infection has a small, but definite, risk of death from acute liver failure. The risk of becoming a chronic carrier is 6–10%; approximately 25% of these carriers develop chronic persistent hepatitis or chronic active hepatitis.[9] A small percentage of these persons go on to develop cirrhosis or liver cancer.

When a RN first assistant is stuck with a needle used for a high-risk patient whose HBV serology is unknown or is exposed to a blood splash onto nonintact skin or a mucous membrane, the problem must be addressed. An attempt should be made to detect HBV serologic markers from the patient's blood. Difficult decisions can be avoided if the high-risk hospital personnel, such as the RN first assistant, receive the HBV vaccine. The full series of three inoculations provides more than 90% protection. With implementation of the

TABLE 4-1

Control and Prevention of Hepatitis

	Hepatitis A	**Hepatitis B**	**Non-A, Non-B Hepatitis**
Precautions for employees with hepatitis	*Handwashing;* restrict from work 1-2 weeks after onset of jaundice	*Handwashing;* glove-wearing with patient contact	*Handwashing;* glove-wearing with patient contact
Pre-exposure prophylaxis	Not available	HBV vaccine to all high-risk employees	Not available
Postexposure prophylaxis	ISG* 0.02 ml/kg IM within 2 weeks of potential exposure	HBIG† 0.06 ml/kg IM plus HBV vaccine IM	ISG* 0.06 ml/kg IM

* Immune serum globulin.

† Hepatitis B immune globulin.

1991 Occupational and Safety Health Administration (OSHA) regulations, health care employers are required to provide HBV immunizations (as well as protective equipment and procedures to prevent the transmission of HBV, AIDS, and other blood-borne diseases). Female RN first assistants who are reluctant to get the vaccine for themselves, but who plan to have children in the future, should be aware of the high rate of vertical transmission of HBV to newborns and the higher rate of chronic carrier state, risk of cirrhosis, and incidence of liver cancer that infected newborns must face.

TYPE C HEPATITIS

Since serologies for Type A and Type B hepatitis have become available, it has become apparent that other hepatotropic viruses also can cause clinical hepatitis. A third type of hepatitis, often referred to as non-A, non-B hepatitis (NANB), probably has more than one virus in its group. Epidemiologic studies have revealed two clinical syndromes. The one studied most to date has been associated with blood transfusions. Posttransfusion hepatitis is estimated to be caused by the hepatitis C virus (HCV) 90% of the time. The incubation period can be from 2 to 10 weeks and can result in the carrier state, cirrhosis, and occasional fatality. Approximately 300,000 cases of NANB posttransfusion virus occur annually, making it the most common hospital-acquired viral disease in the country.

A serologic test to detect antibody to HCV is now available. Because HCV can be spread by a needle stick from an asymptomatic chronic carrier, RN first assistants and their perioperative colleagues are at risk from percutaneous and mucosal inoculation. The precautions for HCV are the same protective measures that should be followed for all blood-borne diseases. Although it remains to be proven in clinical studies, it is recommended that immune globulin be given within 7 days after needle/scalpel exposure from a known HCV patient.

TYPE D HEPATITIS

The delta hepatitis virus (HDV) requires the presence of HBV as a "helper" in its replication. Therefore, persons who test positive for HBsAg are at risk for HDV. The clinical course of coinfection is similar to that of acute HBV; if HBV becomes chronic, so will HDV. During early infection, HDV may be diagnosed by the presence of hepatitis D antigen; during or after infection, a laboratory test for immunoglobin M-specific delta antibody (anti-HDV) may be used for diagnosis.[10] The HBV vaccine provides protection against HDV, as does the use of universal precautions for blood-borne pathogens.

HERPES VIRUS

DNA viruses belonging to the herpes group—especially the herpes simplex viruses (HSVs)—have been of concern to perioperative personnel in the past few years. HSV is divided into two types. Type I has a propensity for infection on the face and lips; type II generally causes genital infection. Some crossover between sites occurs. Although medications such as acyclovir control the clinical symptoms and suppress relapses, medical science has yet to find a cure for this relapsing mucocutaneous viral infection. Health care personnel can contract this infection on the hands in the form of a herpetic whitlow through direct contact with a patient's oral, vaginal, or cutaneous lesions. As long as the glove/gown barrier is kept intact, the risk of this occurring should approach zero.

ACQUIRED IMMUNE DEFICIENCY SYNDROME

The viral infections of greatest anxiety and concern to perioperative personnel are acquired immune deficiency syndrome (AIDS) and the opportunistic organisms to which the AIDS patient usually succumbs. AIDS results from an RNA retrovirus, human immunodeficiency virus (HIV), that destroys the $CD4^+$, or T-helper, lymphocytes. The $CD4^+$ lymphocyte coordinates various important immunologic functions. Loss of these functions results in a progressive impairment of the immune response, leaving the victim defenseless against numerous opportunistic infections, including an aggressive form of Kaposi's sarcoma and *Pneumocystis carinii* pneumonia, the most common serious opportunistic infections diagnosed in AIDS patients. The epidemiology of HIV parallels the epidemiology of HBV in that it is spread by blood products, intimate sexual contact, and shared needles of illicit drug users. Like HBV, HIV has been isolated in many body secretions, such as tears and saliva.

A great concern has been that exposure to AIDS patients, their body secretions, or their internal organs during surgical intervention might transmit the virus through a needle or scalpel stick. But although the transmission model has been compared to that of HBV, there is a difference. When a drop of blood or saliva of a patient with HBV is examined microscopically, large numbers of viral particles can be seen. Epidemiologic studies have clearly substantiated, therefore, that one can contract HBV from needle or scalpel stick exposure. But this is not the case with HIV. Single drops of body fluids from AIDS patients do not contain large numbers of virus particles, and studies to date reveal no risk of contracting HIV from such an exposure. It appears that to contract HIV one needs to have either a large viral exposure, such as from a contaminated blood transfusion, or repeated sexual contact with an infected person. The acquisition of this virus may be even more complex.

Laboratory experiments indicate that HIV has a difficult time entering a $CD4^+$ lymphocyte unless the lymphocyte is activated by recurrent antigenic stimulation. This is thought to be the reason that the major risk groups are still homosexual men, illicit intravenous drug users, heterosexual partners of drug users and of bisexual males, hemophiliacs receiving large amounts of blood products, and newborns of infected mothers. In a Centers for Disease

Control (CDC) longitudinal study of 1,700 paramedical personnel who have had needle stick and other secretion contacts, none of the study participants has contracted AIDS even after a 5- to 7-year incubation period. In other prospective studies, the incidence of subsequent seroconversion in persons who received needle stick injuries from needles used in AIDS patients appeared to be less than 0.5 %.[11,12]

Based on these kinds of studies, the CDC has issued guidelines for health workers whose employment involves contact with AIDS patients. These guidelines emphasize that the risk of acquiring HBV is greater than that for HIV and that recommendations for preventing HBV should also effectively prevent HIV. If indicated, zidovudine (AZT) prophylaxis should begin as soon as possible following the HIV exposure.

CONTROLLING OCCUPATIONAL RISK

In 1991, the Occupational Safety and Health Administration (OSHA) published its final Bloodborne Pathogens Standard. The key provisions of this standard have been clear to perioperative personnel for some time. In its intent to provide a workplace that is free from recognized hazards, OSHA requires that health care facilities meet the minimum standards for universal precautions. Such standards encompass engineering controls, work practices, and personnel protective equipment, coupled with employee education. Both employers and employees are required to be in compliance with the standard. Part of the new regulation requires all health care employers to provide HBV immunizations; there are also requirements for postexposure procedures to prevent further transmission while guaranteeing treatment and confidentiality.

Key provisions of the OSHA Bloodborne Pathogens Standard include the following:

- ☐ identification of tasks that carry a risk of transmission and the employee groups that perform them
- ☐ development of written exposure control plans to control risks, which include universal precautions, work practice and engineering controls, medical waste management, sharps safety, and the use of warning labels
- ☐ provision of personal protective equipment
- ☐ a plan for monitoring compliance
- ☐ documentation of employee education
- ☐ no-cost provision of HBV vaccine to all health care workers who have occupational risk for exposure, with specific procedures for postexposure evaluation and follow-up.[13]

RN first assistants must be thoroughly familiar with the OSHA requirements, all elements of universal precautions, and institutional protocols. They should also participate in ongoing research and evaluation of perioperative protective barriers. One study has suggested that stretching and shearing of gowns, especially during intracavity procedures involving deep penetration of the hands and arms to manipulate tissue, contributes to damage to a surgical gown's fibers.[14] The authors recommend double-gloving by the RN first assistant during all major surgical procedures; protective shields where power saws, drills, and irrigation are used; and specific techniques for sharps safety. Sharps safety is extremely important. In the CDC's 1990 prospective observational study of 1,382 surgical procedures, there were 99 sharps injuries, most from suture needles; 88 of the 99 injuries occurred in surgeons, with 28 (32%) recontacting the patient's wound.[15]

Recommendations for precautions like those of the CDC and OSHA share the objective of minimizing exposure of personnel to blood and body secretions from patients, regardless of whether the patient is known to be infected. The RN first assistant should always use appropriate barrier precautions to prevent skin and mucous membrane exposure. Gloves should be worn for any contact with blood, body fluids, mucous membranes, nonintact skin, or soiled items, and the gloves should be changed after each contact. A 1988 study on the in-use integrity of latex and vinyl procedure gloves indicated that there were leakage defects in 2.7% of latex gloves and 4.1% of vinyl gloves; following wearing that mimicked routine patient care activities, 3.3% of the latex gloves showed penetration, compared to 53.5% of the vinyl gloves.[16] Studies of surgical gloves in operations lasting more than 3 hours found that nearly one-third of the gloves were punctured.[17] In the future, surgical gloves of greater strength and greater continuing integrity will become the standard; until then, RN first assistants may opt for double-gloving. Masks and protective eyewear or face shields should be worn to prevent exposure of mucous membranes of the eye, mouth, and nose. Frequent handwashing is essential, even after gloves are removed.

The RN first assistant should also consider protection by surgical technique to minimize the risk of blood exposure and percutaneous injury. The following suggestions for modifying surgical technique should be considered.[18] Wire sutures should be abandoned in favor of safer alternatives. Even large-bore suture material can cause shearing lacerations without damaging the surgical glove; care should be taken when closing an abdominal wound under tension. The RN first assistant should avoid blind suturing techniques where the tip of a surgical needle is palpated for localization. Needles should be removed from sutures before tying. Passing sharps is a hazardous activity; a basin may be used for the exchange of scalpels and used needles. Such a "hands-free" technique for transferring any instrument sharp enough to puncture a glove may also be accomplished by having the scrub person place a magnetic pad or drape between himself or herself and the surgeon and RN first assistant. This area is considered the neutral zone; the scrub person places the sharp instrument there, verbally notifying the surgeon or RN first assistant as the instrument is placed. The RN first assistant and surgeon pick up and return instruments to this zone. This way, the RN first assistant, surgeon, or scrub person do not touch the instrument at the same time.[19] Surgical adjuncts, such as the electrosurgical unit and stapled anastomoses and skin, should be considered to reduce the use of surgical blades and needles. The RN first assistant should be constantly and vigilantly aware of how sharp instruments and needles are being used.

When the RN first assistant routinely uses appropriate surgical technique and barrier precautions during invasive (or other patient care) procedures, the prevention of transmission of blood-borne pathogens is minimized, both from patient to health care worker and from health care worker to patient.

SUMMARY

In aiming to prevent postoperative wound infection, the RN first assistant has a great deal of control and influence over events in the surgical environment. The RN first assistant, along with perioperative colleagues, must have as a primary focus the control of the numbers and types of microorganisms present during surgery. Although not all of the activities involved with minimizing bacterial hazards are carried out directly by the RN first assistant, the RN first assistant must know and understand the principles involved and the techniques by which these principles are effected. Familiarity with standards and recommended practices, with current text and journal readings, and with guidelines promulgated by external agencies is essential to the safe care of the surgical patient. The goal—freedom from infection—is only as tenable as the knowledge base and competent practice of the surgical team members.

REVIEW QUESTIONS

1. Surgical wound infections account for 20% of
   a. monthly morbidity and mortality reports
   b. the CDC profile in U.S. infection rates
   c. high risk pool infections
   d. nosocomial infections
2. Between 60% and 80% of all surgical wound infections
   a. are necrotizing fasciitis
   b. occur above the fascial plane
   c. are the result of exogenous contamination
   d. result from the patient's own pathogens
3. Skin provides a first line of defense; the opening of the skin, either surgically or traumatically, potentiates
   a. an immunocompromised host
   b. infection
   c. the need for antibiotic therapy
   d. a slower rate of epidermal proliferation

4. An outcome goal for the nursing diagnosis High Risk for Infection might be
   a. the patient's wound will be aseptically closed
   b. the team will use proper handwashing
   c. T:98°, P:90, R:18, no rales or ronchi
   d. the patient will demonstrate progressive healing at the wound site
5. Risk factors associated with wound infection depend on
   a. endogenous factors such as associated disease processes
   b. endogenous factors such as environmental sanitation
   c. exogenous factors such as compromised immune system
   d. exogenous factors such as insufficient leukocytes
6. A pathogenic microorganism that relies on toxin production is
   a. staphylococcus
   b. streptococcus
   c. diphtheria
   d. rickettsiae
7. Antibody-coated capsules from such organisms as *Hemophilus* are fixed with complement and sequestered by the
   a. leukocytes
   b. spleen
   c. humoral immune system
   d. thymus gland
8. An obligate cellular parasite
   a. is competitively inhibited
   b. becomes virulent in antibody-deficient patients
   c. uses the host metabolism for growth and reproduction
   d. can live outside the host in antibody-complement
9. Which of the following organisms is frequently isolated in surgical wound infections?
   a. herpes virus
   b. *S. epidermidis*
   c. *Clostridium*
   d. non-spore-forming streptococci
10. Prophylactic antibiotics are usually not indicated in
    a. clean wounds
    b. clean-contaminated wounds
    c. patients who undergo surgery in an aseptic environment
    d. patients without identifiable risk factors
11. To achieve a significant reduction in the numbers of colonic flora before bowel surgery
    a. mechanical cleansing is sufficient
    b. antimicrobial agents are required
    c. drugs that suppress anaerobic organisms are administered
    d. parenteral antibiotics are required to permeate the lumen

12. Unless the patient has an allergy to it, the antibiotic likely to be selected for systemic prophylaxis before surgery is
    a. ampicillin
    b. gentamicin
    c. cefazolin
    d. erythromycin
13. A route of transmission for the hepatitis B virus (HBV) is
    a. fecal-oral
    b. body fluids
    c. percutaneous
    d. perinatal
14. Following exposure to HBV, the RN first assistant should receive immune serum globulin
    a. as soon after inoculation as possible
    b. within 2 days
    c. within the incubation period of the particular strain
    d. within a few weeks
15. The hepatitis virus most often implicated in posttransfusion hepatitis is
    a. type A
    b. type B
    c. type C
    d. type D
16. An important transmission precaution for herpes viruses is
    a. anti-HDV immunization
    b. gloves and gown
    c. acyclovir
    d. immune globulin
17. While on discharge planning rounds, the RN first assistant spends some time with an AIDS patient who is going home that day. An important goal is that the patient be knowledgeable about methods to prevent transmission of HIV to others. Which response indicates that the patient has a correct understanding?
    a. "I'll wait to donate blood until 5 years after my therapy with AZT."
    b. "I should avoid casual contact with my friends."
    c. "I need to wear a mask and gloves when I come in for my postop check-up."
    d. "I shouldn't donate my blood, sperm, or organs."
18. OSHA's Bloodborne Pathogens Standards require written exposure control plans that include
    a. universal precautions
    b. enzyme-linked immunosorbent assays for at-risk work groups
    c. Westin blot assays for symptomatic patients
    d. gown/glove barrier precautions
19. Based on studies of surgical gloves, RN first assistants may opt to
    a. use latex gloves only
    b. use vinyl gloves only
    c. change gloves every 3 hours
    d. double-glove

20. A technique for transferring sharp instruments on the field that minimizes the potential for injury is the
    a. no-needle technique
    b. single-use technique
    c. hands-free technique
    d. blind-suturing technique

Answers

1. d	6. c	11. b	16. b
2. b	7. b	12. c	17. d
3. b	8. c	13. c	18. a
4. d	9. b	14. a	19. d
5. a	10. a	15. c	20. c

REFERENCES

1. Hiestand, S. Farr, S. Infection Control in the Future. Infection Control Rounds, 15:3, 1991
2. Infection control update. ASEPSIS II:19, 1989
3. Hiestand, S. Farr, S. Infection Control in the Future. Infection Control Rounds, 15:3, 1991
4. Roth RR, James WD: Microbiology of the skin. J Am Acad Derm, 20: 367–381, 1989
5. Meakins JL: Prophylactic antibiotics. Care of the Surgical Patient, Volume I, Perioperative Care. Scientific American Medicine, 3-1–3-10, 1991
6. Nichols RL: Bowel preparation. Care of the Surgical Patient, Volume I, Perioperative Care. Scientific American Medicine, 4-1–4-10, 1991
7. Ibid, p 4-6
8. ANA News, December 2, 1991
9. Grau PA: Are you at risk for hepatitis B? Nursing 91, 21:45–46, 1991
10. Lisanti P, Talotta D: Hepatitis update: the delta virus. AORN J, 55:790–800, 1992
11. Condon RE, Quebbeman EJ: Preparing the operating room. Care of the Surgical Patient, Volume I, Perioperative Care. Scientific American Medicine, 5-7–5-8, 1991
12. Kuhls TL, Viker S, Parris NB, Garakian A, Sullivan-Bolyai, Cherry JD: Occupational risk of HIV, HBV, and HSV-2 infections in health care personnel caring for AIDS patients. Am J Pub Health, 77:1306–1309, 1987
13. Lynch P: Preventing occupational transmission of bloodborne pathogens: What does OSHA expect? Infection Control Rounds, 15:1–3, 1992
14. Hubbard MS, Wadsworth K, Telford GL, Quebbeman EJ: Reducing blood contamination and injury in the OR: a study of the effectiveness of protective garments and OR procedures. AORN J, 55:194–201, 1992
15. Russell B: Summary of CDC meeting to discuss invasive procedures under consideration for designation as exposure-prone and not exposure-prone, November 4, 1991
16. Korniewicz DM, Laughon BE, Butz A, Larson E: Integrity of vinyl and latex procedure gloves. Nurs Res, 38:144–146, 1992
17. Beck WC: A hole in the surgical glove: A change in attitude. ACS Bull, 74(4):16, 1989
18. Report of the Subcommittee on AIDS of the ACS Governor's Committee on Surgical Practice in hospitals: ACS Bull, 76(11):17–21, 1991
19. Fox V: Clinical issues: Passing surgical instruments, sharps without injury. AORN J 55:264, 1992

BIBLIOGRAPHY

Classen DC, Evans S, Pestotnik SL, Horn SD, Menlove RL, Burkee JP: The timing of prophylactic administration of antibiotics and the risk of surgical wound infection. N Eng J Med, 326:281–286, 1992

Dienstag JL: Non-A, non-B hepatitis. Gastroenterology, 84:439–462, 743–768, 1983

Kuo G, Choo QL, Alter HJ, et al: An assay for circulating antibodies for a major etiologic virus of human non-A, non-B hepatitis. Science, 244: 3–5, 1989

Position Statement on Post-Exposure Programs in the Event of Occupational Exposure to HIV/HBV. ANA, September 6, 1991.

Wright JG, McGee AJ, Chyatte D, Ransohoff DF: Mechanisms of glove tears and sharp injuries among surgical personnel. JAMA 266:1668–1671, 1991

5 The Diagnostic Process

Jane C. Rothrock

The diagnostic process involves recognizing, identifying, localizing, and evaluating information provided by and about the patient. The history and physical examination begin the diagnostic process; they are the central foci around which diagnosis and subsequent treatment revolve. The RN first assistant most often will target the history on a specific patient complaint. The patient complaint guides the physical examination. Taken together, the data obtained from the history and physical examination are clustered, grouped, and analyzed. The RN first assistant makes a tentative diagnosis regarding the body structures and processes most likely involved. Diagnostic tests follow.

The RN first assistant's commitment to focusing on the individual patient as a whole requires that assessment cover physical parameters, self-care behaviors, health promotion, culture and values, family and social roles, and developmental tasks. Both subjective data—what the patient says during the history—and objective data—what the RN first assistant observes by inspecting, palpating, percussing, and auscultating during the physical examination—form the initial patient data base.

EVALUATION FOR ELECTIVE SURGERY

Preoperative assessment of the patient scheduled for elective surgery begins with the history and physical examination. Both of these assessment components focus on the patient's presenting complaint while at the same time screening for risk factors and any related patient problems. Once the history and physical are completed, a tentative diagnosis is established and appropriate screening and diagnostic tests are obtained to confirm the diagnosis. Any concomitant risk factors or conditions are stabilized or corrected; this will determine whether surgery is delayed or whether the patient's operative risk is acceptable.

OBTAINING THE HISTORY

Obtaining the patient's history may be the initiation of the relationship between the RN first assistant and the patient. Each patient must be treated as a unique individual. The purpose of the history is to learn about the patient as the nurse-patient relationship is established. The organization of the data derived from the patient's history may reflect both a nursing model and a medical model. The RN first assistant relies on a medical model when working interdependently with the surgeon in the diagnosis and treatment of disease; a nursing model is used with the medical model to focus assessment on core nursing problems.[1] A common foundation of knowledge regarding the patient facilitates collaboration between the RN first assistant and health care team.

A health history has several components, each with a specific purpose. The history's structure is widely accepted: chief complaint, present problem, past medical history, family history, social/experiential history, and systems review.[2] This chronologic and detailed structure elicits information about a wide range of variables that may affect the patient's health status. Chart 5-1 presents these components for an adult patient.

Before conducting a patient history, the RN first assistant should quickly review the patient's medical record. This review yields a "snapshot" of the patient, providing demographic and other information. By knowing the patient's name and some background information, the RN first assistant is able to set a tone of courtesy, interest, and helpfulness. The environment for the interview should be quiet, afford privacy, and be comfortable for both the RN first assistant and the patient. Note-taking should be done in brief, short phrases or words; it should not distract attention from the patient or from following the patient's leads. Asking general questions at the beginning of the interview (*e.g.*, "What brings you here today?", "How can we help you?") allows the patient freedom of response. The RN first assistant follows the patient's lead by actively listening and watching for important cues. The RN first assistant may guide the patient by using facilitation (encouragement without specifying the topic), reflection (a repetition of the patient's words to encourage further information), clarification (a request for the meaning of a statement), and empathic confirmation (a response that indicates understanding and acceptance).

Interviewing and communicating with a patient, and the family or significant other if present, is further guided by an understanding of theories of stress and coping, human growth and development, and patient confidentiality. Patients have the expectation, and the right to expect, that their confidentiality and privacy will be maintained. Treating patients with dignity and

(text continues on page 86)

CHART 5-1

Comprehensive History: Adult Patient

Date of History

Identifying Data, including age, sex, race, place of birth, marital status, occupation, and religion.

Source of Referral, if any, and the purpose of it

Source of History, such as the patient, a relative, a friend, the patient's medical record, or a referral letter

Reliability, if relevant

Chief Complaints, when possible in the patient's own words. ("My stomach hurts and I feel awful.") Sometimes patients have no overt complaints; ascertain their goals instead. ("I have come for my regular checkup" or "I've been admitted for a thorough evaluation of my heart.")

Present Illness. This is a clear, chronological narrative account of the problems for which the patient is seeking care. It should include the onset of the problem, the setting in which it developed, its manifestations, and any past treatments. The principal symptoms should be described in terms of (1) location, (2) quality, (3) quantity or severity, (4) timing (*i.e.*, onset, duration, and frequency), (5) the setting in which they occur, (6) factors that have aggravated or relieved them, and (7) associated manifestations. Relevant data from the patient's chart, such as laboratory reports, also belong in the present illness, as do significant negatives (*i.e.*, the absence of certain symptoms that will aid in differential diagnosis).

A present illness should also include patients' responses to their own symptoms and incapacities. What does the patient think has caused the problem? What are the underlying worries that have led to seeking professional attention? ("I think I may have appendicitis.") And why is that a worry? ("My Uncle Charlie died of a ruptured appendix.") Further, what effects has the illness had on the patient's life? This question is especially important in understanding a patient with chronic illness. "What can't you do now that you could do before? How has the backache, shortness of breath, or whatever, affected your ability to work? . . . your life at home? . . . your social activities? . . . your role as a parent? . . . your role as a husband, or wife? . . . the way you feel about yourself as a man, or a woman?"

Past History

General State of Health as the patient perceives it

Childhood Illnesses, such as measles, rubella, mumps, whooping cough, chicken pox, rheumatic fever, scarlet fever, polio

Adult Illnesses

Psychiatric Illnesses

Accidents and Injuries

Operations

Hospitalizations not already described

Current Health Status

Although some of the variables grouped under this heading have past as well as current components, they all have potential impact on current health and possible health-related interventions.

Allergies

Immunizations, such as tetanus, pertussis, diphtheria, polio, measles, rubella, mumps, influenza, hepatitis B, *Hemophilus influenzae*, type b, and pneumococcal vaccine

(continued)

CHART 5-1
Comprehensive History: Adult Patient *(continued)*

Screening Tests appropriate to the patient's age, such as hematocrits, urinalyses, tuberculin tests, Pap smears, mammograms, stools for occult blood, and cholesterol tests, together with the results and the dates they were last performed

Environmental Hazards, including those in the home, school, and workplace

Use of Safety Measures, such as seat belts and other methods related to specific hazards

Exercise and Leisure Activities

Sleep Patterns, including times that the person goes to bed and awakens, daytime naps, and any difficulties in falling asleep or staying asleep

Diet, including all the dietary intake for a recent 24-hour period and any dietary restrictions or supplements. Be specific in your questions. "Take yesterday, for example. Starting from when you woke up, what did you eat or drink first? . . . then what? . . . and then?" Ask specifically about coffee, tea, cola drinks, and other caffeine-containing beverages.

Current Medications, including home remedies, nonprescription drugs, vitamin/mineral supplements, and medicines borrowed from family or friends. When a patient seems likely to be taking one or more medications, survey one 24-hour period in detail. "Let's look at yesterday. Starting from when you woke up, what was the first medicine you took? How much? How often in the day did you take it? What are you taking it for? What other medicines . . . ?"

Tobacco, including the type (smoked, *e.g.*, cigarettes, or smokeless, *e.g.*, chewing tobacco or snuff), amount, and duration of use, *e.g.*, cigarettes, a pack a day for 12 years

Alcohol, Drugs, and Related Substances

Family History

The age and health, or age and cause of death, of each immediate family member (*i.e.*, parents, siblings, spouse, and children); data on grandparents or grandchildren may also be useful

The occurrence within the family of any of the following conditions: diabetes, tuberculosis, heart disease, high blood pressure, stroke, kidney disease, cancer, arthritis, anemia, headaches, epilepsy, mental illness, alcoholism, drug addiction, and symptoms like those of the patient

Psychosocial History

An outline or narrative description that captures the important and relevant information about the patient as a person:

Home Situation and Significant Others. "Who lives at home with you? Tell me a little about them . . . and about your friends." "Who helps you when you are sick, or need assistance?"

Daily Life, from the time of arising to bedtime. "What is a typical day like? What do you do first? . . . Next?"

Important Experiences, including upbringing, schooling, military service, job history, financial situation, marriage, recreation, retirement

Religious Beliefs relevant to perceptions of health, illness, and treatment

The Patient's Outlook on the present and on the future

Review of Systems

General. Usual weight, recent weight change, any clothes that fit tighter or looser than before; weakness, fatigue, fever

Skin. Rashes, lumps, sores, itching, dryness, color change, changes in hair or nails

Head. Headache, head injury

Eyes. Vision, glasses or contact lenses, last eye examination, pain, redness, excessive tearing, double vision, blurred vision, spots or specks, glaucoma, cataracts

CHART 5-1
Comprehensive History: Adult Patient *(continued)*

Ears. Hearing, tinnitus, vertigo, earaches, infection, discharge; if hearing is decreased, use of hearing aids

Nose and Sinuses. Frequent colds; nasal stuffiness, discharge, or itching; hay fever, nosebleeds, sinus trouble

Mouth and Throat. Condition of teeth and gums, bleeding gums, dentures if any and how they fit, last dental examination, sore tongue, dry mouth, frequent sore throats, hoarseness

Neck. Lumps, "swollen glands," goiter, pain or stiffness in the neck

Breasts. Lumps, pain or discomfort, nipple discharge, self-examination

Respiratory. Cough, sputum (color, quantity), hemoptysis, wheezing, asthma, bronchitis, emphysema, pneumonia, tuberculosis, pleurisy; last chest x-ray film

Cardiac. Heart trouble, high blood pressure, rheumatic fever, heart murmurs; chest pain or discomfort, palpitations; dyspnea, orthopnea, paroxysmal nocturnal dyspnea, edema; past electrocardiogram or other heart tests

Gastrointestinal. Trouble swallowing, heartburn, appetite, nausea, vomiting, regurgitation, vomiting of blood, indigestion; frequency of bowel movements, color and size of stools, change in bowel habits, rectal bleeding or black tarry stools, hemorrhoids, constipation, diarrhea; abdominal pain, food intolerance, excessive belching or passing of gas; jaundice, liver or gallbladder trouble, hepatitis

Urinary. Frequency of urination, polyuria, nocturia, burning or pain on urination, hematuria, urgency, reduced caliber or force of the urinary stream, hesitancy, dribbling, incontinence; urinary infections, stones

Genital

Male. Hernias, discharge from or sores on the penis, testicular pain or masses, history of sexually transmitted diseases and their treatments; sexual preference, interest, function, satisfaction, and problems

Female. Age at menarche; regularity, frequency, and duration of periods; amount of bleeding, bleeding between periods or after intercourse, last menstrual period; dysmenorrhea, premenstrual tension; age at menopause, menopausal symptoms, postmenopausal bleeding; if the patient was born before 1971, exposure to DES (diethylstilbestrol) from maternal use during pregnancy; discharge, itching, sores, lumps, sexually transmitted diseases and their treatments; number of pregnancies, number of deliveries, number of abortions (spontaneous and induced); complications of pregnancy; birth control methods; sexual preference, interest, function, satisfaction; any problems, including dyspareunia

Peripheral Vascular. Intermittent claudication, leg cramps, varicose veins, past clots in the veins

Musculoskeletal. Muscle or joint pains, stiffness, arthritis, gout, backache; if present, describe location and symptoms (*e.g.*, swelling, redness, pain, tenderness, stiffness, weakness, limitation of motion or activity).

Neurologic. Fainting, blackouts, seizures, weakness, paralysis, numbness or loss of sensation, tingling or "pins and needles," tremors or other involuntary movements

Hematologic. Anemia, easy bruising or bleeding, past transfusions and any reactions to them

Endocrine. Thyroid trouble, heat or cold intolerance, excessive sweating; diabetes, excessive thirst or hunger, polyuria

Psychiatric. Nervousness, tension, mood including depression; memory

Source: Bates, B: A Guide to Physical Examination, 5th Edn, 1991

preserving their privacy is one of the ethical standards of a professional.[3] The AORN's Standards of Perioperative Professional Performance further clarify this responsibility by noting that the nurse acts as patient advocate, maintaining patient confidentiality and delivering care that is nonjudgmental, nondiscriminatory, and sensitive to cultural, racial, and ethnic diversity while preserving patient autonomy, dignity, and rights.[4]

Theories of Stress and Coping

Various nursing models can serve as frameworks for understanding stress, coping, and adaptation. Whichever model is chosen to guide nursing practice, the RN first assistant may consider stress to be a state produced by some change in the internal or external environment that the patient perceives as threatening, challenging, or damaging to his or her sense of well being. Each patient is unique in his or her perception of a stressor and in the adaptive mechanisms used to cope with it. Coping has both cognitive and behavioral aspects; the ability to cope effectively is influenced by the patient's resources. Important coping resources include health, energy, problem-solving skills, social skills, support, and the ability to access and afford external resources. Figure 5-1 provides a simplified diagram of the stress and coping process.

Ineffective coping results when the patient is unable to manage internal or external stressors adequately.[5] The patient may verbalize an inability to cope or may use defense mechanisms inappropriately; for example, defensive coping (repeated projection of falsely positive self-evaluation in response to underlying perceived threat to positive self-regard) and ineffective denial (minimization or disavowal of symptoms or situations detrimental to health). The following outcome criteria and nursing interventions by the RN first assistant may be selected with patients exhibiting ineffective coping:

> Desired outcomes: The patient will verbalize feelings, identify coping patterns and their consequences, identify personal strengths, accept support through the nursing relationship, make decisions, and follow through with appropriate actions.
>
> RN first assistant interventions:
>
> 1. Determine causative and contributing factors.
> 2. Assess for risk factors for poor coping.
> 3. Validate the patient's present coping status.
> 4. Teach constructive problem-solving techniques.
> 5. Assist the patient to develop appropriate strategies based on personal strengths and previous experiences.
> 6. Assist the patient in coping with recent diagnosis, as appropriate.
> 7. Initiate referrals as indicated.[6]

Human Growth and Development

Maturational factors are also relevant when obtaining the patient history. A holistic nursing framework acknowledges the patient's developmental stage, appraises the patient's requisite life tasks, values and reinforces the patient's strengths and assets, and assists the patient in determining problems or dom-

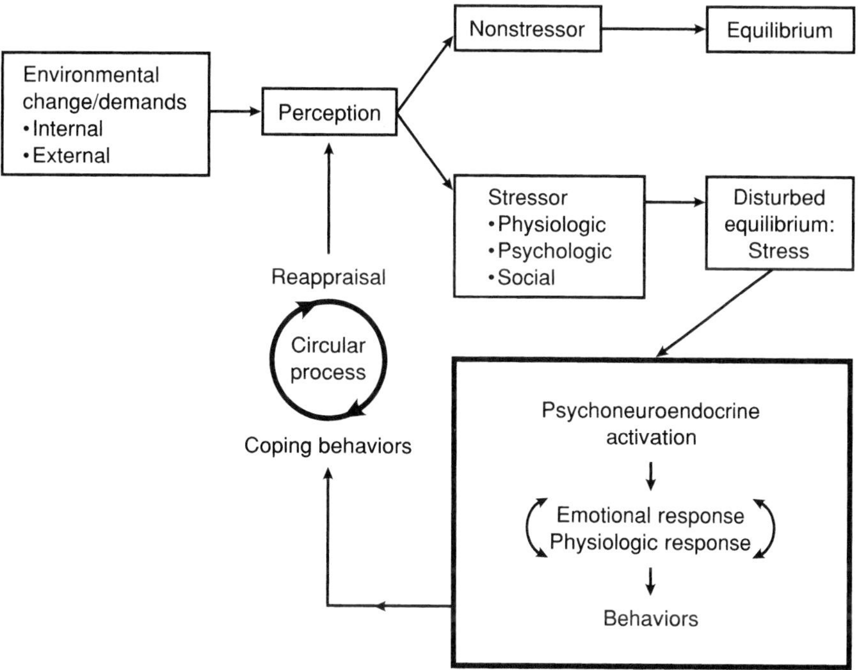

FIGURE 5-1

The stress-coping model. When an environmental change is perceived by the brain as stressful, psychoneuroendocrine activation occurs, eliciting emotional and physiologic responses manifested in objective and subjective behaviors. As the individual copes, using his own resources and social supports, reappraisal will recur again and again, providing feedback to the perception of the situation. *Source: Smeltzer, S, Bare B: Brunner & Suddarth's Textbook of Medical Surgical Nursing, 7th Ed. Philadelphia: JB Lippincott, 1992.*

inant issues. Various nurse experts have built on Erikson's stages of development; Chart 5-2 summarizes these stages for the adult patient.

Skills in obtaining a history must be flexible and sensitive. It is not only the symptoms themselves that must be understood; the personal and cultural meanings attached to them are also important in fully understanding the patient. Most health care facilities have forms that specify the content of the history. Although such forms can be useful, the RN first assistant should be guided just as much by what the patient says and the interview skills necessary to elicit this information.

PERFORMING THE PHYSICAL EXAMINATION

The RN first assistant uses four routine techniques during physical examination: inspection, palpation, percussion, and auscultation. These techniques are discussed in general in this section; the RN first assistant will need to

CHART 5-2

Erikson's Stages of Development for Adults

Stage	Age	Tasks	Lack of Achievement
Early Adult	20–45	Intimacy vs. Isolation Increases independence Establishes career Forms intimate bonds Chooses mate, significant other Sets up, manages household Establishes social support Assumes civic/ community responsibility Initiates parenting Develops meaningful life philosophy	Avoids intimacy Is isolated Is promiscuous Exhibits "character problems" Repudiates relationships
Middle Adult	40–65	Generativity vs. Stagnation Adjusts to physical changes Reviews/redirects career Develops hobby/leisure activity Helps children/aging parents	Is egocentric Is nonproductive Becomes an early invalid Exhibits self-love Becomes impoverished Is self-indulgent
Late Adult	60+	Integrity vs. Despair Adjusts to physical and health changes Forms new roles Adjusts to retirement, loss of income Develops activities that enhance self-worth, usefulness	Feels that time is too short Feels that life has no meaning Has lost faith in self/others Wants second chance Lacks spirituality Fears death

Adapted from: Jarvis, C. (1992). Physical Examination and Health Assessment. Philadelphia: W.B. Saunders Co, 36–40 and Grimes, J. & Burns, E. Health Assessment in Nursing Practice. (1987). Boston: Jones and Bartlett Publishers, Inc., 531.

modify and adapt them to specific body systems. Chart 5-3 provides an overview of a comprehensive physical examination.

INSPECTION

Inspection involves detailed observation; it begins with initial patient contact. Throughout the history and examination, the RN first assistant should observe

(text continues on page 90)

CHART 5-3

Overview of a Comprehensive Examination

General Survey. Observe the general state of health, stature and habitus, and sexual development. Weigh the patient, if possible. Note posture, motor activity, and gait; dress, grooming, and personal hygiene; and any odors of body or breath. Watch the patient's facial expressions and note manner, affect, and reactions to the persons and things in the environment. Listen to the patient's speech and note state of awareness or level of consciousness.

Vital Signs. Count the pulse and respiratory rate. Measure the blood pressure and, if indicated, the body temperature.

Skin. Observe the skin and its characteristics. Identify any lesions, noting their location, distribution, arrangement, type, and color. Inspect and palpate the hair and nails. Study the patient's hands.

Begin your assessment of the skin with the exposed areas—the hands, forearms, and face. Continue it as you examine other body regions such as the thorax, abdomen, genitalia, and limbs.

Head. Examine the hair, scalp, skull, and face.

Eyes. Check visual acuity and, if indicated, the visual fields. Note the position and alignment of the eyes. Observe the eyelids and inspect the sclera and conjunctiva of each eye. With oblique lighting, inspect each cornea, iris, and lens. Compare the pupils and test their reactions to light. Assess the extraocular movements. With an ophthalmoscope, inspect the ocular fundi.

Ears. Inspect the auricles, canals, and drums. Check auditory acuity. If acuity is diminished, check lateralization (Weber test) and compare air and bone conduction (Rinne test).

Nose and Sinuses. Examine the external nose, and with aid of a light and speculum inspect the nasal mucosa, septum, and turbinates. Palpate for tenderness of the frontal and maxillary sinuses.

Mouth and Pharynx. Inspect the lips, buccal mucosa, gums, teeth, roof of the mouth, tongue, and pharynx.

Neck. Inspect and palpate the cervical lymph nodes. Note any masses or unusual pulsations in the neck. Feel for any deviation of the trachea. Observe the sound and effort of the patient's breathing. Inspect and palpate the thyroid gland.

Back. Inspect and palpate the spine and muscles of the back. Check for costovertebral angle tenderness.

Posterior Thorax and Lungs. Inspect, palpate, and percuss the chest. Identify the level of diaphragmatic dullness on each side. Listen to the breath sounds, identify any adventitious sounds, and, if indicated, listen to the transmitted voice sounds.

Breasts, Axillae, and Epitrochlear Nodes. In a woman, inspect the breasts with her arms relaxed and then elevated, and then with her hands pressed on her hips. In either sex, inspect the axillae and feel for the axillary nodes. Feel for the epitrochlear nodes.

By this time you have examined the patient's hands, surveyed the back, and, at least in women, made a fair estimate of the range of motion at the shoulders. Your examination of the anterior thorax will include inspection of additional musculoskeletal structures. Use these observations, together with the patient's history and ease of movement throughout the examination, in deciding whether or not to continue with a full musculoskeletal examination.

If you need to do a more complete musculoskeletal examination, it is convenient to examine the hands, arms, shoulders, neck, and jaw while the patient is still in the sitting position. Inspect and palpate the joints and check their range of motion.

Breasts. Palpate the breasts, while at the same time continuing your inspection.

Anterior Thorax and Lungs. Inspect, palpate, and percuss the chest. Listen to the breath sounds, any adventitious sounds, and, if indicated, transmitted voice sounds.

(continued)

CHART 5-3
Overview of a Comprehensive Examination *(continued)*

Cardiovascular System. Inspect and palpate the carotid pulsations. Listen for carotid bruits. Observe the jugular venous pulsations, and measure the jugular venous pressure in relation to the sternal angle.

Inspect and palpate the precordium. Note the location, diameter, amplitude, and duration of the apical impulse. Listen at the apex and the lower sternal border with the bell of a stethoscope. Listen at each auscultatory area with the diaphragm. Listen for physiologic splitting of the second heart sound and for any abnormal heart sounds or murmurs.

Abdomen. Inspect, auscultate, and percuss the abdomen. Palpate lightly, then deeply. Try to feel the liver, spleen, kidneys, and aorta.

Rectal Examination in Men. Inspect the sacrococcygeal and perineal areas. Palpate the anal canal, rectum, and prostate. If the patient cannot stand, examine the genitalia before doing the rectal examination.

Genitalia and Rectal Examination in Women. Examine the external genitalia, vagina, and cervix. Obtain Pap smears. Palpate the uterus and the adnexa. Do a rectovaginal and rectal examination.

Legs. Inspect the legs, assessing the:

Peripheral Vascular System. Note any swelling, discoloration, or ulcers. Palpate for pitting edema. Feel the dorsalis pedis, posterior tibial, and femoral pulses, and, if indicated, the popliteal pulses. Palpate the inguinal lymph nodes.

Musculoskeletal System. Note any deformities or enlarged joints. If indicated, palpate the joints and check their range of motion.

Neurologic System. Observe the muscle bulk, the position of the limbs, and any abnormal movements.

Musculoskeletal System. Examine the alignment of the spine and its range of motion, the alignment of the legs, and the feet.

Peripheral Vascular System. Inspect for varicose veins.

Genitalia and Hernias in Men. Examine the penis and scrotal contents and check for hernias.

Screening Neurologic Examination. Observe the patient's gait and ability to walk heel-to-toe, walk on the toes, walk on the heels, hop in place, and do shallow knee bends. Check for pronator drift and do a Romberg test. Assess the strength of the grip and of the vertically raised arms. Look for winging as the arms are lowered.

Check the deep tendon reflexes and plantar responses.

Assess sensory function by testing pain and vibration in the hands and feet, light touch on the limbs, and stereognosis in the hands.

Source: Bates, B: A Guide to Physical Examination, 5th Edn, 1991

for and note the patient's body posture and stature, gait and stance, body movements, speech patterns, body temperature, skin color and moisture, any unusual odor, and general state of nutrition. Preliminary observations provide basic information that can influence the remainder of the examination. Unlike other physical examination techniques, inspection continues throughout the examination. With this kind of continuity, the RN first assistant constantly subjects to confirmation or dispute what is "seen" about the patient.

The right and left side of the body should be compared; they should be nearly symmetrical.

As the RN first assistant gains clinical practice in inspection, visual acuity and sense of sight become trained to focus in on detail. Specific inspection will be directed to the focused part of the physical examination. During focused inspection, good lighting, adequate patient exposure, and certain instruments may be required.

PALPATION

Palpation involves "feeling" through the use of touch. The RN first assistant confirms points noted during inspection, assessing temperature, texture (roughness, smoothness), size, swelling, rigidity, lumps or masses (motility and configuration), and presence of tenderness or pain. Different parts of the hand are better suited to certain assessment parameters. The fingertips are tactile discriminators, good for noting skin texture, swelling, pulsatility, consistency, moisture, and shape of lumps or masses. To further detect the position, shape, or consistency of a mass, a gentle grasping of the fingers is used. The dorsum (back) of the hand or fingers, where the skin is thinner than on the palms, is best for assessing temperature. The ulnar surface of the hand or palmar aspect (base) of the fingers is best for detecting any vibrations.

Palpation should be slow and systematic. The hands should be warmed before touching the patient. Light palpation, gently pressing in to a depth up to 1 centimeter, is used for most of the physical examination. Heavy, continuous pressure will blunt the sense of touch. Any tender areas should be palpated last. Bimanual palpation, the use of both hands to capture or envelop a body part or structure, is used in breast or pelvic examination. Deep palpation, pressing in to a depth up to 4 centimeters, is used for specific structures, such as abdominal organs. During deep palpation, intermittent pressure is often better than one continuous palpation.

PERCUSSION

The hands are also used for percussion, wherein the application of a physical force translates into sound. The "feel" and sound assist in depicting location and size by a change in the percussion note between two borders and in determining the density of a structure by a characteristic note. Figure 5-2 shows the procedure for a right-handed RN first assistant; a left-handed RN first assistant should reverse the hand positions.

The distal phalanx of the middle finger (sometimes referred to as the pleximeter) of the nondominant hand is placed firmly on the body surface being percussed. The remaining fingers and palm either gently rest or are raised off the surface to prevent dampening of sound vibrations. A sharp, rapid, light tap with the middle finger (sometimes referred to as the plexor) of the dominant hand, or the index and middle fingers together, is made using wrist action. Thus, in this technique one finger acts as the hammer, and the other acts as the striking surface. The shoulders and elbow should remain sta-

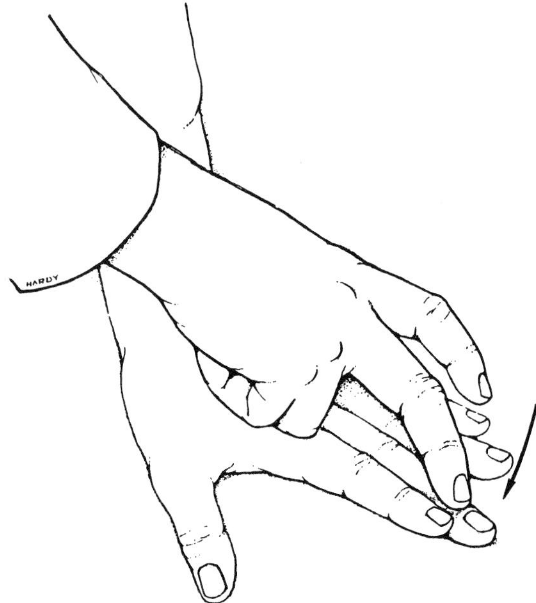

FIGURE 5-2
Percussion technique. The middle finger of the right hand strikes the terminal phalanx of the middle finger of the left hand. *Source: Smeltzer S, Bare B: Brunner & Suddarth's Textbook of Medical-Surgical Nursing. 7th Ed. Philadelphia: J B Lippincott, 1992.*

tionary; the downward snap of the striking finger (or fingers) should originate from the wrist. The tap of the "hammer finger" should be quick. The finger strikes, the wrist snaps back, and the finger is lifted off by this wrist action to prevent dampening the sound. The striking finger should hit at right angles to the stationary finger, with just enough force to achieve a clear note. The thickness of the body part being percussed is a factor in determining this force. Percussion tones usually arise from vibration 4 to 6 centimeters deep in body tissue. A stronger percussion stroke may be required for patients who are obese or have a very muscular body wall.

The sound produced by percussion reflects the density of the underlying structure. From the least to the most dense, these sounds are called tympany (over air-filled viscus), hyperresonance (over lungs with an abnormal amount of air, as with emphysema), resonance (over normal lung tissue), dullness (over dense organs), and flatness (no air present, as over thigh muscle).[7] Changes in sound assist in mapping the location and size of an organ and in detecting superficial masses. The RN first assistant should evaluate the amplitude (intensity), pitch (frequency), quality, and duration of the sounds heard. Percussion may elicit pain if an underlying structure is inflamed. A percussion instrument, such as a percussion hammer, is used to elicit deep tendon reflexes.

AUSCULTATION

The final technique in physical assessment, auscultation usually is accomplished through the use of a stethoscope. The diaphragm of this instrument has a flat edge used to auscultate high-pitched sounds, such as heart, breath, and bowel sounds and friction rubs and crepitus. The diaphragm should be warmed and then placed firmly against the patient's skin. Firm placement will leave a slight ring on the skin when the diaphragm is removed. The stethoscope's bell endpiece detects soft, low-pitched sounds such as heart murmurs, stenotic arteries, venous hums, and bruits. The bell is held lightly against the skin with only enough pressure to form a seal. The RN first assistant uses the stethoscope to listen for intensity (loudness), frequency (pitch), and quality (overtone). Special applications of auscultation depend on specific organ systems.

PREOPERATIVE TESTING

Demands for quality, effectiveness, appropriateness, and cost containment have altered past practices of prescribing a battery of routine screening tests for surgical patients. In the 1990s, preoperative testing should be based on clinical relevance. The RN first assistant should understand each test's predictive value in detecting a disease or condition and its specificity in confirming whether the patient has the disease or condition. Appendix II provides a review of common diagnostic tests and their significance.

INFORMED CONSENT AND PATIENT SELF-DETERMINATION

Consent, per se, is an agreement reached between a physician and a patient, resulting from a discussion between them.[8] A consent form provides evidence of such an agreement. Informed consent implies that the patient and physician discussed the proposed procedure and reasons for it, its inherent risks and benefits, and any treatment alternatives. The physician is responsible for this discussion. The RN first assistant is held to a nursing standard of care requiring that the nurse advise a superior or the physician if the nurse has reason to believe that consent was not obtained or was not adequately "informed."

A patient's right to self-determination is protected through the informed consent process. This process requires that the patient be capable of giving consent, understand the advantages and disadvantages of consenting, and not be coerced.[9]

The Patient Self-Determination Act (PSDA) further enunciates patients' rights to make decisions concerning their medical care. The PSDA requires that all health care institutions participating in Medicare and Medicaid maintain written policies and procedures to inform adult patients of their rights to formulate advance directives (written instructions, such as durable power of attorney), to document on the medical record whether or not they have executed advance directives, to ensure compliance with state laws regarding advance directives, and to provide education for staff members and the public concerning advance directives.[10] The RN first assistant should review these institutional policies and procedures, as well as the written information that must be provided to patients on admission.

Part of the RN first assistant's patient assessment should include the patient's emotional status, values orientation, and willingness and capability to execute an advance directive. Diplomacy, compassion, sensitivity, and empathy may be required when negotiating between the patient, family, and health care staff in implementing PSDA protocols.[11]

CONCLUSION

Trust, respect, and empathy underpin the creation of a therapeutic relationship between the RN first assistant and the patient. Productive communication that is free of imposed values or judgments facilitates the health assessment process. People communicate in a variety of ways, and the RN first assistant must listen actively to understand what the patient is really saying. As the RN first assistant collects subjective and objective data about the patient, the health state is assessed to uncover and diagnose health problems. At the same time, the patient's strengths and health assets are acknowledged and nurtured. Relevant data should be fit into the patient's developmental stage. The rapport built during the history and physical examination establishes and facilitates the continuing RN first assistant-patient relationship.

REVIEW QUESTIONS

1. Subjective data are obtained
   a. as the RN first assistant develops from novice to expert
   b. from what the patient says
   c. as part of the RN first assistant's intuition
   d. as the RN first assistant observes the patient
2. One of the most important points to keep in mind during a history is
   a. that each patient is an individual
   b. to make use of some of the time to teach correct health behaviors
   c. that using a preprinted form expedites the process
   d. that it should result in an index of operative risk
3. It is common, and desirable, to describe which component of the health history in the patient's own words?
   a. source of referral
   b. chief complaint
   c. history of present illness
   d. current health status

4. Relevant data from the patient's chart, such as laboratory reports, belong in which section of the history?
   a. chief complaint
   b. history of present illness
   c. current health status
   d. past history
5. As part of a holistic framework, during the psychosocial history the RN first assistant will query the patient regarding
   a. use of alcohol, drugs, and related substances
   b. age and health/cause of death of immediate family members
   c. cultural and religious beliefs
   d. exercise and leisure activities
6. To allow the patient some freedom of response, it is helpful to begin the history interview by
   a. providing information about the RN first assistant's role on the health care team
   b. having the patient complete a health questionnaire
   c. reassuring the patient that all information will be kept confidential
   d. asking general, open-ended questions
7. A useful interviewing technique that repeats the patient's words to encourage further information is termed
   a. facilitation
   b. reflection
   c. clarification
   d. empathic confirmation
8. The AORN Standards of Professional Performance set the expectation that the RN first assistant will
   a. assist the patient in adapting to stressors
   b. preserve the patient's autonomy, dignity, and rights
   c. make referrals when the patient requires access to external resources
   d. interpret relevant findings in the context of the patient's growth and development
9. A utilitarian definition of stress views it as a patient state produced by
   a. some change in the internal or external environment
   b. inability to cope
   c. psychoneuroendocrine activation
   d. cognitive perception and behavioral change
10. A desired patient outcome for a nursing diagnosis of Ineffective Coping might be
    a. assess for risk factors
    b. teach constructive problem-solving
    c. minimize symptoms; focus on positive results of treatment
    d. verbalize feelings and personal strengths

11. The usual sequence in physical examination is
    a. inspection, percussion, palpation, auscultation
    b. inspection, palpation, percussion, auscultation
    c. palpation, inspection, auscultation, percussion
    d. auscultation, palpation, percussion, inspection
12. Focused visual attention best describes the technique of
    a. auscultation
    b. palpation
    c. percussion
    d. inspection
13. Information from resonance sounds is obtained through
    a. auscultation
    b. palpation
    c. percussion
    d. inspection

Column A lists findings from palpation. Column B lists the areas of the hand that are most sensitive to a specific finding. Match the finding (Column A) with the appropriate area of the hand (Column B).

Column A - Finding	*Column B - Area of the hand*
14. _______ skin texture	A. Fingertips
15. _______ pulsatility	B. Dorsum
16. _______ temperature	C. Ulnar surface
17. _______ consistency	
18. _______ vibrations	
19. _______ swelling	
20. _______ shape of mass/lump	

21. Light palpation presses in to a depth up to
    a. 1 centimeter
    b. 3 centimeters
    c. 4 centimeters
    d. 6 centimeters
22. During percussion, the middle finger of which hand is used to perform a light, rapid tap
    a. dominant
    b. nondominant
23. The percussion tone expected over normal lung tissue is
    a. dullness
    b. flatness
    c. resonance
    d. tympany

24. The _______ of the stethoscope should be placed _______ against the patient's skin
    a. diaphragm; lightly
    b. diaphragm; firmly
    c. bell; firmly
    d. bell; flatly
25. The Patient Self-Determination Act enunciates the patient's right to
    a. read and obtain a copy of his or her medical record
    b. be informed of the inherent risks and benefits of treatment
    c. a private and confidential physician relationship
    d. make decisions regarding his or her medical care

Answers

1. b	6. d	11. b	16. b	21. a
2. a	7. b	12. d	17. a	22. a
3. b	8. b	13. c	18. c	23. c
4. b	9. a	14. a	19. a	24. b
5. c	10. d	15. a	20. a	25. d

REFERENCES

1. Jarvis C: Physical Examination and Health Assessment. Philadelphia, WB Saunders, 1992
2. Seidel HM, Ball JW, Dains JE, Benedict G: Mosby's Guide to Physical Examination. St. Louis, CV Mosby, 1987
3. Glidewell B: Confidentiality and Professionalism Go Hand-In-Hand (Video). American Hospital Association, 1989
4. Association of Operating Room Nurses: AORN Standards and Recommended Practices. Denver, Association of Operating Room Nurses, 1992
5. Carpenito LJ: Nursing Diagnosis: Application to Clinical Practice. Philadelphia, JB Lippincott, 1992
6. Ibid, pp 278–280
7. Brunner LS, Suddarth DS: Textbook of Medical Surgical Nursing, p 63. Philadelphia, JB Lippincott, 1988
8. Horty J, Webb P: Informed consent: Nurse as troubleshooter. OR Manager, 6(2):10–11, 1990
9. Carpenito, p 573
10. Murphy EK: Advance directives and the Patient Self-Determination Act. AORN J, 55:270–272, 1992
11. Weber G, Kjervik DK: The Patient Self-Determination Act: The nurse's proactive role. J Prof Nurs, 8:6, 1992

6 Perioperative Patient Preparation

Jane C. Rothrock*

As part of perioperative nursing, the RN first assistant is involved with the patient preoperatively, intraoperatively, and postoperatively. In a practice setting providing optimum continuity of care, the RN first assistant and patient would establish a relationship that originated at the time the decision for surgical intervention was made. The RN first assistant would begin patient assessment, identify and assist the patient to meet learning needs, initiate dialogue and plans for home care, and work in partnership with the patient to see that he or she was prepared emotionally, physically, spiritually, and in whatever other way the patient needed preparational assistance. In the operating area, be it an acute care setting or ambulatory surgery, the RN first assistant would assist in admitting the patient to the operating room and then engage in patient care throughout the surgery as needed. The RN first assistant would accompany the patient to the PACU, give a nursing report, and follow the patient through the hospital stay, making home visits if necessary and seeing the patient postoperatively in the office. This chapter reviews preoperative education, admission to the operating room, skin preparation, and creation of a sterile field with surgical barriers.

PREOPERATIVE PATIENT EDUCATION

A prevalent mechanism for designating the role and domain of nursing, and nursing knowledge, is the use of nursing diagnoses. This classification system

* *In the first edition of this book, this chapter was titled Perioperative Skin Preparation and Draping and was written by Lillian H. Nicolette.*

provides nurses with a common frame of reference in providing and directing patient care and identifies what nurses will be accountable for. As defined by the North American Nursing Diagnosis Association (NANDA), a nursing diagnosis is a clinical judgment about individual, family, or community responses to actual or potential health problems/life processes. Nursing diagnosis provides the basis for selecting nursing interventions to achieve outcomes for which the nurse is accountable.[1]

There are five types of nursing diagnosis: actual, high risk, possible, wellness, and syndrome. Actual nursing diagnoses must be clinically validated by identifiable characteristics. In 1992, NANDA changed the former terminology of "potential" nursing diagnosis to high risk; this diagnostic category is used when the nurse makes a clinical judgment that a particular patient is more vulnerable to develop a problem than are others in a similar situation. Possible nursing diagnoses describe suspected problems for which additional data are required. Wellness diagnoses describe a transition from one level of wellness to a higher level. Syndrome diagnoses are clusters of actual or high risk nursing diagnoses that are predicted to be present because of a certain event or situation.

KNOWLEDGE DEFICIT AND ANXIETY

Most RN first assistants would begin their approach to patient education with the nursing diagnosis Knowledge Deficit. This state exists when a patient exhibits a deficiency in cognitive knowledge or psychomotor skills regarding his or her condition or treatment plan. The RN first assistant must not assume that a knowledge deficit is present; the patient should verbalize a lack of knowledge or skills, request information, express an inaccurate perception regarding surgery or required care, or incorrectly perform a care requisite. The patient and family/significant others should be involved in identifying areas of learning need and skill mastery, and patient/family teaching should correspond to these needs. Too often, nurses have assumed and directed what the patient should know without determining what the patient needs or wants to know. Such assumptions are not part of a nursing plan that respects the patient as an individual who is capable of self-determination and participation in the plan of care.

The term "care" is used in different ways in nursing. In some instances nurses "take care of"; this is an act of tending for another or doing something for the other. "Caring for" is often expressed in terms of physical needs. Care can also be "caring about"; in this sense, it is an attitude or emotional investment in another person. "Taking care" indicates a caution or concern, a guarding against harm, as in prevention of injury. The care processes engaged in by the RN first assistant may involve comforting, supporting, providing direct helping behaviors, assisting with coping and stress reduction, or offering empathy or compassion. As part of his or her care, the RN first assistant should understand that caring is an interpersonal experience involving moment-to-moment human encounters between two people. Patient education may involve taking care of dressings until the patient can perform self-dressing changes; it may involve caring about the patient's anxiety and fears; and it may involve taking care that the patient does not suffer an injury or harm due to lack of instruction.

It has been suggested that rather than Knowledge Deficit, a more appropriate nursing diagnosis for surgical patients is Anxiety related to insufficient knowledge of preoperative routines, postoperative exercises/activities, or postoperative alterations/sensations.[2] Anxiety should be confirmed by patient verbalization or the nurse's observation of anxious behaviors, such as restlessness, inability to concentrate and retain information, increased verbalization, poor eye contact, facial tension, extraneous movements, quivering voice, and tremulousness. This vague uneasiness that characterizes anxiety is usually due to the situational event of surgery and its perceived threats. The RN first assistant seeks to intervene by providing information related to preparation for, need for, and expectations for diagnostic studies, the surgical procedure, postoperative treatment regimens, and follow-up care.

RN FIRST ASSISTANT INTERVENTIONS

Patient education can occur in various settings by various methods. It may be through discussion, printed materials, video, computer disk, or demonstration; it may be planned or spontaneous; it may be formal or informal. Whichever method is selected, certain general premises of adult education should guide the RN first assistant in planning and delivering patient education.

At the outset, the RN first assistant should determine what the patient needs to know and wants to know. Because the patient may not know exactly what information he or she needs, it is helpful to ask about past experiences with surgery and positive or negative perceptions. Directed questions such as "Can you tell me what you are most concerned about?" may help the patient focus on worries and fears. This focused assessment will assist the RN first assistant and patient in determining sources of anxiety and direct some of the teaching content. These content areas should be agreed on between the RN first assistant and the patient. A teaching plan is developed around these areas; the plan should take into consideration the patient's level of understanding of the planned surgical procedure and its associated events, as well as the patient's level of education and preferred learning style. It is desirable to involve the patient and family/significant others in developing content area; there may be an area not identified by the patient that is of concern to a family caregiver.

Teaching should begin with the most relevant and important information, with simple but clear explanations. At appropriate intervals, the RN first assistant should have the patient restate information or demonstrate what has been taught. Positive reinforcement and affirmation are important; the RN first assistant should not assume that a patient knows that he or she is doing something correctly or well. Pacing during education is important; too much information in too little time is liable to stimulate anxiety, not reduce it. Providing written material can reinforce verbal teaching. The patient and family/significant other can refer to such written material and identify areas that are still unclear. It is critical to listen actively to a patient and redesign material to incorporate any concerns or anxieties. As necessary, and with the patient's agreement, the RN first assistant should initiate appropriate referrals to other assistive resources.

OUTCOME CRITERIA: KNOWLEDGE DEFICIT AND ANXIETY

Establishing and evaluating outcomes is part of the accountability associated with nursing diagnoses. By knowing what is expected to result from a nursing intervention and determining whether this expectation was achieved, the RN first assistant validates that the problem is either resolved or that further intervention is required. Appropriate outcome criteria for the nursing diagnosis "Anxiety related to insufficient knowledge of perioperative events might include the following":

The patient will verbalize what to expect during the perioperative period.
The patient will demonstrate postoperative regimens and home care requirements.
The patient will relate/report less anxiety following teaching.

ADMISSION TO THE OPERATING ROOM

Whether the patient is an ambulatory surgery patient or an inpatient, the RN first assistant should make every attempt to greet the patient on his or her arrival in the surgical suite. In the holding area, the RN first assistant may assist the holding area nurse in the routine admission procedures of patient identification, operative site/side verification, allergy verification, and so forth. The RN first assistant should take the time to briefly review the patient's medical record for any recent reports that have not previously been reviewed and to assess the patient's emotional status. The rapport begun during the history, physical examination, and patient education sessions will facilitate the ongoing interpersonal relationship between the RN first assistant and the patient.

The RN first assistant should also remain with the patient for preanesthesia preparation. (See Chapter 7, Anesthesia and Patient Positioning, for more information.) As an experienced perioperative nurse, the RN first assistant is invaluable to the patient, anesthesia staff, and perioperative nursing colleagues during insertion of lines, transfer to the OR bed, and anesthesia induction. This versatility and multidimensional nursing role are critical and essential contributions of a RN first assistant. Because the RN first assistant is well-acquainted with patient care routines, productivity is enhanced, patient care quality improved, and risk managed.

SKIN PREPARATION

All surgical patients have a high risk for infection related to impaired skin and tissue integrity. The RN first assistant's skill and knowledge of the origin of and containment methods for exogenous microorganisms by antiseptic skin preparation aid in protecting the patient from serious complications of wound infection.

Vitalized tissue has enormous resistance to infection. It takes a significant microbial deposit in the tissue to cause an infection; when bioburdens of 10^5 microorganisms per cubic millimeter are left in wounds, wound infection rates increase dramatically. Bacteria are commonly found on skin surfaces, especially in the moist areas of the axillae, the mouth, and the perineum. These areas are ideal incubators for microbes. Other body areas such as the trunk and extremities have negligible numbers of microbes. On the other hand, exposed body parts such as the face, hands, and feet can harbor up to 10^3 microorganisms per cubic millimeter. These bacteria are commonly found on the top, horny layer of the skin and around the entrance to hair follicles. For these reasons, the effectiveness of an antimicrobial chemical agent is critical to microbial destruction on the skin. Through proper skin antisepsis, the RN first assistant can rid the skin of these superficial microbes.

ANATOMY AND PHYSIOLOGY OF THE SKIN

Intact skin and mucous membranes are the body's first line of defense against infection. The skin has two specific layers: the outer epidermis and the deeper dermis. Stratified squamous tissue that varies in thickness from 0.06 mm to 0.10 mm, the *epidermis* functions as a barrier to protect inner tissues, as a receptor for a range of sensations, and as a regulator of temperature. Essentially avascular, the multiple levels of epidermal cells progressively die as they reach the surface; this tissue layer constantly sheds cells, which are replaced from the dermal layer. The hair follicles and sweat glands pass through the epidermis. The *dermis* is a layer of fibroelastic connective tissue that contains lymphatic vessels, blood vessels, nerves, hair follicles, and sebaceous and sweat glands (Figure 6-1).

Bacteria are prevalent on all skin layers and are categorized as either transient or resident flora. The transient flora are those in loose contact with the skin, such as grease, sweat, and oil particles. Because they are in loose contact, these organisms are easily removed by gentle mechanical friction. The resident flora, on the other hand, are found in and around the glands and hair follicles. They are carried to the surface and shed with perspiration and skin cells. Examples of resident flora include *Staphylococcus epidermidis,* aerobic and anaerobic diphtheroid bacilli, aerobic spore-forming bacilli, aerobic and anaerobic streptococci, and gram-negative rods. Because the surgical incision breaks the continuity of the skin, skin preparation must be directed at removing transient flora and suppressing the activity of resident flora.

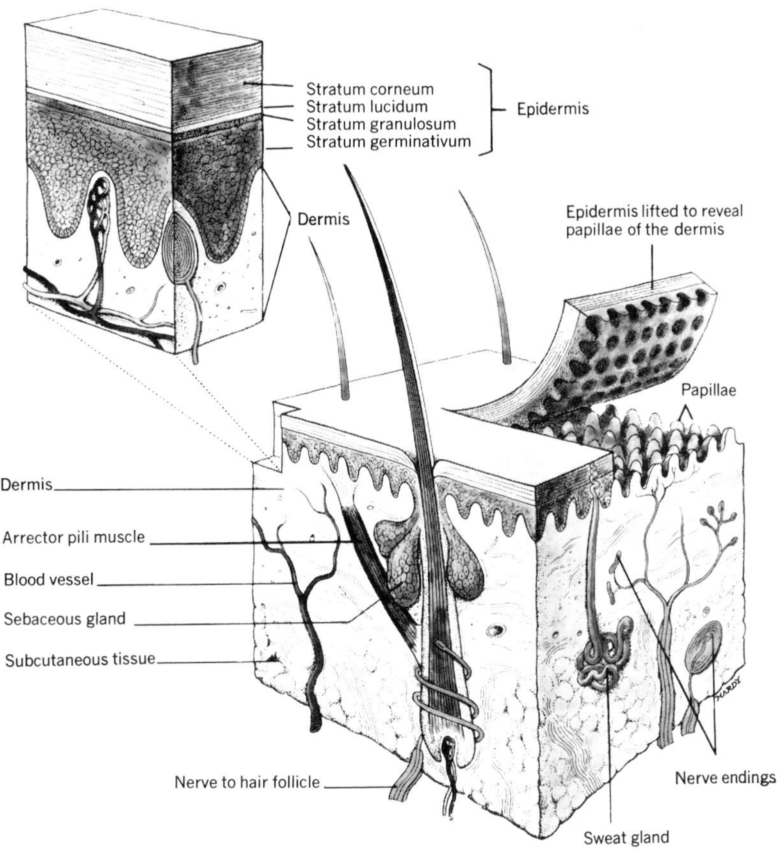

FIGURE 6-1.
Anatomy of the skin. *(From Chaffee EE, Lytle IM: Basic Physiology and Anatomy, 4th ed. Philadelphia, JB Lippincott, 1980)*

OBJECTIVES OF SKIN PREPARATION

General considerations in the preparation of skin include the surgical site, condition of the site, the numbers and kinds of contaminants, skin characteristics, the patient's overall condition, the use of aseptic technique, and the selection of effective antimicrobial agents and application techniques. The primary purpose of perioperative skin preparation is to remove the transient dirt, oil, and microorganisms from the epidermis and to prevent the growth and multiplication of the dermal microbes. According to the Association of Operating Room Nurses' (AORN) *Recommended Practices for Preoperative Skin Preparation of Patients*, three objectives should be met:

1. to remove soil and transient microbes from the skin
2. to reduce the resident microbial count to subpathogenic amounts in a short time with the least amount of tissue irritation
3. to inhibit the rapid rebound growth of microbes.[3]

NURSING DIAGNOSES

Basic nursing diagnoses that guide nursing intervention during skin preparation activities include:

1. High Risk for Infection related to impaired skin integrity: a state in which the patient is at risk to be invaded by an opportunistic or pathogenic agent from external sources[4]
2. High Risk for Injury related to use of chemical agents for skin preparation: a state in which the patient is at risk for harm because of a lack of awareness of environmental hazards[5]
3. Possible Anxiety related to loss of privacy during skin preparation procedures: a state in which the patient experiences a feeling of uneasiness.[6]

OUTCOME CRITERIA

Identification of potential patient problems assists the RN first assistant in planning prevention strategies that offer the patient an injury-free outcome from the nursing activities involved in skin preparation. For the above-listed nursing diagnoses, appropriate outcome criteria might be stated as follows:

The patient will demonstrate progressive healing at the surgical site.
The patient will be free of injury associated with chemical antisepsis.
The patient will relate/report decreased anxiety following measures to promote privacy.

MANAGEMENT OF HAIR IN THE OPERATIVE AREA

The purpose of perioperative skin preparation is to reduce the number of existing microorganisms on skin surfaces and to prevent their entry into the surgical wound. The recommendation that hair not be removed preoperatively is supported by a broad, heterogeneous body of research. Shaving of hair causes skin damage and approximately doubles the incidence of wound infection.[7] If hair removal is absolutely necessary for accurate approximation of wound edges, using sterile clippers in the operating room is suggested.[8] Meticulous care should be taken with the sterile clippers to avoid skin injury and irritation.

The RN first assistant must afford privacy to the patient during hair clipping. The procedure should be performed in a warm, well-lighted environment. Because removed hair and skin debris can act as potential airborne contaminants, removal should not be done in the OR itself, but rather in an area of the suite that facilitates privacy.

Before beginning to clip the hair, the RN first assistant should assess the patient's general skin condition, ensuring that the skin is dry and healthy. Good hand-washing technique and wearing gloves prevent cross-contamination. Hair removal should be documented in the patient's record.

ANTIMICROBIAL AGENTS FOR SKIN PREPARATION

The numbers and kinds of microorganisms cultured from wounds vary according to wound classification, wound location, host susceptibility and resistance, and other endogenous and exogenous factors. *Staphylococcus aureus* and *Staphylococcus epidermidis* are highly implicated in wound infection. Gram-negative aerobes are frequently seen. Studies indicating the kinds and numbers of microorganisms found in wound sepsis form the basis for the selection criteria for antimicrobial agents. Groah listed six criteria that should characterize agent effectiveness:

1. act rapidly
2. not require cumulative action
3. have broad-spectrum activity
4. be minimally harsh on the skin
5. be nontoxic
6. inhibit rapid rebound growth of microbes.[9]

Antimicrobial agents from which the RN first assistant might select are described in the following sections.

Iodine and Iodine-Containing Compounds

Masterson recommended painting the skin with povidone-iodine (10% available povidone iodine and 1% available iodine) and letting it dry. If the surgical area contains intertriginous folds or the umbilicus, the same solution should be used to mechanically cleanse these areas.[10] Iodine-containing agents are bactericidal against gram-negative and gram-positive organisms, providing microbicidal activity for up to 8 hours. The combination of an iodine complex plus a detergent, such as found in the iodophors, produces an excellent cleansing agent. The slow release of iodine following application of an iodine-containing solution, often referred to as paint, provides sustained antisepsis at the operative site. Iodine-containing compounds should not be wiped off following final application; the bactericidal activity is prolonged by the slow release of free iodine as the antiseptic agent dries and gradually fades. This brown stain outlines the prepped area in Caucasian patients, clearly demarking for the RN first assistant the anatomically aseptic landmarks. Pooling of iodine solutions at the bedlines can cause skin maceration and chemical contact dermatitis; absorbent towels should be placed at the bedlines of the prepped area prior to prepping and carefully removed at the conclusion of skin preparation.

For a conscious patient, the RN first assistant is often concerned about the discomfort of cold antiseptic solutions. Labels on povidone-iodine solutions should be read to determine whether warming is advised. Heating in a closed container can decrease iodine concentration in the solution, decreasing its effectiveness. Heating in an open container can result in water evaporation, resulting in increased iodine concentration.

Chlorhexidine Gluconate

This agent offers a broad spectrum of bactericidal action. It is highly effective against a variety of organisms. It has a relatively low skin reaction history with patient use and maintains microbial inhibition for up to 4 hours after application. It is colorless and does not stain skin or clothing. These latter properties are considered highly desirable in certain surgeries, especially in aesthetic surgery, and in certain practice settings, such as the ambulatory surgical unit.

Ethyl Alcohol

Used in a 70% solution, alcohol may be applied as a degerming agent. It is bactericidal for many gram-negative and gram-positive organisms. However, alcohol coagulates tissue protein and cannot be applied on open wounds or mucous membranes. Its potential flammability needs to be considered; pooling must not occur, and surrounding table covers must not become saturated, especially when an electrosurgery unit is being used as a surgical adjunct. Consideration also must be given to the storage of potentially flammable solutions in the operating room.

Triclosan

This is a broad-spectrum antimicrobial agent combined with oils and lanolin to provide a detergent effect. It is safe for use around the eyes, but develops a cumulative suppressive action only after prolonged use.

TECHNIQUE FOR PREPARING THE SURGICAL SITE

Policies and procedures for skin antisepsis vary according to institutional protocol and physician preference. Nonetheless, the broad general principles of reducing the microbial count in the shortest time, suppressing regrowth, using aseptic technique, and attending to patient safety and privacy are applicable to any practice setting.

Before initiating any skin prep procedure, the RN first assistant should verify landmarks denoting skin preparation for the intended surgical procedure. The next step is to inspect the patient's skin, noting any irritation, rashes, abrasions, or localized infection. Skin prep accessories vary, but usually will include gloves, forceps, sponges, absorbent towels, cotton applicators, and solution cups. Maintaining a separate table for skin prep is the best approach, confining and containing instruments and supplies used on the skin so that there is no transfer from the prep table to the sterile instrument table. Once antiseptic solutions have been poured and sterile gloves have come in contact with the patient's operative site, they are considered clean but not sterile.

If a disposable prep tray is used, it may or may not contain prep solution. If prep solution needs to be added to disposable or in-house setups, an adequate but not wasteful amount of solution should be poured. After doing this, the RN first assistant dons sterile gloves and tucks absorbent towels at the bedline. These towels absorb excess solution to prevent possible skin excoriation and chemical contact dermatitis from pooled solution.

Cleansing begins with the detergent solution, proceeding in a circular fashion from clean to dirty. If an abdominal prep includes the umbilicus, the umbilicus is considered potentially contaminated. Some detergent is squeezed into the umbilicus, and the prep is begun immediately outside it. As the rest of the abdomen is prepped, the antiseptic softens the detritus. The umbilicus should be cleansed last, then the sponge discarded. Cleansing is done to rid the skin of transient microorganisms; a gentle mechanical action is all that is necessary to remove these loosely attached bacteria. As the sponge reaches the wound periphery, it is discarded; a sponge that reaches the bedline should not be brought back to the incision site.

In many instances, only antimicrobial "paint' is applied. A sponge forceps may be used for this application. The sponge on the forceps is dipped in the solution, gently squeezed of excess, and applied to the skin in a circular fashion from incision line to periphery. A prepped area should not be retraced. The solution should be applied at least twice. After application, the bedline towels are removed and gloves and prep table contents are disposed of. The paint is allowed to dry on its own while draping takes place.

There are some exceptions to the standard skin prep principles. Infected or draining wounds, open trauma, body orifices, or ostomy sites are considered potentially contaminated areas. For surgical interventions that involve such a contaminated site, the prep technique is reversed. Skin antisepsis begins with the peripheral areas and moves circularly to the center. If a skin graft is being done, the recipient site is considered the contaminated site. If more than one incision is being made, it is safest to use separate prep trays to minimize any cross-contamination.

The goal for the patient during skin antisepsis can be stated as: The patient will be free from any adverse conditions resulting from skin preparation. The criteria by which this goal is judged include the selection of an agent that rapidly decreases bacterial counts, allows for quick application and prolonged activity, does not cause skin irritation or sensitivity, is not rendered ineffective by alcohol or the presence of organic matter, and is easily removed from skin and fabrics. Patient privacy is considered throughout the preparatory process. Documentation includes hair clipping, if done, the anatomically prepped area, the prep agent, and the skin condition before and at completion of the procedure.

DRAPING THE OPERATIVE SITE

Draping is the procedure of covering the patient and surrounding areas with a sterile barrier to create and maintain an adequate sterile field during surgery. The role of the barrier material used in operating room gowns and drapes has received a good deal of attention in the nursing literature, especially with the development of synthetic and new reusable materials. The type and quality of barrier material have been suggested as important factors in the development of wound infection following surgery. The physical and bacteriologic barrier characteristics of draping materials, as well as environmental considerations in the disposal of biohazardous waste, need to be considered by the RN first assistant when participating in the selection of barrier materials.

As in many perioperative patient procedures, in draping the surgical patient common nursing diagnoses are used as the basis for nursing actions. Consideration must be given to providing a sterile, safe environment for surgical intervention, as well as one that is comfortable and private for the conscious patient. The risk for infection, possible loss of dignity, and possible anxiety all characterize patient problems for which nursing interventions might be developed.

QUALITIES OF BARRIER MATERIAL

Barrier materials are considered a key factor in the effort to decrease airborne contamination of the surgical wound. With the disrupted integrity of the patient's skin, the risk for infection is greatly increased. The proper use of surgical drapes and the creation of a sterile field are essential protective measures against this threat of infection. The RN first assistant initiates patient care measures by using surgical drapes to create a wide margin of sterility between the operative site and the surrounding unsterile area. Principles of infection control guide the RN first assistant and surgical team in creating the sterile field. The goal is to interrupt the transmission of microorganisms by establishing an aseptic area through the use of surgical barriers that isolate the operative site.

The materials used to create the sterile field will vary according to physician preference, agency policy, and characteristics of the operative site. The selection of a barrier material must be guided by a thorough knowledge of the criteria that characterize an effective barrier. These materials must be resistant to blood, body fluids, and aqueous solutions; must remain intact for the duration of the surgical procedure; should be nonabrasive and lint-free; should not possess memory; and should be drapable, easily fitting the contours of the patient and equipment. Dyes, often used to reduce glare, should be nontoxic. Material must be antistatic, meeting the standards of the National Fire Protection Association. It must also be sufficiently porous to allow temperature regulatory mechanisms to function to keep body temperature normothermic. The safety and efficacy of the material should be documented by manufacturer's performance standards.

Reusable Drapes

Reusable barrier materials are usually composed of chemically treated 100% cotton with a 288-thread count per square inch. These materials are porous, eliminating heat buildup. They should be used with nonpenetrating clamps. These materials are considered advantageous in terms of institutional cost. They have a number of disadvantages, however. Consideration must be given to the amount of time, personnel, and equipment needed to reprocess reusable drapes. They must be inspected for holes, washed after every use, refolded, sterilized, and stored. Heavily soiled drapes present contamination hazards to the personnel who must handle them. Additionally, hospital laundering systems must be effective in reducing the pathogenic organisms that colonize the surface and interstices of cotton drapes. A system must be devised for tracking the numbers of times these drapes are reprocessed, for their barrier effectiveness can diminish with repeated use. Manufacturer's standards in defining barrier quality and reprocessing limitations must be strictly adhered to.

Single-Use Drapes

Since the wick phenomenon was first shown to be a potential mechanism in microbial transport and subsequent wound infection, efforts have been undertaken to improve the barrier qualities of draping materials. The evolution of synthetic, disposable draping systems has resulted in the production of soft, lint-free, nonirritating, static-free, flame-resistant, and moisture-resistant materials. Many of these disposable drapes have an inner layer of spunbonded fibers that have been frozen and broken, resulting in a web of right-angled fibers that retard microbial migration. The outer layer of the disposable drape has properties similar to cloth. These drapes have the advantage of being lightweight, easily handled, and time-saving. Standardization of product line and consistency of packaging are additional benefits. Nonetheless, disposable drapes have disadvantages in terms of environmentally safe disposal, cost, inventory levels, and storage space.

DRAPING TECHNIQUES

Whether using reusable cotton drapes or disposable synthetic drapes, the RN first assistant will encounter various types of drapes. Draping is a procedure in which the RN first assistant must be an expert.

In draping the patient, one of the most familiar steps will be applying the towel drape, used to demarcate and limit the operative parameters. The conventional four-towel method uses four surgical towels placed around the operative site. These may be fully opened or folded in half lengthwise and placed next to the skin. If reusable, the towel should be secured with nonperforating towel clamps. The disposable draping towel has an adherent sticky strip for fixation.

Some surgeons prefer a plastic incise drape to the use of four towels. If a plastic incise towel drape is used, two sterile team members are required. The drape, made of impermeable polyvinyl with adhesive on one side, is carefully applied and pressed firmly into place; a sterile rolled towel or lap sponge may be used to minimize air pockets and wrinkles. These self-adhering draping materials may be used instead of the towel drape, in combination with the towel drape, as aperture drapes, or as plastic sheets. They are controversial in terms of claims for microbial inhibition. Advocates of this type of drape claim that its advantage is in preventing lateral migration of skin microorganisms. In opposition are those who claim that the heat and moisture buildup under the draped area promotes microbial growth. Some of the larger plastic drapes are available with antimicrobial agents impregnated into the drape. Plastic incise drapes are commonly used in orthopedics and implant surgery, where their usefulness is apparent in keeping the implant from any contact with skin surfaces. These drapes are also helpful in isolating surgical anatomy where a high occurrence of microorganisms is expected, such as with stomas.

Following application of towels or plastic incise drapes, a large fenestrated sheet may be applied. Fenestrated sheets are most commonly used in surgical interventions of the abdomen, chest, flank, and back. The fenestration is modified in terms of length and width to accommodate approaches to the abdomen, thyroid, breast, kidney, hip, and perineum. The fenestrated sheet is placed over the towels and incision site. The drape should be of adequate size to provide a wide margin of sterility between the operative site and surrounding unsterile areas.

PRINCIPLES OF ASEPTIC TECHNIQUE IN DRAPING

The procedure for draping the patient follows principles of basic aseptic technique. Drapes should be handled as little as possible. The sterile field should be kept in view throughout the draping procedure. The RN first assistant must protect the gown and gloves from coming in contact with unsterile, undraped areas. Maintaining an adequate distance from unsterile areas, cuffing hands with drapes, and walking around the patient rather than leaning over an unsterile area are all ways of protecting the sterile self. The drape must be controlled during the draping process by holding it in its compact shape, to prevent it from unfolding or flipping down. The drape must be carried above waist level. Once placed on the patient, the drape is unfolded from center to periphery. The edges of the drape that fall below bed level are considered unsterile. Once the drape is placed, it cannot be moved. If a sterile drape becomes unsterile, or if sterility is questionable, the drape should be replaced.

All members of the surgical team are responsible for maintaining the integrity of the sterile field during the operative procedure. The RN first assistant, along with circulating and scrub person colleagues, monitors this integrity. Movements of team members are carefully coordinated as the nursing team provides a method of confining and containing supplies and instruments used in patient care.

Basic principles of aseptic technique guide the RN first assistant during patient draping procedures. Knowledge of the existing body of literature regarding barrier materials is essential in product selection and application. Professional development should include both a current knowledge base and a willingness to participate in nursing research that continues to evaluate barrier materials, both reusable and disposable, and their effectiveness in reducing surgical wound infections.

CONCLUSION

A genuine bond of communication and caring underpins the relationship between the RN first assistant and the surgical patient. The patient's participation in this relationship should be active; the patient should understand, to the extent desired, the nature of perioperative events and participate with the RN first assistant in developing a teaching plan and meeting its objectives. Because infections that develop in clean surgical wounds are primarily caused by exogenous microbial sources, proper preparation of the patient's skin before the surgical incision is one of the most important ways to decrease infection in clean operations. The most commonly used antimicrobial agents for skin antisepsis are the iodophors. The RN first assistant must use a skin preparation technique that prevents chemical injury. Sterile drapes are then applied to define and maintain the sterile field during the operative procedure. Drapes should preserve their barrier characteristics, even when wet. The sterile field must be closely monitored for integrity during the procedure. Prevention of wound infection is a multifaceted, ongoing process that requires the RN first assistant to pay particular attention to details of technique. The RN first assistant's commitment to preventing any potential adverse consequences for the patient, however, makes meticulous technique a naturalized component of skill proficiency.

REVIEW QUESTIONS

Answer questions 1–10 in relation to the following patient situation: Mrs. Thomas is scheduled for a modified left mastectomy. She is a morning admission. RN first assistant Hutt is meeting her for the first time to complete a perioperative assessment and begin patient education.

1. Following the assessment, RN first assistant Hutt begins to develop a teaching plan with Mrs. Thomas. Which of the following would be most appropriate for inclusion in the teaching plan?
   a. the possibility of a skin graft
   b. dimpling and nipple changes
   c. incisional approaches to breast lesions
   d. use of a closed wound suction drain
2. As RN first assistant Hutt is explaining the surgical skin preparation, she notices that Mrs. Thomas is clenching and unclenching a tissue and has tears in her eyes. What would RN first assistant Hutt's most appropriate response/action be at this point?
   a. suggest that they stop the discussion for awhile
   b. ask Mrs. Thomas to pay attention
   c. recognize Mrs. Thomas' apparent distress and ask if she wants to talk about what she is feeling
   d. simply continue with the discussion
3. An actual nursing diagnosis represents a state that has been clinically validated by major defining characteristics. Mrs. Thomas exhibits symptoms from the emotional category. Which of the following symptoms would RN first assistant Hutt look for from the cognitive category?
   a. trembling
   b. inability to concentrate
   c. inability to relax
   d. self-depreciation

4. A focused assessment for the nursing diagnosis "Anxiety" includes a determination of the patient's usual _______ behaviors. To do this, RN first assistant Hutt might ask "How do you usually handle (the particular situation)?"
   a. coping
   b. lifestyle
   c. communication
   d. religious
5. If major defining characteristics of a nursing diagnosis are present, it is what type of nursing diagnosis?
   a. actual
   b. potential
   c. high risk
   d. possible
6. An appropriate nursing intervention during patient education is to explain
   a. reason for, anticipated outcome, and risks involved in the surgical procedure
   b. type of anesthesia and the patient's ASA classification
   c. perioperative routines, reasons for them, and their importance
   d. postoperative complications and their expected incidence
7. For Mrs. Thomas, which of the following would most likely best meet learning needs for discharge planning?
   a. providing written materials for her to read
   b. continuing one-on-one encounters with RN first assistant Hutt
   c. receiving a referral to an assistive resource
   d. participating in a group session with other mastectomy patients
8. An expected outcome of a teaching plan for Mrs. Thomas' anxiety related to knowledge deficit of perioperative routines would be that she
   a. has a good cry and gets it out of her system
   b. verbalizes her anxiety
   c. thanks RN first assistant Hutt for her assistance
   d. verbalizes anticipated routines and what to expect
9. The use of outcome criteria and their evaluation is an indication of RN first assistant Hutt's
   a. understanding of the nursing process
   b. accountability for patient care
   c. participation in medical effectiveness initiatives
   d. compliance with quality indicator development
10. If outcome criteria are met, RN first assistant Hutt will indicate on Mrs. Thomas' plan of care that
    a. anxiety has been ruled out
    b. goals and interventions are appropriate
    c. goals and interventions need revision
    d. a goal has been achieved; discontinue that portion of the plan
11. Skin bacteria are most commonly distinguished as
    a. resident or transient
    b. pathogenic or nonpathogenic
    c. parasitic or commensalist
    d. endogenous or exogenous

12. When a patient is at risk to be invaded by an opportunistic or pathogenic agent from an external source, then
    a. prophylactic antibiotics should be initiated
    b. the nursing diagnosis "High Risk for Infection" is present
    c. repeated preoperative showers with an antimicrobial are recommended
    d. the surgery should be postponed until the patient's status improves
13. According to AORN Recommended Practices for Preoperative Skin Preparation
    a. iodine-containing compounds are the most effective preparation agents
    b. a paint, not a detergent, should be used if a plastic incise drape will be applied
    c. one of the objectives of skin preparation is to inhibit rapid rebound growth of microbes
    d. soil and transient microbes should be eliminated from the dermis
14. There is a broad body of research that indicates that hair at the operative site should
    a. not be removed unless absolutely necessary
    b. be shaved as close to the time of surgery as possible
    c. be removed in a wide margin near the incision site with a depilatory
    d. be removed in the operating room after the patient is anesthetized
15. If hair must be removed from the operative site, then
    a. a razor with a recessed blade should be used
    b. the patient should do this in a private area
    c. it should be done immediately before wound closure
    d. sterile clippers should be used
16. For the awake patient, the antimicrobial skin agent should be warmed
    a. in a closed container
    b. in an open container
    c. only after consulting manufacturer's recommendations
    d. in a sterilizer
17. To prevent chemical contact dermatitis, the RN first assistant should
    a. place absorbent towels at the bedlines
    b. test for skin reaction before application
    c. use antimicrobial agents only on intact skin
    d. blot the area dry following application
18. Which of the following agents carries a disadvantage because it develops a cumulative suppressive action only after prolonged use?
    a. alcohol
    b. Hibiclens
    c. triclosan
    d. Betadine
19. If both a detergent and a paint are being used to prepare the skin, which is applied first?
    a. detergent
    b. paint
    c. the order is inconsequential
    d. these agents should not be used in combination

20. A general maxim for preoperative skin preparation is
    a. start at the bedline, squaring off the area to be prepped
    b. progress from clean to dirty
    c. start in the center; progress to the periphery
    d. the 5-minute scrub should suffice
21. Documentation of skin preparation should include
    a. the patient's consent for hair removal
    b. area prepped and agent used
    c. skin condition before and after preparation
    d. both b and c
22. When participating in the institution's selection of barrier materials, the RN first assistant should consider
    a. recommending antiseptic-impregnated incise drapes
    b. delegating this purchasing decision
    c. environmental disposal of biohazardous waste
    d. conducting a survey of local community standards
23. A prime consideration in selecting any barrier material for perioperative use is that it meet what standards?
    a. NFPA
    b. OSHA
    c. ACS
    d. CDC
24. If towel drapes do not have an adhesive backing, what should be used to secure them?
    a. allis
    b. skin staple
    c. nonperforating towel clamp
    d. simple silk suture
25. Drapes should be
    a. unfolded from periphery to center
    b. unfolded towards a sterile person, then away
    c. handled as little as possible
    d. replaced at frequent intervals

Answers

1. d	6. c	11. a	16. c	21. d
2. c	7. b	12. b	17. a	22. c
3. b	8. d	13. c	18. c	23. a
4. a	9. b	14. a	19. a	24. c
5. a	10. d	15. d	20. b	25. c

REFERENCES

1. Carpenito LJ: Nursing Diagnosis: Application to Clinical Practice, p 6. Philadelphia, JB Lippincott, 1992

2. Ibid, p 152
3. Association of Operating Room Nurses: Recommended Practices for Perioperative Skin Preparation of Patients, III:18-1–18-4.3. *In* AORN Standards and Recommended Practices, Denver, Association of Operating Room Nurses, 1992
4. Carpenito, p 503
5. Ibid, p 525
6. Ibid, p 657
7. Alexander JW, Dellinger EP: Surgical infections and choice of antibiotics. In DC Sabiston and HK Lyerly, Textbook of Surgery: Pocket Companion, pp 99–107. Philadelphia, WB Saunders, 1992
8. Masterson BJ: Skin preparation. In Care of the Surgical Patient, p 2-4. Scientific American Medicine, New York, NY, 1990
9. Groah LK: Operating Room Nursing, Perioperative Practice, p 208. Norwalk, CT, Appleton & Lange, 1990
10. Masterson, p 2-2

7 Anesthesia and Patient Positioning

Jane C. Rothrock*
Robert H. Sculthorpe

ANESTHESIA

The discovery and refinement of anesthesia and its administration have made important contributions to the advancement of surgery. The first public demonstration of anesthesia administration took place at Massachusetts General Hospital in 1846. The scientific merits of this technique were not readily accepted, however, and it was not until many years later that anesthesiology became an academic discipline in medicine. Following the rapid advances in the specialty after World War II, anesthesia now includes subspecialties in such areas as pediatrics, cardiothoracic surgery, neurosurgery, critical care, and pain management. Contemporary anesthesia practice includes quality improvement efforts and clinical reviews that collect data on anesthesia indicators and performance criteria to optimize the safety and quality of anesthesia administration.

GENERAL ANESTHESIA

General anesthesia may be produced by volatile inhalation agents or by intravenous agents. Although the mechanisms differ, each agent produces a reversible modulation of synaptic communication between neurons (Figure 7-1). Simply put, the central nervous system functions via neuronal transmis-

* *In the first edition, part of this chapter (in original Chapter 12) was written by Mark L. Phippen.*

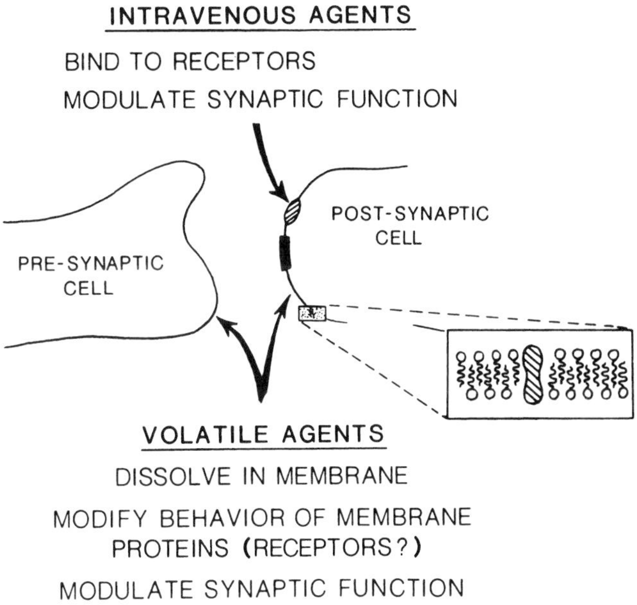

FIGURE 7-1
Diagram of the synaptic mechanisms of general anesthesia. Anesthesia results from the reversible modulation of synaptic communication between neurons. Most intravenous agents bind to receptors and influence the effects of neurotransmitters. Volatile agents influence membrane function by causing physico-chemical changes within membrane lipids and proteins. *(From Barash et al: Clinical Anesthesia, 2nd ed. Philadelphia, JB Lippincott, 1992.)*

sion at synaptic junctions. A chemical neurotransmitter is released from the presynaptic ending, travels across the synaptic cleft, and binds to a receptor site on the postsynaptic membrane. When this receptor site is occupied, changes occur in the postsynaptic cell. These changes differ according to drug—receptor interactions, but commonly effect amnesia, analgesia, and control of sympathetic response. Thus, perception of pain is altered, memory of events are dampened while a medically induced state resembling sleep occurs, and reflexes are depressed such that the normal sequence of pain-triggered withdrawal of a body part and autonomic release of catecholamines is suppressed.

The pharmacokinetics of inhalation agents depends on the concentration, partial pressure, and minimum alveolar concentration (MAC) of the particular agent. To achieve the goal of inhalation anesthesia, an adequate partial pressure, or tension, of anesthetic in the brain needs to be developed and maintained. Partial pressure is related to the concentration, or the fraction of an anesthetic, in the gas phase. Partial pressure begins at the delivery hose of the anesthesia machine and exists in gradients until equilibrium is achieved. The MAC of an inhalational agent is the concentration of that agent in alveolar gas which is necessary to prevent movement in 50% of patients during a routine surgical procedure. For inhalation agents, the potency is commonly expressed as the MAC. The MAC of an inhaled agent can be increased or decreased by selected factors. Increased temperature (hyperthermia), drugs that increase catecholamine release (for example, MAO inhibitors, cocaine, ephedrine), hypernatremia, and chronic abuse of ethanol all may increase the MAC. On the other hand, increased age, decreased temperature (hypothermia), narcotics (and opioid agonist-antagonist analgesics), catecholamine depleters (such as reserpine), hypoxia ($PaCO_2$ greater than 90 mm Hg, PaO_2

less than 38 mm Hg), anemia with a hematocrit under 10%, metabolic acidosis, and various other physiologic or pharmacologic factors all can decrease the MAC of an agent. The lower the MAC, the more potent the agent.

The onset and duration of action of an inhalation anesthetic agent depends on the agent's absorption, distribution, metabolism, and elimination. An ideal inhalation anesthetic would provide rapid and predictable onset and recovery, be easy to administer, yield easily discernible signs of its depth, and possess a high safety margin for a wide variety of patients. Table 7-1 lists commonly used inhalation agents.

TABLE 7-1

Inhaled Agents of General Anesthesia

Agent	Administration	Advantages	Disadvantages	Implications
Enflurane (Ethrane)	Inhalation	Rapid induction and recovery Potent analgesic Not explosive or flammable	Respiratory depression may develop rapidly along with EEG abnormalities Not compatible with epinephrine	Observe for possible respiratory depression. Administration with epinephrine may cause ventricular fibrillation.
Halothane (Fluothane)	Inhalation; special vaporizer	Not explosive or flammable Induction rapid and smooth Useful in almost every type of surgery Low incidence of postoperative nausea and vomiting	Requires skillful administration to prevent overdosage May cause liver damage May produce hypotension Requires special vaporizer for administration	In addition to observation of pulse and respiration postoperatively, it is important that blood pressure be monitored frequently.
Isoflurane (Forane)	Inhalation	Rapid induction and recovery Muscle relaxants are markedly potentiated	Profound respiratory depressant	Respirations must be monitored closely and supported when necessary.
Nitrous oxide (N_2O)	Inhalation (semiclosed method)	Induction and recovery rapid Nonflammable Useful with oxygen for short procedures Useful with other agents for all types of surgery	Poor relaxant Weak anesthetic May produce hypoxia	N_2O is most useful in conjunction with other agents with longer action. Observe precautions with "other agents."

(Adapted from Smeltzer, Bare: Brunner & Suddarth's Textbook of Medical-Surgical Nursing, 7th ed. Philadelphia, JB Lippincott, 1992.)

To promote patient comfort and speed of anesthesia induction, anesthesia is often begun with an intravenous agent. An inhalation agent is then introduced in a concentration sufficient for toleration of endotracheal intubation. Supplemental doses of sedatives and relaxing drugs may also be administered. Once the patient has been intubated, anesthesia may be maintained by the inhalation agent alone or by a combination of inhalation agent and adjuvant agents. A current practice involves combining inhaled drugs with adjuvants such as sedatives, opioids, and other drugs that have central nervous system effects. Referred to as "balanced" anesthesia, this method uses adjuvants that provide sedation and amnesia, suppress reflexes, and rapidly induce unconsciousness and relaxation for intubation; anesthesia is maintained by the inhalation agent. Muscle relaxation is provided by the intravenous administration of neuromuscular blocking agents (see Table 7-2).

POSITIONING THE ANESTHETIZED PATIENT

Positioning the surgical patient has far-reaching implications for the patient's well-being; the potential for complications is great. A thorough knowledge of the principles of positioning and of the equipment involved is a prerequisite for this patient care activity. The RN first assistant is concerned not only with preventing physical and psychogenic injury in a general sense, but also with providing interventions that address the individual patient's situation.

Each patient has special needs that are identified in the course of the RN first assistant's nursing assessment. When the collected data have been analyzed, a plan of care is designed to meet the identified patient needs. Using this plan, the RN first assistant works with the other members of the surgical team to place the patient in a position that provides optimum exposure at the operative site while ensuring patient safety. In this chapter, the RN first assistant's contributions to efficient and effective patient positioning are presented in a collaborative problem framework.

POSITIONING AS A COLLABORATIVE PROBLEM

Positioning the patient for surgery is an interdependent function performed by the surgical team. All team members, including the surgeon, anesthetist/anesthesiologist, RN first assistant, and registered nurse circulator, share the responsibility for this function. Nursing practice often involves the nurse in collaborative relationships with other health care professionals. Positioning the anesthetized patient is an example of such a collaborative relationship. The RN first assistant brings knowledge of important nursing interventions to positioning the patient without injury; however, the act of positioning requires collaboration. It is rarely an independent nursing function.

Carpenito has developed a "bifocal clinical practice model" that classifies certain nursing situations as collaborative problems. In her definition, collaborative problems are certain physiologic complications that nurses monitor to

TABLE 7-2

Muscle Relaxants

Muscle Relaxant	Action	Advantages	Disadvantages	Uses and Comments
Nondepolarizing Neuromuscular Blocking Agents				
Tubocurarine chloride (Tubarine)	Peaks at 30–60 min	50%–70% excreted unchanged in 3–6 hr	Histamine-like reaction Hypotension Increased airway resistance Skin erythema	Contraindicated with history of allergy, asthma
Gallamine (Flaxedil)	1/5 as potent as curare Lasts 25% shorter than curare Blocks vagal ganglia in heart	All excreted unchanged	Tachycardia	Used well with cyclopropane or halothane
Pancuronium bromide (Pavulon)	Similar to curare but 5 times more potent Duration, 60–85 min	Safe; stable Good muscle relaxant Reversible by neostigmine and atropine		Excellent for situations requiring complete relaxation Avoid with myasthenia gravis or renal disease Avoid with patients sensitive to bromide
Vecuronium bromide (Norcuron)	Blocks depolarization	Facilitates endotracheal intubation; good muscle relaxant	Prolonged dose-related apnea	Related to Pavulon Well tolerated in patients with renal failure
Depolarizing Neuromuscular Blocking Agents These mimic the action of acetylcholine at the neuromuscular junction. Acetylcholine is discharged almost immediately on release → repolarization of muscle takes place. When depolarizing neuromuscular blocking agents are used, skeletal muscle depolarizes.				
Succinylcholine (Anectine; Sucostrin)	Onset is rapid: 1 min Duration: 4–8 min	Ideal for endotracheal intubation, fracture reduction; treatment of laryngospasm	Contraindicated for patients with low pseudocholinesterase On second IV injection, bradycardia and various dysrhythmias May cause fasciculations of the muscles and pain	Used to treat laryngospasm, status asthmaticus, and toxic reactions to local anesthetic drugs
Decamethonium bromide (Syncurine)	Onset: 30–40 sec Duration: 15–20 min	Excreted unchanged by kidney	Some fasciculation of muscle: jaw masseter muscles; posterior calf muscles Difficult to reverse its action	Produces depolarization of end plate region

(From Smeltzer, Bare: Brunner & Suddarth's Textbook of Medical-Surgical Nursing, 7th ed. Philadelphia, JB Lippincott, 1992.)

detect onset or changes in status. Nurses manage collaborative problems using physician-prescribed and nursing-prescribed interventions to minimize the complications of the events.[1] The RN first assistant continues to make independent decisions with collaborative problems. The difference is that in nursing diagnoses, the RN first assistant prescribes the definitive interventions to achieve a desired patient outcome; but with collaborative problems, such prescriptions come from both medicine and nursing. The same steps of the nursing process—assessment, diagnosis, outcome identification, planning, implementation, and evaluation—are involved. However, the nature of a collaborative problem is such that it will probably occur with a specific treatment. Thus, the sequelae of patient positioning (the treatment) become, in a collaborative problem framework, potential complications; these are designated throughout the chapter as "PCs."

SUPINE POSITION

Even though supine is considered the least stressful of positions, patients in this position may experience significant physiological changes. In a supine position, posterolateral chest movement is restricted, causing a 9.5% reduction in vital capacity. The abdominal organs, which have a tendency to lie against the upper wall of the abdomen in the supine position, restrict diaphragmatic excursion. Particularly during anesthesia induction, patients can experience a decrease in mean arterial pressure, heart rate, and peripheral resistance; however, cardiac output and stroke volume will increase. Significant venous pooling in the legs results from reduced venous pressure. This in turn will cause a decrease in circulating blood volume. Depending on patient status, there is potential for the position-induced hypotension to cause a decrease in tissue perfusion. To complicate matters, the surgical position, as well as other variables such as anoxia, duration of surgery, and fluid and electrolyte imbalance, may cause cardiac dysrhythmias.

These potential complications should not be considered as inherent attributes of only the supine position. Rather, they are potential complications common to all surgical positions. Certainly the RN first assistant must exercise extreme caution with all positions because, depending on the variables of the situation, the surgical position might be the initiating factor leading to a devastating consequence.

No matter what the position, if a general or regional anesthetic is administered, the patient will lose all or some physiologic ability to cope with the stresses and strains associated with surgical positioning. Once the patient is anesthetized, pain and pressure receptors that alert an awake person to impending anatomic compromise will be temporarily altered. Consequently, it will be easy to extend or abduct an extremity or joint beyond the normal range of motion and thus cause injury to the joint, as well as to ligaments, tendons, and muscles.

When a patient is awake and standing, the lower extremities, trunk, and vertebral muscles are in a dynamic state of tone. This muscle tone decreases in a horizontal position. During surgery, the anesthetized state causes muscular relaxation, which leads to the loss of tone of opposing muscle groups. Under normal conditions, muscle tone, which is an anatomic coping mechanism, guards against joint damage and muscle stretch and strain. Because of this, the RN first assistant should be very cautious if resistance to range of motion is encountered. There is always the chance of peripheral nerve and blood vessel damage, especially when sensitive areas are placed on hard surfaces or limbs are misaligned. One of the most common injuries is to the brachial plexus. When arms are placed at the sides during surgery, there is less likelihood of an injury resulting from hyperabduction. However, misalignment or compression of the arms against the operating room bed may result in radial, median, or ulnar nerve damage. The elbows are especially susceptible to compression injury; the RN first assistant should adequately pad the elbows to prevent the potential complication of ulnar nerve injury.

If it is necessary to extend the patient's arms during the positioning process, the RN first assistant must exercise extreme caution and ensure that the arms remain at less than a 90-degree angle from the body. Another aspect of the brachial plexus problem is rotating the head and neck in the opposite direction to an arm, which along with suspending an arm by the wrist (a frequent occurrence during the prepping of an upper extremity) may cause pressure on the brachial plexus and lead to injury. The RN first assistant should also be aware that nerve damage is not the only injury caused by hyperabduction of an arm; another potential complication is occlusion or compression of the subclavian and axillary arteries.

To prevent injury from a fall, patients should be secured to the operating room bed with a safety strap. To avoid undue pressure and its consequences, the strap should be placed 2 inches above the knees. Tension on the strap should be just sufficient to ensure stability; the strap should never be secured too tightly. To avoid damage to the popliteal area, the RN first assistant should ensure that items such as a pillow or rolled sheet are not placed *directly* under the knees.

Certain patients do not tolerate the stresses of the flat-lying supine position. Obese patients experience stress in this position due to a relatively low blood volume-to-weight ratio, increased cardiac output (which is further increased in the supine position), systemic and pulmonary vasculature resistance, pulmonary arterial pressure, and left ventricular filling pressure.[2] As if this were not enough, obesity—particularly 100% or more over normal weight—will cause the patient to breathe approximately 40% to 50% harder, which in turn increases oxygen consumption by up to 11%.[3]

The Lawn Chair Modification

Instead of a flat-lying supine position, Martin recommends the lawn chair position (contoured supine), especially for patients receiving a regional or local anesthetic.[4] As was mentioned earlier, when the patient is horizontal, body weight is unequally distributed over the occiput, scapulae, sacrum, and heels. This, in addition to the major joints being out of neutral alignment, can make lying flat on the operating room bed distressful for the awake patient. Unfortunately, even though the padded operating room bed helps reduce some of the pressure on sensitive areas, it is not considered the epitome of comfort. No matter how well the bed is padded, if the joint positions remain unchanged, the awake patient will rapidly become uncomfortable. If the operating room bed is adjusted so that it resembles a lawn chair or a contour chair, weight is distributed along the full length of the dorsal body surface. Additionally, gentle flexion occurs at the hips and knees, allowing these joints to be placed in a more neutral position (see Figure 7-2). Easier abdominal closure is another positive aspect of the lawn chair position. When the hips are flexed, the distance between the xiphoid process and pubic area is decreased, reducing the stretch on the anterior abdominal musculature.

To place the patient in the lawn chair position, the RN first assistant elevates the back of the operating room bed by turning the back control a full three turns (approximately 15 degrees) and lowers the foot section by turning the control handle three full reverse turns (again, about 15 degrees).

Pressure Ulcers

Pressure ulcer development is a potential and insidious complication of surgical positioning. A pressure ulcer is any lesion caused by unrelieved pressure

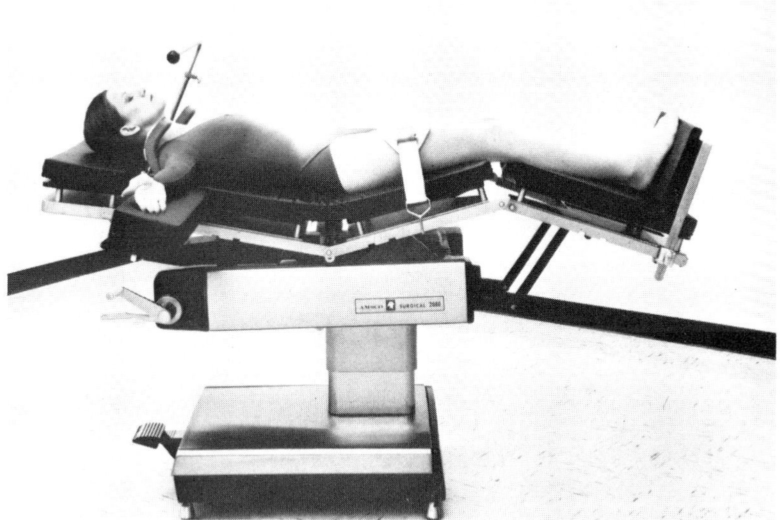

FIGURE 7-2
The contoured supine position is established by arranging the surface of the operating room bed so that the trunk-thigh hinge is angulated about 15 degrees and the thigh-knee hinge is angulated at a similar amount in the opposite direction. In this, termed the lawn chair (or contour chair) position, the patient lies comfortably with hips and thighs each gently flexed. *(Photo courtesy of American Sterilizer Company, Erie, PA.)*

resulting in damage to the underlying tissue.[5] All patients are candidates for this potential complication. In patients of normal weight, each surgical position results in an unequal distribution of body weight. In the supine and sitting positions, pressure areas are the occiput, scapulae, elbows, sacrum, and heels. Obesity increases this pressure and makes a patient even more susceptible. No matter what the position or weight of the patient, the RN first assistant should remember that surgical positioning may be the initiating stressor that leads to pressure ulcer development.[6] Research indicates that there are certain vulnerable patient populations for which the RN first assistant must exercise even greater care.

Individual patient characteristics, type of surgery, and length of surgery have all been implicated in pressure ulcer development. Elderly surgical patients have less fat and muscle to equally distribute pressure. This is true also for very thin, cachetic patients. Surgical patients with inadequate dietary intake of protein and calories, especially a protein deficit as manifested by a preoperative albumin level below 3.0 gm/dl, have been found to have an increased incidence of pressure ulcer development.[7] Sacral pressure ulcer development has been identified in patients undergoing vascular surgery lasting over 4 hours.[8] Other researchers postulate that the amount of pressure at the heels and sacrum on an operating room bed using standard padding is enough to cause necrosis in an anesthetized, immobile patient if surgery exceeds 2 hours.[9] Perioperative patients with prolonged immobility or inactivity, such as quadriplegic patients or elderly patients with fractures, are also at higher risk.

Pressure ulcers usually occur over bony prominences at "points of contact." Several systems to grade or stage the degree of tissue damage have been used in nursing. In most classification systems, a Stage I pressure ulcer is a nonblanchable erythema of intact skin, representing epidermal and dermal damage prior to deeper tissue involvement. However, in surgical patients, it has been hypothesized that pressure ulcers may develop in a reverse order. That is, they may develop initially in muscle and subcutaneous tissue and then progress outwards. Prolonged pressure, combined with shear stress, has been described as a "closed pressure sore."[10] Instead of a nonblanchable erythema, pressure ulcers may present as bluish-purple ecchymoses.

In light of this research, RN first assistants should know risk factors for pressure ulcer development and plan patient positioning accordingly. In general, all patients undergoing anesthesia and surgery are at risk due to their decreased mobility, activity, and sensory perception. Additional risk factors are present depending on the length of surgery (immobility), hypotension, decreased tissue perfusion, dehydration, hypothermia, and hyperthermia.[11] These factors are compounded in patients who are age-extreme, cachetic, or obese and those with metabolic or vascular problems, edema, or concurrent infection. The more risk factors identified, the more protection the patient needs.

The RN first assistant should pay particular attention to bony prominences when positioning the patient. Because skin injury due to friction and shearing forces is a significant potential complication, turning and transfer techniques that lift rather than pull should be used. Protective padding should be used at bony prominence contact points. Similarly, positioning devices such as pillows or foam should be used to keep bony prominences from pressing on one another. Patients at high risk for pressure ulcer development should be placed on an operating room bed with a pressure-reducing device such as an air-and-gel mattress or gel mattress overlay.[12] The patient should be draped for moisture resistance. The RN first assistant should make every effort to prevent pooling of skin preparation solutions or surgical drainage. The patient should be kept dry; if this is questionable, underpads or absorbent materials should be placed to keep the skin dry.

Potential Complications: Supine Position

PC: Pressure Injury
PC: Impaired Tissue Perfusion
PC: Neuropathy

Positioning Goals And Criteria: Supine Position

During the perioperative period, the patient will not experience any of the following complications related to the supine position: impaired skin integrity, impaired tissue perfusion, or alterations in postoperative kinesthetic perception. There will be no signs of:

1. pressure ulcer formation at susceptible pressure sites
2. tingling, numbness, cramping, pain or aches in joints; weakness and stiffness in the extremities
3. pain or discomfort on adduction, abduction, flexion, and extension of extremities.

The patient's bony prominences should be assessed when the patient is placed on the operating room bed and removed from the bed. Because it is not unlikely that a reddened area will be present at dependent pressure sites, another evaluation should be made on discharge from the recovery area to distinguish pressure ulcer development from reactive hyperemia. The best evaluation of outcome criteria for pressure ulcer development would take place 3 days postoperatively to assess for deep pressure ulcers.[13]

Positioning Requirements: Supine Position

The RN first assistant should ensure that the following nursing interventions are accomplished while placing the patient in the supine position:

1. padding pressure sites (scapulae, sacrum, elbows, occiput and heels)
2. applying a safety/body strap
3. providing positioning devices to maintain normal body curvature (neck, small of back, knees)
4. maintaining normal body alignment
5. protecting arms (armboard/arms secured at sides; elbows protected).

REVERSE TRENDELENBURG POSITION

The reverse Trendelenburg position is a modification of the supine position. In this position, head elevation is selected to facilitate surgical exposure or to improve venous drainage from the wound. A slight reverse Trendelenburg position is commonly used in endoscopic access to the upper abdomen, as it displaces viscera downward and away from the operative site. On the other hand, certain neurosurgical procedures require marked head elevation. Reverse Trendelenburg may be achieved either by tipping the entire chassis of the operating room bed or by modifying the lawn chair position (foot section of the bed lowered, bed flexed, back section of the bed raised). When the lawn chair position is used, the patient's thighs should be gently flexed and the knees bent so that the legs are horizontal and nearly at the level of the heart; this prevents prolonged knee extension and stretch injury to the sciatic nerve. With the bed-tilt or lawn chair position, a padded footboard is attached to the operating room bed to prevent caudad slippage and plantar flexion. The heels and soles of the foot should be padded. If neck extension is required to facilitate surgical exposure, a small pad may be placed under the upper thoracic spine; this permits the neck to be extended as the shoulders drop dorsally. The head, neck, and cervical spine should be supported in a straight line. Patients with limited dorsiflexion due to cervical neck limitations need careful positioning to prevent severe postoperative neck pain.

Potential Complications: Reverse Trendelenburg Position

PC: Pressure Injury
PC: Impaired Tissue Perfusion in the lower extremities
PC: Neuropathy
PC: Hypotension

Positioning Goals and Criteria: Reverse Trendelenburg Position

During the perioperative period, the patient will not experience any of the following complications related to reverse Trendelenburg positioning: impaired skin integrity, impaired tissue perfusion, or alterations in postoperative kinesthetic perception. There will be no signs of:

1. pressure ulcer formation at susceptible sites
2. edema, discoloration, temperature change, phlebitis, thrombosis, venous stasis, or ulcerations in the lower extremities
3. tingling, numbness, cramping, pain or aches in joints; weakness and stiffness in the upper extremities
4. pain or discomfort on adduction, abduction, flexion, and extension of the upper extremities
5. nerve injuries, especially to the ulnar or sciatic nerves
6. blood pressure change during positional adjustment.

Positioning Requirements: Reverse Trendelenburg Position

The RN first assistant should ensure that the following nursing interventions are accomplished while placing the patient in the reverse Trendelenburg position:

1. padding pressure sites (scapulae, sacrum, elbows, soles, and heels)
2. attaching a padded footboard
3. applying an antithromboembolic device
4. protecting the upper extremities with padding and toboggan-like arm protectors
5. supporting normal body curvatures (knees, lumbar area)
6. ensuring gradual and slow position changes.

TRENDELENBURG POSITION

The Trendelenburg position, another modification of the supine position, enhances exposure of the surgical field in lower abdominal and pelvic surgery. This position is especially important with the increasing use of endoscopic access to the lower abdominal and pelvic structures. It lowers arterial perfusion at the surgical site, which in turn results in less bleeding. In addition, the vascular gradient from the wound to the heart reduces vascular ooze and improves venous drainage at the surgical site. The anesthetist/anesthesiologist will find the Trendelenburg position helpful, especially if there is the possibility of the patient regurgitating during induction of or emergence from anesthesia. This position also facilitates the insertion of needles and catheters into dependent neck veins that become engorged as a result of the change in the angle of the operating room bed.[14]

There are numerous disadvantages to the Trendelenburg position, however. If the angle of the operating room bed is too extreme, the abdominal viscera, which will be lying against the diaphragm, may move in and out of the operative field during assisted ventilation. At a minimum, this will be disturbing to the surgeon and the RN first assistant. Theoretically, it could cause inadvertent damage, especially while the team is ligating, suturing, or cutting. Also, the Trendelenburg position enhances the central venous return of blood and preserves cardiac output. As a result, it becomes more difficult to recognize blood loss during surgery. This potential disadvantage can be dealt with by estimating and restoring blood volume deficits before the patient is returned to a level position. Fortunately, the surgical team can compensate for many of the disadvantages associated with the Trendelenburg position. Even so, numerous potential complications are associated with the position.

Potential Complications: Trendelenburg Position

PC: Hypotension
PC: Impaired Gas Exchange
PC: Hypovolemia
PC: Atelectasis
PC: Venous Thrombosis
PC: Neuropathy
PC: Pressure Injury
PC: Postoperative Discomfort

Of all these potential complications, the RN first assistant should be especially alert for neuropathy. Nerves particularly susceptible to injury are those in the upper portion of the body, especially the brachial plexus. Pressure and stretching frequently cause brachial plexus injury to the patient in the Trendelenburg position, especially when shoulder braces are used. In such cases, the clavicles may be inadvertently depressed into the retroclavicular spaces, resulting in pressure on the nerve roots. When the patient's head is turned to the side, additional stretching of the nerve roots on the opposite side occurs and may result in injury. Finally, if an arm is externally rotated, abducted, or hyperextended, the head of the humerus may damage the plexus. The best way to prevent this potential injury is to avoid using wrist straps or shoulder braces. If shoulder braces are essential, then the RN first assistant must remember that padding, although certainly necessary, will not prevent injury. Braces should not be placed over the clavicles, but rather should be placed at the acromioclavicular junction. In the event that an arm is extended on an armboard, the opposite shoulder should be positioned against the brace.

Like the reverse Trendelenburg position, the Trendelenburg position has the potential to cause shearing force, which may lead to pressure injury. This potential danger does not justify the use of restraining devices, such as shoulder braces and wrist straps. The best intervention is a specially designed mattress, such as a Hewer mattress, which has a nonslip surface. This mattress is ribbed and has bolsters to fit the neck, the lumbar area of the back, and the ankles.

Responsibility for the patient's surgical position does not end when the RN first assistant scrubs and dons gown and gloves. As with all other surgical positions, the RN first assistant must be cognizant throughout the surgical procedure of the possible complications associated with the particular position being used. For the Trendelenburg position, a good rule of thumb is the greater the tilt, the greater the potential for injury. A head-down tilt of 10 to 20 degrees is usually sufficient for exposure. In the event that more tilt is requested to provide better exposure, the RN first assistant's immediate reaction should be not compliance, but rather investigation. The alternative to ineffective retraction is not necessarily more tilt. Perhaps more vigorous retraction is needed, or maybe a different retractor should be used.

Positioning Goals and Criteria: Trendelenburg Position

During the perioperative period, the patient will not experience any of the following complications related to surgical positioning: severe hypotension, hypovolemia, hypoventilation, impaired skin integrity, venous thrombosis, neuropathy, or postoperative discomfort. There will be no signs of the following:

1. pressure ulcer formation at susceptible pressure sites
2. tingling, numbness, cramping, pain, or aches in joints; weakness and stiffness in the upper and lower extremities
3. inability to resume preoperative patterns of ambulation
4. pain or discomfort when abducting, adducting, flexing, and extending the upper and lower extremities
5. atelectasis, hypovolemia, or hypoxemia
6. neuropathy or brachial plexus injury.

Positioning Requirements: Trendelenburg Position

The RN first assistant should ensure that the following nursing interventions are accomplished while placing the patient in the Trendelenburg position (see Figure 7-3):

1. arranging with the surgical suite manager for the placement of a special friction mattress (Hewer type) on the operating room bed
2. coordinating with the surgical team for the Trendelenburg position to be used only if absolutely necessary (The decision should be made after the peritoneal cavity is opened and the surgeon determines that the position will enhance surgical exposure.)
3. placing the patient on the operating room bed with the cephalad tips of the patellae opposite, or footward of, the metal leg-thigh hinges of the operating room bed, to minimize pressure on the calves and knee joints if the foot section of the operating room bed is angled downward
4. ensuring that any ankle straps used are well padded
5. avoiding extending the armboards more than 90 degrees from the patient's body
6. if a vaginal prep or an indwelling urinary catheter insertion is required, gently positioning the patient in a frog-leg position, without leaning or placing pressure on the thighs

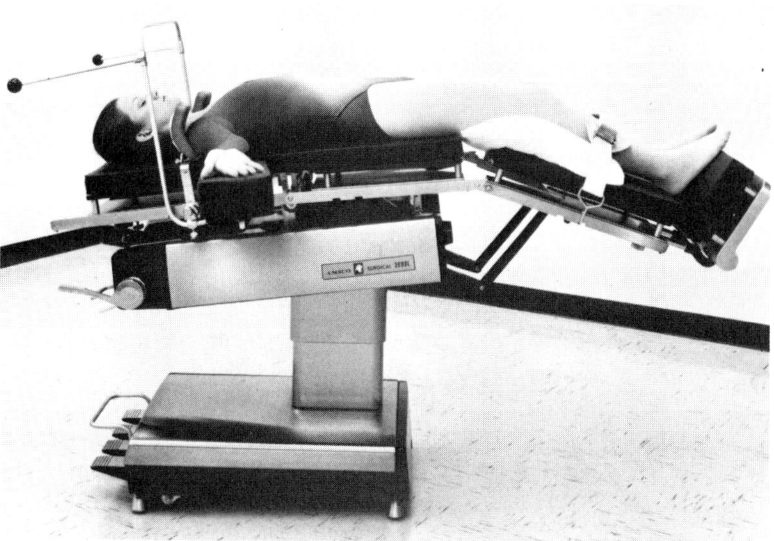

FIGURE 7-3

The Trendelenburg position, with 10 to 15 degrees of head-down tilt, is more common in modern surgery than is the former traditional steep tilt. Bent knees and an ankle restraint retain the patient in the tilt position without shoulder braces as long as the flexed knee joint is placed sufficiently caudad of the leg-thigh hinge of the operating room bed top so that the adjacent firm edge of the depressed leg section of the bed cannot indent the patient's calf. *(Photo courtesy of American Sterilizer Company, Erie, PA.)*

7. following the vaginal prep, ensuring that the mattress area beneath the prep site is dry
8. performing all positional changes gradually and slowly

LITHOTOMY POSITION

The lithotomy position presents hazards to the musculoskeletal, integumentary, respiratory, and cardiovascular systems. Potential complications include venous stasis, decreased respiratory effectiveness, hypotension, lower extremity compartment syndrome, joint damage, and nerve injury.[15,16] When the patient's legs are elevated, the thighs press against the abdomen. This may result in increased intraabdominal pressure with a subsequent reduction in diaphragmatic movement. In both normal-weight and obese patients, the consequence of such pressure is increased pulmonary blood volume, resulting in engorgement of lung tissue, which then reduces compliance. An 18% decrease in vital capacity and a 3% decrease (14% with a 10-degree Trendelenburg position) in tidal volume also result from the lithotomy position.[17]

Circulation is also affected. In addition to venous pooling in the lumbar region, vascular compression might occur throughout the lower extremities due to positioning equipment and in the groin due to thigh flexion. Patients with varicose veins are particularly susceptible to venous stasis; to reduce venous stasis, antithromboembolic devices are very helpful, especially if the procedure will take longer than 15 minutes.[18] Another effect on circulatory status is reduced blood volume in the legs. As the patient's legs are lowered at the completion of the procedure, between 500 and 600 ml of blood drains into the legs from the torso; severe hypotension may result if this maneuver is not carried out slowly and carefully.

Nerve injury can result from stretching or compression; capillaries surrounding the nerve may rupture, leading to necrosis.[19] Obturator nerve injury is a potential complication of the lithotomy position with acute flexion of the thighs, resulting in postoperative patient complaints of sensory disturbances along the medial aspect of the thigh and inability to abduct the extremity.[20] The saphenous nerves are also susceptible to injury, especially from misplaced or unpadded stirrups along the medial aspect of the knee and lower leg. If the saphenous nerve is injured, the patient suffers loss of sensation to the medial aspect of the legs. Damage to the peroneal nerve may cause footdrop; the lateral aspect of the knee must be protected from compression. With care, the saphenous and common peroneal nerves are easily protected; it is a matter of placing ankle-strap stirrups well to the outside of the legs and allowing no contact between the legs and the stirrups. In the obese patient or the patient who is difficult to position, foam padding around the knees offers a measure of protection. The sciatic nerve may be damaged if the legs are not abducted simultaneously; the femoral head may compress the sciatic nerve against the ischial tuberosity.[21] This nerve may also be overstretched if the thigh is hyperflexed at the hip or if a flexed thigh is externally rotated to its maximum range of motion.[22]

Before initiating the lithotomy position, the RN first assistant should adjust the height of ankle-strap stirrups to the length of the patient's legs. This prevents pressure at the knees and on the lumbar spine (which, incidentally, should have been padded). Additionally, symmetry is a positioning priority. The consequence of asymmetry in the lithotomy position may be injury. Symmetry should be verified by ensuring that the patient's pelvis is level on the operating room bed and that the torso and head, as well as hips, knees, and feet, are in a straight line. Also, the perineum should be in line with the longitudinal axis of the operating room bed; the buttocks should not extend beyond the break of the bed.

With ankle-strap stirrups, the patient's legs are elevated together and then flexed, simultaneously, at a 90-degree angle to the abdomen. To accomplish this maneuver, each leg is grasped by the sole of the foot with one hand while the other hand supports the leg near the knee. While supporting the legs, the knees are flexed. Next, the padded feet are placed in the stirrup slings with one set of loops around the soles at the area of the metatarsals and the other set around the ankles. The result should be hips that are symmetric and calves that are parallel with the operating room bed. If more abduction is needed for better exposure, this should be accomplished by flexing or externally rotating the hips, not the knees. The hips are supported with one hand while the legs and feet are gently extended. It is extremely important to prevent excessive abduction and uncontrolled hyperextension when ankle-type stirrups are used. These devices have been implicated in many nerve injuries, most likely because of their inability to control abduction of the thigh.[23]

There are many leg-support devices that might be selected instead of the ankle-strap stirrup. Calf-support devices may place the patient at greatest risk for compartment syndrome, because the entire weight of the leg is supported in one area. When heel and calf support devices are used, this problem is somewhat reduced. Total leg support systems are more frequently used for prolonged, complex procedures requiring abdominal-perineal access.

Another very important consideration is protecting the arms and hands. If these are left at the sides and extended beyond the operating room bed break, they can be injured while lowering and raising the foot of the bed. Alternative methods of protecting the patient's hands and arms include folding the arms across the abdomen and securing them with a towel or placing the arms on armboards. When armboards are used, extreme care must be exercised, especially if the patient requires realignment or repositioning on the operating room bed. Performing such a maneuver without consideration for the extended arms can be harmful to the patient. The arms could be hyperextended, resulting in injury to the brachial plexus. Consequently, if repositioning is necessary, the arms should be placed across the abdomen during the maneuver.

Potential Complications: Lithotomy Position

PC: Impaired Postoperative Mobility
PC: Neuropathy

PC: Impaired Tissue Perfusion
PC: Decreased Cardiac Output
PC: Pressure Injury
PC: Postoperative Discomfort
PC: Compartment Syndrome

Positioning Goals and Criteria: Lithotomy Position

During the perioperative period, the patient will not experience any of the following positioning-related complications: impaired mobility, decreased cardiac output and tissue perfusion, impaired skin integrity, altered postoperative kinesthetic perception, or postoperative discomfort. Discomfort in patients who have been in the lithotomy position may increase over time; to evaluate this goal, discomfort should not be measured only on the first postoperative day.[24] There will be no signs of the following:

1. inability to resume preoperative patterns of ambulation
2. tingling, numbness, cramping, pain, or aches in joints; weakness and stiffness in the upper and lower extremities
3. inability to abduct, adduct, flex, and extend the upper and lower extremities without experiencing pain or discomfort
4. edema, discoloration, temperature change, phlebitis, thrombosis, venous stasis, or ulcerations in the lower extremities
5. hypotension, increased pulse rate, or compromised venous integrity
6. pressure ulcer formation at susceptible pressure sites
7. postoperative discomfort
8. self-concept distress.

Positioning Requirements: Lithotomy Position

The RN first assistant will ensure that the following nursing interventions are accomplished while placing the patient in lithotomy position (see Figure 7-4):

1. placing protective padding under dependent pressure sites
2. applying antithromboembolic devices
3. avoiding excessive hip abduction and external rotation
4. taking steps to maintain privacy and preserve dignity
5. placing the arms on armboards angled 10 to 15 degrees from the operating room bed, verifying with the patient that his or her arms are comfortable
6. placing the arms across the chest in the event that the patient must be realigned on the bed, with realignment done by lifting, not pulling
7. ensuring adequate padding of leg-support stirrups; for ankle-strap stirrups, using a wide foot strap and padding the feet and ankles before placement in the stirrups
8. simultaneously elevating the legs, with each person supporting the foot with one hand and the leg just under the knee with the other hand and flexion of the knees as the hips are flexed
9. checking the patient for symmetry by ensuring that the pelvis is level and the torso and head, as well as the hips, knees, and feet, are in a straight line
10. providing adequate protection to prevent inadvertent wetting of the sheet and mattress beneath the patient's sacrum and buttocks
11. closely monitoring instrument placement on the draped surgical field, avoiding placement in the groin area

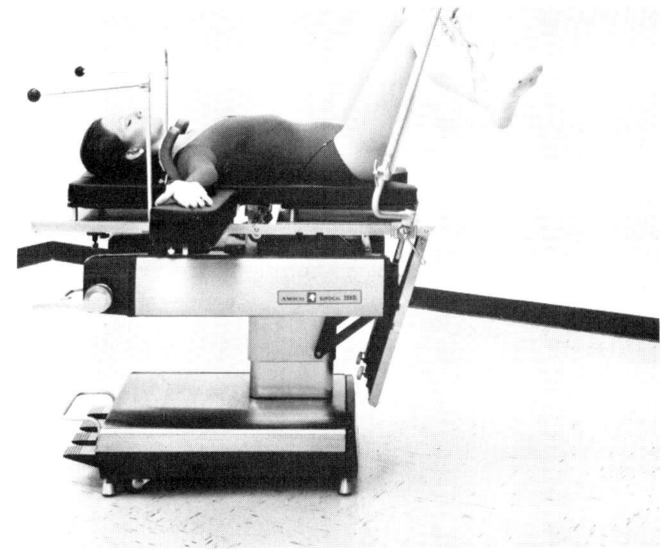

FIGURE 7-4
In the lithotomy position, the thighs are flexed slightly more than 90 degrees on the abdomen, and the knees are flexed enough to bring the lower legs nearly parallel to the operating room bed top. Arms are placed on armboards (or across the abdomen or at the patient's sides; not shown here). Frequently, some degree of head-down tilt is added; well-padded shoulder braces, placed over the acromioclavicular joints, prevent the patient from shearing forces caused by slipping cephalad. *(Photo courtesy of American Sterilizer Company, Erie, PA.)*

12. for a patient with mobility limitations, considering awake positioning to prevent joint/muscle strain
13. ensuring that no one leans on the inner aspects of the patient's thighs, thus causing strain on the joints, ligaments, and muscles of the hips and knees.

PRONE POSITION

The prone position presents a significant challenge to the RN first assistant; it affects the patient's cardiovascular, respiratory, integumentary, musculoskeletal, and neurologic systems. With proper positioning, relatively few cardiovascular problems should arise. However, there is a possibility that pressure may be exerted against the inferior vena cava and femoral veins, in which case hypotension may occur, causing blood to seek another pathway, such as the perineal venous plexus and the veins of the vertebral column. This outcome would not be conducive to maintaining adequate cardiac output or systemic blood pressure. In addition, the increased blood flow through the veins of the vertebral column may result in excessive intraoperative blood loss.

Correct prone positioning, barring intervening variables, should result in few respiratory problems. Torso support, from the clavicles to the iliac crests, prevents the weight of the body against the abdominal wall curtailing movement of the diaphragm, limiting tidal volume, and resulting in hypoventilation. Without such support, the surgeon's and RN first assistant's jobs will be more difficult because the restricted abdominal wall will cause the patient's entire back to move with every inflation of the lungs. When the patient is properly positioned, not only will respiratory efforts be enhanced, but the back will remain almost motionless from level T10 down, even if the anesthetist/anesthesiologist engages in vigorous ventilation.

The prone position and its modifications can cause neurologic injuries. Especially susceptible is the brachial plexus, which may be damaged by stretching during turning and pressure from inadequate or improperly placed support devices. The lateral femoral cutaneous nerves may be injured by compression against the pelvic support device. When the anesthetist/anesthesiologist turns the patient's head, care must be exercised to protect the facial motor nerves over the infraparotid area. Ulnar nerves are easily damaged by pressure if they are placed against the sharp edges of support devices. The nerves and tendons of the dorsa of the feet are prime targets for injury when they rest on the edge of the operating room bed.

Other areas of potential injury are the female breasts and male genitalia. The breasts or the penis and scrotum may become twisted and compressed. The ears, shoulders, iliac crests, knees, and toes are susceptible to pressure. The RN first assistant must exercise caution and avoid undue manipulation of the joints, particularly in the upper extremities. Dislocation of the shoulder is a very real possibility.

The most crucial aspect of the prone position is the act of turning the patient. Some anesthetists/anesthesiologists prefer anesthetizing the patient on the operating room bed; others prefer that the patient be intubated and relaxed and then turned from the gurney to the bed. Before turning the patient on the operating room bed, the head of the bed may be lowered 5 to 10 degrees to facilitate the return of blood from the lower part of the body while the upper part is being turned. In either method, extreme care must be taken with vascular access lines, catheters, monitoring leads, and breathing tubes to maintain their patency and prevent dislodgement.

The anesthetist/anesthesiologist coordinates patient turning so that control is maintained over respiratory and cardiovascular status while the head and neck are kept in the correct position. As a part of the planning process, the RN first assistant should arrange for an adequate number of people to turn the patient. At least three persons are needed, not including the anesthesia team member.

Smith provided a concise and detailed description for placing the patient in the prone position from the supine position.[25] The steps are as follows:

1. Move the patient on his back toward one side of the operating room bed and roll him onto one side. Two persons should make the lift from back to side, one at the shoulders and one at the hips, and they should move both parts at the same speed. The anesthetist/anesthesiologist keeps the face in the proper plane. Now the patient is in the lateral decubitus position with one arm under his body and close to his uppermost side. At least one person should "receive" the body on the other side of the bed.
2. The patient is rolled into the three-fourths turn position; the under arm is then freed of his weight, moved to a position behind him, and lowered over the side of the operating room bed as soon as this can be done without putting stress on the shoulder. The uppermost arm is swung forward to hang free over the other side of the bed.
3. Next, the hips and shoulders are lifted back toward the starting edge of the bed to return the patient to the middle of it.

4. As the turn is completed, the person controlling the shoulders has an arm under the chest, pulling the patient back toward the middle of the bed. This arm must continue to hold the upper part of the patient off the bed while the anesthetist/anesthesiologist gets the head into a safe position, reconnects the anesthesia machine, ventilates the patient vigorously for a few breaths, and measures the blood pressure. Only then can the attendant's supporting arm be removed from under the chest and the patient's "down" arm be lowered.
5. At this point the patient is prone, with his head turned to one side and both arms hanging down beside the bed, which is in a 5- to 10-degree head-down position. Now supporting devices for the pelvis and chest can be applied, or any other planned modification of the prone position can be effected.
6. Only after all movement is finished is it advisable to move the operating room bed back to the horizontal position.

Of course, there are other methods for turning a supine patient to the prone position. The most appropriate method should be chosen by the anesthetist/anesthesiologist with input from the surgeon, RN first assistant, and circulating nurse. Whatever the method used, extreme caution must be exercised to avoid injuring the patient.

Potential Complications: Prone Position

PC: Hypoventilation
PC: Pressure Injury
PC: Postoperative Discomfort
PC: Neuropathy

Positioning Goals and Criteria: Prone Position

During the perioperative period, the patient will not experience any of the following complications related to surgical positioning: hypoventilation, pressure injury, neuropathy, or postoperative discomfort. There will be no signs of the following:

1. increase in pulse rate and significant fluctuations in blood pressure (as reported by the anesthetist/anesthesiologist and related to positioning), cyanosis, or oliguria
2. edema, discoloration, temperature change, phlebitis, thrombosis, venous stasis, or ulcerations in the lower extremities
3. pressure ulcer formation at susceptible pressure sites
4. tingling, numbness, cramping, pain, or aches in joints; weakness and stiffness in the upper and lower extremities
5. inability to abduct, adduct, flex, and extend the upper extremities without experiencing pain or discomfort
6. inability to resume preoperative patterns of ambulation.

Positioning Requirements: Prone Position

The goal of nursing intervention is to control and modify the potential for complications from the prone position or one of its variations. The RN first assistant ensures that the following nursing interventions are accomplished while positioning the patient in prone position:

1. applying antithromboembolic devices
2. placing a ventral chest support system (such as a support frame or 9-inch-diameter body rolls) from the acromioclavicular joints to the iliac crests, verifying that the abdomen is not compressed
2. padding all potential pressure sites
3. placing a small pillow at the pubis to help protect the genitalia; after positioning, checking the genitalia to ensure they are not distorted or compressed; checking the integrity of a urinary catheter, if appropriate
4. checking the breasts to ensure that they are in a neutral or medial position without stretch on the nipples
5. using positioning devices to protect the eyes and ears and prevent neck torsion
6. supporting the feet with a pad or pillow placed under the anterior surface of the legs and ankles to prevent pressure injury to the toes and plantar flexion
7. checking the skin to ensure that it is not stretched over the ventral chest support device(s)
8. rotating the arms by lowering them toward the floor and swinging them upward in a natural arc so that they lie beside and beyond the top of the head either on angled armboards or at the patient's side; preventing compression of any part of the arm against the side of the operating room bed
9. applying a gluteal safety restraint; checking that the restraint is not placed tightly.

LATERAL POSITION

In the simple lateral position (lateral decubitus), which is used for thoracic surgery, vital capacity is reduced by 10% and tidal volume by 8%. Additional position modifications made for kidney surgery will cause a 14.5% reduction in vital capacity. These reductions occur as a result of restricted chest expansion and altered pulmonary blood-to-gas exchange ratios. Also, the pulmonary blood flow is usually not distributed evenly throughout all parts of the lungs, resulting in a dependent lung that may be well-ventilated but poorly perfused.[26]

The lateral position causes blood pooling in the dependent extremities. In addition, there are deviations in blood pressure. In the left lateral position, arterial pressure can drop by as much as 24 mm Hg; in the right lateral position, the drop may be up to 33 mm Hg. It is thought that the right lateral position causes the drop in pressure by obstructing the flow of blood through the vena cava. Also, there may be interference with cardiac action because of a possible shift in heart position.

In the lateral position the dependent brachial plexus is vulnerable to injury because of the weight of the body pressing on the arm and axilla, causing excessive stretching of the plexus. Other nerves susceptible to injury from the lateral position are the median, radial, ulnar, and peroneal. The RN first assistant should pay particular attention to protecting the common peroneal nerve, which leaves the posterior aspect of the knee and travels laterally around the head of the fibula. Sufficient padding must be placed under the dependent knee and upper leg to protect this vulnerable nerve; footdrop may result from improper positioning.

Like all positions, the lateral position puts significant pressure on selected dependent body surfaces. The RN first assistant needs to pay close attention to protecting the hips, legs, and ankles. The weight from the upper leg may press on the lower leg; this can be minimized with the proper use of pillows. The dependent hip, especially in the area of the great trochanter major of the femur, is highly susceptible to pressure; special padding is warranted for this highly sensitive area.

Placing the patient in the lateral position, whether for a kidney procedure or for a thoracic procedure, requires a team of at least four people. As in the prone positioning procedure, the anesthesia team member leads the maneuvers, coordinating each positional change, controlling the patient's head and neck, and maintaining respirations. Before turning, the patient is placed in the supine position on the operating room bed. If a "beanbag" or other moldable support system is being used to stabilize the trunk and prevent forward or backward rolling, it is placed on the bed before patient transfer. All bed surfaces need to be at an equal height; it may be necessary to pad the head and foot portions of the bed when beanbags are used. Once the patient is supine on the operating room bed, one arm is extended on an armboard, and the other arm is placed at the side. Following induction of general anesthesia, the anesthetist/anesthesiologist turns the patient's head toward the side.

To position the patient in the lateral position, the RN first assistant and circulating nurse stand on the patient's side, and another team member stands at the foot of the operating room bed. With the anesthetist/anesthesiologist controlling the patient's head and neck, the RN first assistant places an arm under the neck to the shoulder, the circulating nurse places an arm under the thighs to the hip, and the fourth team member grasps both ankles. On cue from the anesthesia team member, the RN first assistant and circulating nurse simultaneously lift and pull the patient's side up and into position. At the same time, the fourth team member flexes the lower leg at both the hip and knee for stabilization and places a pillow between the legs. Meanwhile, the anesthetist/anesthesiologist supports the head with a small pillow or several folded towels. Careful alignment of the head and spinal column prevents lateral flexion of the neck and stretching injury to the cervical sympathetic chain.[27] Both arms are flexed at the elbow. The upside arm may be placed in a holding device or placed on a padded Mayo stand; the arm is positioned forward and cephalad. Excessive traction or abduction of the arm must be avoided to prevent brachial plexus injury. Next, as the RN first assistant and circulating nurse gently lift the patient, the fourth team member places an axillary roll or pad near the axilla, under the upper chest. The purpose of this chest support is to relieve pressure on the head of the dependent humerus, axillary nerve, and artery, as well as to allow more room for respiratory excursion. Checking the radial pulse in the dependent arm is a good way to determine whether pressure has been obviated by axillary support.

After the patient is side-lying, further modifications may be made for access to the retroperitoneal space. This is accomplished by positioning the iliac crest just below the kidney elevator of the operating room bed. The anesthetist/anesthesiologist raises the kidney elevator and flexes the bed. If the patient has been properly positioned, the area between the twelfth rib and the iliac crest will be elevated. The anesthetist/anesthesiologist then brings the patient's shoulder slightly forward and flexes the arm so that it rests on the mattress, near the face. The entire bed is then tilted downward toward the head, making the operative site horizontal. For the lateral kidney position, the RN first assistant and circulating nurse may attach padded kidney rests to the operating room bed; the short rest is placed at the back and a long rest in the front. If the patient is obese, the RN first assistant should ensure that tissue folds do not extend over the end of the kidney rest. Restraints should also be placed over the hips and right leg. A strap placed over the calf helps to secure the legs. If restraints are placed too tightly, pressure areas may result. When closure begins, the RN first assistant should request that the kidney elevator be lowered and the bed returned to a horizontal position. This will facilitate closure.

Potential Complications: Lateral Position

PC: Pressure Injury
PC: Neuropathy
PC: Impaired Postoperative Mobility

Positioning Goals and Criteria: Lateral Position

During the perioperative period, the patient will be free from evidence of positioning-related pressure injuries, alterations in postoperative kinesthetic sensory perception, and impaired postoperative mobility. There will be no signs of the following:

1. pressure ulcer formation at susceptible pressure sites
2. tingling, numbness, cramping, pain, or aches in joints; weakness and stiffness in the upper and lower extremities
3. inability to adduct, abduct, flex, and extend the upper and lower extremities without experiencing pain or discomfort
4. inability to resume preoperative patterns of ambulation.

Positioning Requirements: Lateral Position

The RN first assistant will ensure that the following nursing interventions are accomplished while placing the patient in the lateral position (see Figure 7-5):

1. ensuring adequate personnel to turn the patient
2. placing a large pillow between the legs
3. placing protective padding under the dependent ankle, elbow, knee, and hip, or using a moldable support system
4. positioning the upper extremities to add stability and protect pressure areas and neurovascular bundles
5. applying a securing device over the hip without stretching the underlying skin
6. placing the head on a small pillow or other device to maintain alignment with the spinal column
7. placing a small axillary pad under the upper chest, near the dependent axilla.

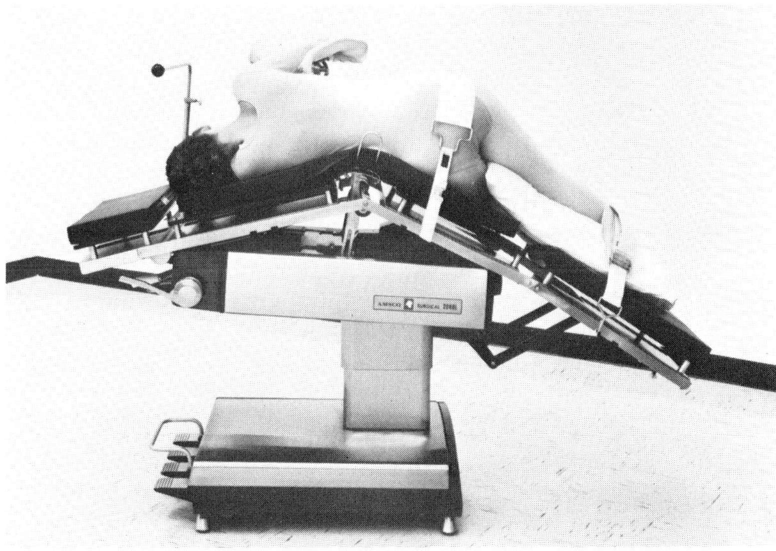

FIGURE 7-5
The lateral position for kidney procedures adds the use of an elevated rest under the downside iliac crest to increase the amount of lateral flexion and improve access to the upside kidney. Careful stabilizing precautions should be taken to prevent the patient from shifting on the operating room bed such that the elevated rest impedes ventilation of the downside lung. *(Photo courtesy of American Sterilizer Company, Erie, PA.)*

THE SITTING POSITION

The sitting position presents the RN first assistant with a major challenge. It is both technically difficult to achieve and physiologically stressful. The potential for inadvertent hypotension, if untreated, can lead to cerebral hypoperfusion, resulting in cerebral hypoxia. The anesthetist/anesthesiologist plays a major role in preventing this complication, especially through the use of pharmacologic agents; however, the RN first assistant also plays a significant role. Application of antithromboembolic devices or an antigravity suit will facilitate venous return and reduce the tendency toward venous pooling in the lower extremities.

Cardiac dysrhythmias in seated, anesthetized patients may occur and must be distinguished as either perfusing or nonperfusing. Nonperfusing dysrhythmias are accompanied by or cause a drop in perfusion pressure; they require urgent treatment to prevent cerebral ischemia. They are frequently associated with surgical manipulation; cessation of the manipulation may terminate the dysrhythmic episode. Perfusing dysrhythmias are usually unaccompanied by hypotension. They may be related to surgical stimulation, an air embolism, or hypercarbia. The cause must be identified and treated; frequent arterial blood gas determinations, administration of vasopressors, correction of hypovolemia, air aspiration, and the use of other supportive drugs may be required.[28]

A catastrophic possible complication is a venous air embolism, which can lead to circulatory collapse and death. The anesthetist/anesthesiologist plays a major role in preventing and treating this complication. Essential to prevention and treatment are the placement of a right atrial catheter and the use of a precordial Doppler ultrasonic device. If the complication occurs, the Doppler will assist in diagnosing the event; the catheter will confirm the diagnosis, as well as help to aspirate and remove the embolized air. Because the atrial line is placed while the patient is supine, the position of the catheter may be compromised while the patient is moved from the supine to the sitting position. Once the sitting position is achieved, the location of the catheter tip must be rechecked and adjusted as necessary.

Improper positioning has the potential to affect the integumentary, musculoskeletal, and peripheral nervous systems. Because the body weight will rest on the ischial tuberosities with the patient in the sitting position, there is the potential for the development of pressure injuries. Prolonged extension of the knees may lead to stretch injuries of the sciatic nerves. In addition, there may be significant pressure on the Achilles tendons and the heels; the possibility for the development of footdrop from injury to the sciatic or common peroneal nerve also exists. Preventing these potential complications requires adequate padding at vulnerable pressure sites and the use of a padded footboard. The arms, particularly the elbows, are also susceptible to injury, especially ulnar nerve damage from compression against the side of the operating room bed. Careful support of the elbows on a pillow or pads prevents contact compression.

Positioning must be done with precise teamwork. The patient is usually anesthetized in the supine position; intravenous lines, atrial catheters, arterial lines, esophageal stethoscopes, cardiography leads, urinary catheters, and thermal probes are inserted as required. Antithromboembolic devices are applied. When the anesthesia team is ready, the circulating nurse loosens the restraining strap. The RN first assistant then fully flexes the operating room bed and lowers the foot section approximately 45 to 60 degrees. Next, the back of the bed is slowly elevated while the chassis is lowered; that is, placed in the Trendelenburg position. The foot of the bed should be adjusted to a horizontal, heart-level position. Throughout this process, the circulating nurse stands by the patient to prevent a fall from the bed. During each movement, the anesthetist/anesthesiologist sustains perfusion, monitors blood pressure, and administers vasopressors if necessary.

When the patient is in a full sitting position, the RN first assistant is ready to stabilize the head. After the circulating nurse applies the safety strap, she and the RN first assistant will usually attach the U-frame of the selected head holder to the back rails of the operating room bed. In the event of an air embolus, this will allow the anesthetist/anesthesiologist to lower the back of the bed without compromising head stability. In selected cranial procedures, the U-frame may need to be attached to the side rails on the thigh section of the bed. A padded headrest or skull pin head holder is then applied. Following this maneuver, the bed head section is removed; the shoulders may be stabilized with restraining tapes applied to the U-frame. Once this is accomplished, a careful and complete reassessment is made to ensure that there is adequate padding and protection and that lines and catheters are patent and still correctly located.

Potential Complications: Sitting Position

PC: Hypotension
PC: Air Embolism
PC: Pressure Injury
PC: Dysrhythmia
PC: Neuropathy

Positioning Goals and Criteria: Sitting Position

During the perioperative period, the patient will not experience any of the following complications related to surgical positioning: hypotension, air embolism, pressure injury, dysrhythmias, or neuropathy. There will be no signs of the following:

1. hypotension, increased pulse rate, or compromised venous integrity
2. edema, discoloration, temperature change, phlebitis, thrombosis, venous stasis, or ulcerations in the lower extremities
3. pressure ulcer formation at susceptible pressure sites
4. tingling, numbness, cramping, pain, or aches in joints; weakness and stiffness in the upper and lower extremities
5. inability to abduct, adduct, flex, and extend the upper and lower extremities without experiencing pain or discomfort
6. inability to resume preoperative patterns of ambulation.

Positioning Requirements: Sitting Position

The RN first assistant will ensure that the following nursing interventions are accomplished while placing the patient in the sitting position (see Figure 7-6):

1. applying antithromboembolic devices
2. performing each positioning maneuver slowly, allowing sufficient time for the anesthetist/anesthesiologist to measure blood pressure before performing the next maneuver
3. placing adequate protective padding under the patient
4. attaching a padded footboard to the end of the operating room bed and ensuring that the patient's feet are positioned at a 90-degree angle
5. placing foam padding under each heel
6. resting the patient's elbows on a pillow or pad
7. when stabilizing the patient's back, attaching restraining tape without stretching or pinching the skin
8. after positioning is completed, checking the patient's genitalia to ensure that the scrotum and penis are not twisted or compressed between the legs; checking the patency of all lines to ensure that tubing is not kinked or stretched.

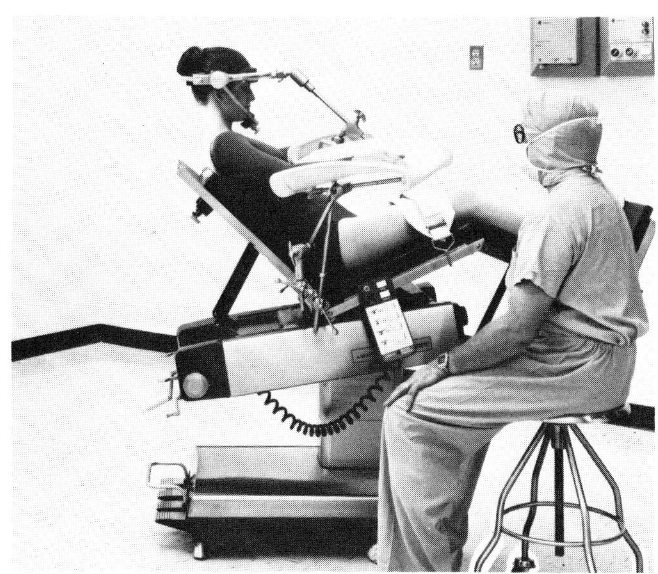

FIGURE 7-6
In a neurosurgical sitting position, the frame of the head-holder is clamped to the side rails of the trunk section of the operating room bed so that patient's torso can be leveled in the event of a venous air embolus at the cervico-occipital operative site. *(Photo courtesy of American Sterilizer Company, Erie, PA.)*

CONCLUSION

Anesthesia produces a state of narcosis, analgesia, relaxation, and reflex loss. Although these are desirable patient states for accomplishing surgical interventions, they put the patient at risk for positional injury. The ordinary protective states of pain, discomfort, and resistance are deliberately obviated, leaving the patient totally dependent on a perioperative team that is well versed in the principles and protocols for safe patient positioning. The RN first assistant, along with the rest of the perioperative team, must consider what the patient can physiologically and structurally tolerate as they seek a position that provides adequate surgical exposure and access. Various surgical positions each have physiologic consequences, and the techniques used to obtain and maintain the position must be selected with these consequences and potential complications in mind.

REVIEW QUESTIONS

1. Communication between neurons occurs at the _______ and is the physiologic basis for CNS function.
   a. excitatory motor endplate
   b. receptor mechanism
   c. biologic membrane
   d. synaptic junctions

2. For inhaled anesthetic agents, potency is commonly expressed as the minimum alveolar concentration (MAC), determined as the necessary alveolar concentration to prevent _______ in 50% of subjects in response to the painful stimuli of surgery.
   a. pain
   b. increased heart rate
   c. movement
   d. the surgical stress response
3. Of the commonly used inhalation anesthetics, which provides not only rapid induction and recovery, but also potent analgesia?
   a. enflurane
   b. halothane
   c. isoflurane
   d. nitrous oxide
4. An ideal neuromuscular blocking agent would probably be nondepolarizing, yet have an onset and duration of action similar to succinylcholine but without which of the following disadvantages?
   a. dose-related apnea
   b. bradycardia and dysrhythmias
   c. allergic, histamine-like reactions
   d. difficult reversal
5. A collaborative problem is usually a physiologic complication that the RN first assistant
   a. delegates to assistive personnel
   b. reports to a physician
   c. monitors for onset or change in status
   d. discovers on review of the medical record
6. RN first assistants manage collaborative problems using
   a. physician-prescribed interventions
   b. nursing-prescribed interventions
   c. medical treatment algorithms
   d. both a and b
7. True or false: In a collaborative problem framework, the nursing process becomes unnecessary.
   a. True
   b. False
8. Using a collaborative problem framework, the RN first assistant refers to the potential sequelae of patient positioning as
   a. interdependent nursing diagnoses
   b. potential patient problems/needs
   c. potential complications
   d. bifocal clinical problems
9. Respiratory consequences of the supine position include
   a. restriction of posterolateral chest excursion
   b. a sequential increase in vital capacity
   c. a serious potential increase in mean arterial pressure
   d. mobile abdominal viscera that gravitate caudad

10. The RN first assistant might consider modifying the standard supine position to increase the comfort of the awake surgical patient to the
    a. recliner position
    b. rocking chair position
    c. lawn chair position
    d. semi-supine position
11. Risk factors associated with pressure ulcer development include
    a. inadequate dietary intake of protein
    b. administration of epinephrine with local anesthesia
    c. cardiopulmonary bypass over 4 hours
    d. an unpadded point of contact exceeding 6 hours
12. Lifting rather than pulling the patient during positional change decreases the potential for injury related to
    a. Stage I pressure ulcers
    b. shearing forces
    c. bony prominence compression
    d. inadequate oxygen to underlying muscle tissue
13. Endoscopic access to the lower abdominal and pelvic structures usually requires that the patient be positioned in
    a. reverse Trendelenburg
    b. low lithotomy
    c. Trendelenburg
    d. high lawn chair
14. Lower extremity compartment syndrome is a potential complication of which position?
    a. reverse Trendelenburg
    b. Trendelenburg
    c. Fowler's
    d. Lithotomy
15. With acute flexion of the thighs, the _______ nerve may be injured, causing _______.
    a. obturator; postoperative sensory disturbance along the medial aspect of the thigh
    b. saphenous; loss of sensation to the medial aspect of the foot
    c. peroneal; footdrop
    d. sciatic; painful hip abduction
16. If additional abduction is required for better exposure in the lithotomy position, the RN first assistant should consider
    a. raising the height of the stirrups
    b. angling the knees closer to the chest
    c. flexing and externally rotating the knees
    d. flexing and externally rotating the hips
17. Ventral chest support devices used in the prone position have the potential to cause injury to what nerve?
    a. obturator
    b. lateral femoral cutaneous

c. saphenous
d. perineal venous plexus

18. The most crucial aspect of the prone position is turning the patient; it is safest to anesthetize the patient on the _______ to prevent injury during turning.
    a. operating room bed
    b. stretcher/gurney
    c. bed from the patient care unit
    d. either a or b
19. At the conclusion of any positioning maneuver, the RN first assistant should check major body areas to ensure that they are
    a. symmetrical and in alignment
    b. adequately restrained
    c. padded with a pillow or foam
    d. nondependent
20. During report to a postoperative patient unit, the RN first assistant should relate
    a. initial response of patient to awake positioning
    b. identification of padded/protected body parts
    c. presence of any abnormal skin conditions
    d. position changes during the procedure

Answers

1. d	8. c	15. a
2. c	9. a	16. d
3. a	10. c	17. b
4. b	11. a	18. d
5. c	12. b	19. a
6. d	13. c	20. c
7. b	14. d	

REFERENCES

1. Carpenito, LJ: Nursing Diagnosis: Application to Clinical Practice, pp 36–45. Philadelphia, JB Lippincott, 1992
2. Martin JT: Positioning in Anesthesia and Surgery, p 30. Philadelphia, WB Saunders, 1987
3. Kneedler JA, Dodge GH: Perioperative Patient Care: A Nursing Perspective, p 464. Boston, Blackwell Scientific, 1987
4. Martin, pp 37–40
5. Bergstrom N: Clinical Practice Guidelines—Managing Pain and Skin Problems. Dallas, Association of Operating Room Nurses Congress, 1992
6. Phippen ML: OR nurse's guide to preventing pressure sores. AORN J 36:207–208, 1982
7. Kemp M, Keithley J, Morreale B, Smith D: Factors That Contribute to Pressure Sore Formation. Anaheim, CA, Association of Operating Room Nurses Congress, 1989
8. Gendron F: Unexplained skin injuries may be pressure sores. OR Manager 2(10):1, 6–8, 1986
9. Vermillion C: OR acquired pressure ulcers. Decubitus 3:26–30, 1990
10. Ibid, p 28
11. Bergstrom, op cit
12. Hoshowsky V: Intraoperative Pressure Sore Prevention (Research poster presentation). Dallas, Association of Operating Room Nurses Congress, 1992
13. Bergstrom, op cit

14. Martin, p 128
15. Martin, pp 41–62
16. Graling PR, Colvin DB: The lithotomy position in colon surgery: Postoperative complications. AORN J 55:1029–1039, 1992
17. Kneedler, pp 467–470
18. Martin, p 48
19. Paschal CR, Strzelecki LR: Lithotomy positioning devices: Factors that contribute to patient injury. AORN J 55:1011–1022, 1992
20. Martin, p 332
21. Smith KA: Positioning principles: An anatomical review. AORN J 52:1196–1208, 1990
22. Paschal and Strzelecki, p 1016
23. Ibid, pp 1018–1020
24. Groom LE, Frisch SR: Sequelae of the intraoperative lithotomy position: A research study. AORN J 50:826–831, 1989
25. Smith RH: The prone position. In Martin JT (ed): Positioning in Anesthesia and Surgery, pp 36–38. Philadelphia, WB Saunders
26. Martin, p 132
27. Martin, p 333
28. Martin, pp 102–103

8 Principles of Tissue Handling

Rudolph C. Camishion
Arthur S. Brown
Richard K. Spence

In the early part of the 19th century, the four most important problems confronting the surgeon were pain, hemorrhage, shock, and infection. In 1842 Crawford Long used ether as a general anesthetic to remove small skin tumors; thus began the solution to the control of pain during surgery. Treatment of hemorrhage by specific therapy had to await the development of blood typing and cross-matching in the early 20th century. Shock is still imperfectly understood. Before the time of Lister, most patients did not survive operative procedures or open traumatic wounds because of infection. With the use of carbolic acid and simple "clean technique," the incidence of wound sepsis dropped precipitously. Eventually, carbolic spray was found to be unnecessary and perhaps even harmful, but better sterile technique evolved and proved to be one of the more important factors in avoiding infection. By the late 1980s, the incidence of wound infection following uncontaminated, clean operations dropped to 1% or less.

Halsted was probably the first American physician to teach that both surgical antisepsis and gentle tissue handling during an operation helped decrease the incidence of wound infection. Adopting and amplifying Theodore Kocher's meticulous bloodless surgical techniques, Halsted developed an approach that mandates the following: tissues should be cut by scalpel or scissors whenever possible rather than bluntly dissected; with sharp dissection, less tissue is injured. Sutures are foreign bodies; the fewer left in the wound, the better. Small bleeding vessels will clot spontaneously if covered with a sponge while the operation proceeds; direct pressure is an effective way to stop bleeding and to provide a clear operating field. The hemostat should clamp only the tissue to be ligated. Clamping and tying large amounts of tissue surrounding blood vessels causes excessive tissue necrosis and produces a fertile culture medium for bacterial growth. Unobliterated or undrained "dead space" in a wound quickly fills with blood or serum, inviting infection by providing bacteria with nutrient material in which to grow.

In the 1880s, when Halsted championed good surgical technique, little was known about the biology of wound healing. To practice surgery in the 1990s, one must have a clear understanding of how wounds heal.

OVERVIEW OF WOUND HEALING

From the moment of injury, whether traumatic or surgically created, the body begins to repair itself. Events are taking place on a biochemical and microscopic level even though no gross changes are noted by the casual observer. Initially, capillaries dilate with resultant increased blood flow to the injured area. Vasoactive substances (*e.g.*, serotonin, histamine, kinins) are released to help promote this vascular response. In addition, platelets are mobilized, and the coagulation cascade is activated to promote hemostasis. Various types of white blood cells—polymorphonuclear leukocytes, monocytes, and macrophages—are also called forth to start the phagocytic process that helps clean the area of foreign matter and debris. A fibrin network is initiated, and coagulum is formed—all part of the body's means of self-preservation.

After the initial inflammatory phase, which can last up to 3 days or so, the second phase of wound healing begins. In this phase the fibroblasts that have migrated into the wound start to produce collagen, the protein that gives the wound its strength. Also at this time, the squamous epithelium begins to migrate and replicate from the basal cell layer to restore the surface anatomy of the skin. Moisture, provided by damp dressings, promotes this epithelial migration and prevents dessication of these newly produced cells.

For optimal collagen synthesis, certain factors should be present in ideal concentrations. Among these are ascorbic acid (vitamin C), oxygen, zinc, amino acids, other vitamins and nutrients, and adequate blood flow. Other generalized conditions can interfere with wound healing. These include malnutrition, anemia, long-term use of anti-inflammatory medications including corticosteroids, systemic illnesses such as malignancy, immunosuppression, and infection. Nevertheless, local factors at the wound site are considered to be more important in the overall healing process than are these other, less alterable conditions.

After the fibroblastic, scar-forming phase, which can last several weeks, the third phase of wound healing begins. Scar maturation and remodeling continue, albeit at a slow pace, for months to years. External forces, such as those provided by pressure garments, can be used to help in this remodeling phase. Maximum tensile strength of a skin and fascia wound is usually achieved at about 6 weeks, although this level of tissue strength never reaches that of unwounded tissue. During the remodeling phase, the wound begins to contract and reorganize along the direction of least resistance. It is necessary, therefore, to apply appropriate splints to counteract this contracting force when such forces could create scar contractures and their subsequent deformities, such as those seen over flexion creases (*e.g.*, elbow, neck, axilla).

PREPARATORY MANEUVERS

Despite the remarkable advances in surgical technology and scientific knowledge, there are no absolute methods at the surgeon's disposal to accelerate the orderly wound healing process. Although careful patient preparation and choice of the appropriate procedure are essential ingredients in a successful operation, a poorly prepared surgeon or assistant can nullify even the most meticulous planning and judgment. To be competent, the RN first assistant must master some basic techniques common to all operations. The RN first assistant's goals are to carefully consider the planned incision, to handle tissues properly, and to possess the requisite manual and intellectual dexterity that will facilitate efficient surgery. With these competencies, iatrogenic tissue injury is reduced and fluid loss through evaporation, tissue drying and dessication, and the amount of time the open wound is exposed to exogenous contamination are decreased. As a result, wound healing is facilitated.

Most surgeons are right-handed. Consequently, most operations have been designed to be done from the patient's right side, to facilitate the use of the surgeon's right hand. The first assistant stands opposite the surgeon. Other assistants stand at the head or the foot with their bodies perpendicular to the surgeon's. Sometimes the surgeon can work better on the patient's left side—for example, during abdominal aortic surgery. Microsurgical procedures are best done with the surgeon and assistant seated. By resting the arms on the operating table, gross motor movement can be minimized. Various magnifying devices, including flip-down loupes, lenses mounted on eyeglass frames, and operating microscopes, are available if needed.

The height of the operating table should reach the level of the surgeon's elbows; the RN first assistant should seek this same position in relation to the table height. This height allows the wrist to be in slight extension, the desired position of function. A table raised too high requires compensatory flexing of the wrists, elongating the long extensors and shortening the long flexors. In this position, these tendons are out of tonic balance, small muscle control in the hands is reduced, and fatigue is increased.

For an operation on a depressed body area or in the mouth or deep cavity, the table is lowered. Lowering the field to below the surgeon's and assistant's elbows allows the wrists to be kept relatively straight or in slight dorsal extension. This position improves dexterity and finger strength. Again, the goal is to seek a table height that does not require the wrists to be in a position of flexion.

Speed is not an essential element of good surgical technique, but it is generally true that the shorter the operating time, the better off the patient. A fast surgeon does not rush. All movements are economical and expertly made.

Economy of time and motion is a principle that guides actions of both surgeon and RN first assistant during all phases of the surgical intervention.

Each operating room usually has two lights—one small, one large—mounted on tracks or swivels above the operating table. Because an operating room table can be moved, it is wise to check that it is centered under the lights before the patient is anesthetized. The best position for the lights is usually along the vertical axis of the patient's body; that is, one light at the head and one at the feet. Lights positioned behind the surgeon or assistant interfere with optimum illumination. In some instances, however, light from behind the surgeon is preferred, as when operating within the mouth (*e.g.*, cleft palate repair). The surgeon and the assistant must learn to stand upright to avoid casting shadows. In cases where the incision is narrow (as in a thoracotomy) or where the structures are deep (as in an abdominal aortic aneurysm), it is wise to wear a headlight to illuminate the operating field.

SURGICAL APPROACHES TO THE ABDOMEN

The abdominal cavity is opened more frequently than any other area by the general surgeon. As with any incision, a primary goal for abdominal incisions is to provide safe access to underlying structures. Abdominal incisions are classified into four groups: rectus, midline, oblique, and transverse (see Figure 8-1).

RECTUS INCISIONS

Made lateral to the midline, rectus incisions can extend from above the umbilicus to the pubis. Paramedian incisions are placed at the medial rectus border; pararectus incisions, at the lateral border; and transrectus incisions, through the muscle belly. Of the three types, the paramedian approach is preferable, because it avoids nerves entering the rectus along its lateral border. Midway between the umbilicus and the pubis at the semicircular line of

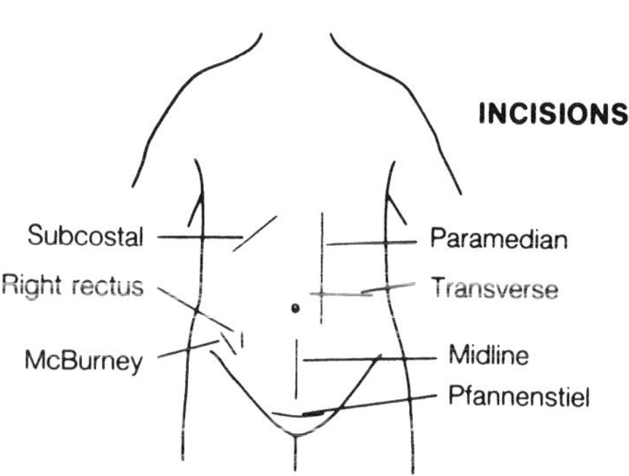

FIGURE 8-1
Incisions of the abdomen. *(Source: The Lippincott Manual of Nursing Practice, 5th Ed. Philadelphia: J.B. Lippincott, 1991.)*

Douglas, the inferior epigastric artery emerges from the peritoneal cavity. Incisions through this point or excessive traction on the muscle may damage the artery, necessitating ligation. Transrectus incisions are bloodier and should be avoided when possible. Advocates of paramedian incisions believe that they produce strong incisions and scars because the wound is closed in three layers. Studies of bursting strength comparing paramedian to midline incisions, however, seem to indicate that the midline approach is stronger.

STANDARD MIDLINE INCISIONS

The standard midline incision offers several advantages. It provides excellent access to all intraperitoneal structures. It is fast and requires less dissection. With one stroke of the scalpel blade above the midline, the surgeon can rapidly and safely open the abdominal cavity by incising skin, subcutaneous fat, linea alba, and peritoneum. By lifting the walls of the abdomen, the surgeon and the assistant can extend the incision quickly under direct vision. If further exposure is needed, the midline incision can be extended as a median sternotomy in the chest. Because the linea alba contains no blood vessels or nerves above the umbilicus, the midline incision is almost bloodless and does not injure nerves. Below the umbilicus, the linea alba is a fine line and may be difficult to locate. Postoperative incisional hernias are more common above the umbilicus than below it, because the single layer closure of the linea alba is weaker than the two-layer closure of the rectus sheath. The inexperienced surgeon has a tendency to bevel the edges of the incision around the umbilicus, which leads to ischemia of the skin. This, in turn, promotes wound infection and poor healing. By keeping the scalpel blade perpendicular to the skin at all times, this problem can be avoided.

OBLIQUE INCISIONS

The most common oblique incisions are the McBurney, the Kocher, and the lower oblique incisions.

McBurney Incision. This standard appendectomy incision is made at the junction of the middle and outer thirds and at right angles to an imaginary line drawn between the anterior superior iliac crest and the umbilicus in the right lower quadrant. The incision is usually 4 to 5 inches long and is made in the direction of the fibers of the external oblique muscle. Muscle layers are split in the direction of their fibers down to the peritoneum. Splitting rather than incising muscles causes less damage and reduces postoperative incisional weakness. Use of the McBurney incision is limited to patients with appendicitis. The mobility of the skin and subcutaneous tissues in the lower quadrant allows the surgeon to place the skin incision below the bikini line. By retracting skin cephalad, the muscles overlying the appendix can be split easily. When the appendix has perforated, it is best to approach it through a McBurney incision, because the incidence of wound infection doubles if a paramedian or midline incision is used.

Kocher Incision. The Kocher, or right subcostal, incision is used to approach the gallbladder. A similar incision can be made on the left side for splenectomy. A chevron incision—right and left subcostal incisions joined across the midline—provides excellent exposure to the stomach, duodenum, pancreas, and portal structures. Oblique incisions take longer because the rectus muscle must be transected. However, they provide much better exposure to structures under the diaphragm than do midline or paramedian incisions.

Lower Oblique Incision. Long, lower abdominal oblique incisions are used in transplant, urologic, and occasionally vascular surgery. These incisions require transection of the abdominal wall and flank musculature, which is best done with electrosurgery to minimize blood loss. Access to deep flank structures, including the aortic vessels, kidney, and retroperitoneal aorta, is facilitated using this approach. If needed, this incision can be extended into the chest to provide access to vessels at the hiatus of the diaphragm. The retroperitoneal approach to the abdominal aorta using this incision may result in fewer postoperative pulmonary problems.

TRANSVERSE INCISIONS

Like oblique incisions, transverse incisions follow Langer's lines of tension in the abdominal wall. Because they are made parallel to nerves and vessels, these structures are rarely injured. Vertical scars, such as those left by midline and paramedian incisions, stretch with time. Transverse scars usually heal with a more pleasing cosmetic result and are less conspicuous with time.

PFANNENSTIEL INCISIONS

Used most often in obstetric and gynecologic surgery, the Pfannenstiel incision combines midline and transverse incisions, offering some advantages of both approaches. The skin and soft tissues are incised transversely below the bikini line, but the compartment is entered by incising the midline fascia. The end result is a strong, deep wound with a cosmetically acceptable superficial closure.

SHARP DISSECTION

Surgical dissection is a complex skill that cannot be learned simply by study. The wide range of tissue composition in the human body requires a variable response in selecting the most appropriate dissection technique. Dissection technique must be suited to the character of the tissue.

DISSECTION WITH THE SCALPEL

Of the various scalpel blades available, the general purpose #10 and #20 blades are used most often for skin incisions. They are designed with a wide blade and a straight cutting surface. Long skin incisions, such as an abdominal midline, are best made with the scalpel held between the thumb and the first two fingers like a violin bow (Figure 8-2). This allows the balance point to pivot on the middle finger while lateral movement is controlled by the index finger and thumb. In this position, the arm moves as a unit from the shoulder; downward pressure is controlled by using the weight of the arm. Sometimes the index finger can be placed directly on the back of the handle. By applying pressure on the top of the handle with the index finger, the depth of the incision can be varied. The scalpel handle is forced against the thenar muscles; lateral and vertical movement is controlled by the wrist.

Fine scalpel dissection depends on control by finger movement. The scalpel is held like a pencil, with the heel of the hand resting firmly on adjacent tissue for stability. One single controlled incision through the skin and subcutaneous tissues is preferred to multiple hesitation cuts. A single, smooth incision with the blade held perpendicular to the skin prevents beveled skin edges and sharply transects blood vessels, which allows them to retract effectively. When speed is mandatory, as in a ruptured abdominal aortic aneurysm or a thoracotomy for cardiac compression, this technique permits rapid, controlled entry into a body cavity.

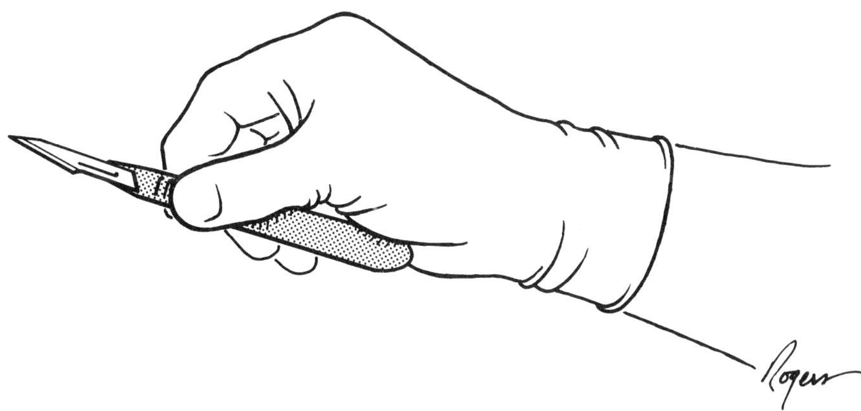

FIGURE 8-2
Long skin incisions, such as the abdominal midline incision, are best made with the scalpel held between the thumb and the first two fingers like a violin bow. Holding the scalpel in this position allows the balance point to pivot on the middle finger while lateral movement is controlled by the index finger and thumb.

For small incisions in the skin or fine structures, the #15 blade is more suitable. The smaller curve concentrates the short cutting surface at the tip of the scalpel blade. Holding the scalpel handle like a pencil, the surgeon has pinpoint control of the cutting surface.

The #11 blade has a sharp, tapered point, making it useful for puncturing rather than incising. It is used most often for puncturing an abscess or a vessel wall. The sharp point of this blade also makes it useful for excising small skin lesions where full-thickness removal is required.

Many other blades are available for use in specialty work. Each is designed for a specific purpose.

Assisting During Scalpel Dissection. In preparation for skin incision, the RN first assistant should stretch and fix the skin. Sponges are useful in aiding this maneuver on a moist skin surface. Once skin tension is achieved, it should not be relaxed unless the surgeon pauses in the stroke or lifts the scalpel. As the incision is started, steadily increasing traction helps open the developing incision. Any inadvertent tightening or relaxing while the scalpel is cutting may result in a misdirected or beveled incision. A beveled skin edge results in uneven closure of skin margins and the risk of necrosis. Additionally, uneven pulling as the incision is deepened causes each sweep of the scalpel to fall in a different line, resulting in a terraced effect and subsequent poor wound healing. A long incision may require two or more resettings of the RN first assistant's hand to improve skin fixation. While resetting, the RN first assistant must be attentive to the surgeon's movements to avoid inadvertent injury from the scalpel when reaching across its path.

SCISSORS DISSECTION

Scissors come in all shapes and sizes, varying by tip (blunt or sharp), blade (straight or curved), and length. The Metzenbaum and Mayo scissors are the most commonly used types. The workhorse of the general surgeon, the Metzenbaum scissors is used for most sharp dissection. The heavier Mayo scissors is most useful in cutting through large or thick structures that would dull the Metzenbaum scissors. Both of these scissors have slightly curved tips and blades, allowing versatility in the angle of approach and the ability to lift and palpate tissue. This is not as possible with straight-tipped scissors. Although sharp dissection with a scalpel blade is an art that can be learned, many surgeons feel more comfortable using good Metzenbaum scissors. Regardless of the instrument used, sharp dissection is preferable to blunt dissection in most situations.

Using A Scissors for Dissection. One of the first things the RN first assistant needs to learn about using scissors is the movement basic to all ringed instruments. By rotating the axis of the forearm, a full range of positions for the tips of the scissors is available. The RN first assistant's body should be turned to maintain the axial relationship between forearm and scissors. For good scissors control, the thumb and ring finger are placed through the rings, with the distal joints of the index and long fingers curling beneath the scissors' shank. This gives three points of fixation against the hand; the index and long fingers provide stability and control the direction of the tips. For extremely dense tissue, it may be necessary to extend the index finger along the shanks behind the scissors' fulcrum; the thumb comes through the ring to press down on one handle. With this grip, more downward pressure is exerted on the tips and blades while cutting.

The most natural and controlled cut is made away from oneself, from right to left. A left-to-right cut may necessitate cocking the wrist and rotating the body. Supination puts slightly more strain on fine hand control. Squeezing the scissors' blades together will enable a clean cut when the instrument is not sharp.

Accurate dissection requires exposure of the structure, good lighting, careful hemostasis, and two-point traction. One of these traction points is often a fixed feature of the anatomy, such as the adhesions between the gallbladder and liver bed. When the gallbladder is gently stretched, the liver bed becomes a fixed point. Stretching tissues allows a clean cut. The anatomy should be clearly exposed to allow dissection under clear vision, which will help prevent injury to adjacent structures. The curve of the scissors follows the curve of the structure under dissection. If the structure is curved, as in a cyst, a small tunnel is created to follow the natural shape. Dissection continues one layer at a time.

Blunt dissection with the Metzenbaum scissors is used to define a natural tissue plane. Pressure is applied to the scissors' rings to keep the cutting edges firmly apposed. Only a gentle spread is needed to open space for a subsequent cut. Any forceful stretching tears adjacent vessels and structures. When the scissors is withdrawn, it is turned 90 degrees and the lower blade is inserted. With the structure held taught to ensure a clean cut, the tip is inserted only to the level of dissection; then the cut is completed in a single smooth motion.

ACCESSORIES USED IN TISSUE HANDLING

The RN first assistant is required to anticipate each step of the surgical procedure, responding to each of the surgeon's moves with the appropriate follow-up move. As the pattern of the surgeon's approach is observed, the RN first assistant anticipates the next move. A flowing synergy develops as move and countermove are synchronized appropriately. This occurs when the RN first assistant knows how to provide good exposure, how to handle tissues, and how to efficiently achieve hemostasis. A number of accessory surgical items are available to the skillful first assistant.

RETRACTORS

Retraction should first and always be gentle to tissue. A retractor that exerts prolonged, excessive pressure destroys cells, injures small vessels, and damages nerves or other structures. A detailed discussion of retractors and retraction is presented in Chapter 9, Providing Exposure: Retractors and Retraction; the basic points are elucidated here. Retractors of all shapes and sizes are available for use in the operating room. Each has been designed for a specific purpose and obviously works best when used appropriately.

Deaver retractors are the most commonly used retractors in abdominal surgery. On this device, the handle is curved and constructed to be held with the hand under the handle, palm up. This keeps the tip of the retractor "toed-in" and lessens the need for strong pulling on the blade to provide retraction. The assistant should be familiar with the various types of specialty retractors. Retractors used in a typical bowel resection include "army-navy" or small Kelly-Richardson retractors to hold back wound edges during the fascial incision. This can also be done with sponges. Once the peritoneal cavity is entered, intestines can be held down in the wound either with retractors or sponges. During closure, a flat, broad plastic wound retractor shaped like a "flounder" holds the intestines out of the way.

Several devices that attach to the operating table are available. These have either separate, articulated metal arms or a large metal ring to hold retractors. The latter sometimes requires placement of opposing retractors to provide adequate exposure. The former, the "Iron intern,"™ pulls against itself and can be positioned without the need for opposing forces. These devices can obviate difficult, inadequate exposure and eliminate the need for extra help. Once in place, the instruments generally do not move, unlike human assistants. The surgeon and assistant can operate quickly without having to stop to readjust a retractor to regain exposure lost by a fatigued assistant.

SPONGES

Sponges are used (1) as padding to keep organs, usually intestine, out of the way, to protect solid organs, like the liver, from retractor injury; (2) to absorb blood, bile, and other sera that collect in the wound; and (3) as packs to provide hemostasis. Sponges should be placed, not shoved, into the wound to provide adequate retraction. The organs to be retracted are held back with the spread fingers of one hand. The opened sponge is placed over the hand with the operator's second hand or long forceps. The deep edge of the sponge is curled under the organs to be retracted at the level of the retroperitoneum. The upper edge of the sponge is tucked under the incision, between the organs and the anterior abdominal wall. Sponges placed in this way will maintain good exposure without the need for back-breaking retracting by the assistant.

Bleeding from individual vessels or rapid, exsanguinating bleeding is best controlled by ligation. Oozing, especially in localized spaces in the retroperitoneum, can be stopped by packing moistened sponges into the area. Using dry sponges increases the risk that the adherent sponge surface will pull away freshly formed clots. The sponges should be left undisturbed for 5 to 10 minutes to allow blood in vessels to clot. Direct pressure over small areas, such as needle holes in vessels, is applied more effectively with the gloved finger without any intervening sponge. When the finger or sponge packing is withdrawn, the RN first assistant should be prepared to control any renewed bleeding.

During a skin incision, the assistant may place a moistened sponge against the opened ends of transected or bleeding vessels. Small clots will usually form in the ends of small vessels after 15–20 seconds of digital pressure. When the sponge is withdrawn, it must be done so as not to dislodge the fresh clot.

In a deep incision or recess, a "sponge on a stick" (a sponge grasped in a packing forceps or similar instrument) may be required to reach the vessel to apply pressure until the surgeon is ready to clamp and ligate it. The RN first assistant holds this "stick sponge" in position until the clamp is in the surgeon's hand. If necessary, the area should be cleared away by suction. When the field is clear and the surgeon ready, the stick sponge is slowly rolled off the vessel to expose it for clamping.

The RN first assistant may also need to remove clotted blood from a wound with a sponge. The sponge should be pressed firmly against the clot with a slight grasping or pinching movement of the fingers. The clot is then lifted away in one single motion. Heavy rubbing movements are avoided. If rebleeding occurs, or when blood is still liquid, the sponge should be used in a gentle blotting action.

A surgical procedure can be made technically easy or difficult on the basis of the incision made and retraction obtained. All too frequently, a surgeon tries to perform an operation through a poorly placed incision rather than extend it or close it and make another incision. Forceful retraction of an inadequate incision can be dangerous. The direction and force of retraction by an assistant must be controlled by the surgeon. Care must be exercised to gain exposure without causing injury. During operations on extremities, a retractor may compress nerve against bone, causing serious injury. In the abdomen, improper retraction can tear the liver or spleen and avulse mesenteric vessels. Injury can be minimized by padding the retractor with a moistened, folded sponge. Sponges used to protect solid organs from retractor injury should be moistened and folded to double or triple thickness, then placed between the retractor blade and the organ. Improper retraction during abdominal operations can inadvertently compress the vena cava, diminishing venous return to the heart and decreasing cardiac output. In a fragile and marginally compensated patient, this could be harmful.

When the bowel must be displaced from the abdominal cavity during a procedure, the intestines must be protected. They may be wrapped with a sponge moistened in physiologic saline solution, but a specially designed plastic intestinal bag is an easier and more desirable means of protection. The bag keeps the intestines together and out of the way while maintaining a humid atmosphere to prevent drying and injury to the serosal surfaces of the bowel. Bowel displaced in this way hangs over the end of the incision and is suspended by its mesentery. This impedes venous return and, if prolonged, may result in injury to the intestinal vascular supply. Frequent observation of the bowel and periodic temporary return of the bowel to the abdominal cavity will help prevent this problem.

ELECTROSURGERY

Used properly, electrosurgery diminishes blood loss and decreases operating time. Dessication of large areas of tissue causes excessive damage and increases wound infection rates. Extensive tissue "frying" with the coagulation current set at maximum is unnecessary. Precise visualization, clamping, and electrosurgical coagulation of individual vessels is preferable. For pinpoint coagulation, short applications of high energy can be used. When blood loss must be kept at a minimum, subcutaneous tissue, fascia, muscle, and viscera can be incised with electrosurgery. Chapter 13, Providing Hemostasis, presents a detailed discussion of using electrosurgery to achieve hemostasis.

WOUND CLOSURE

The goal of wound closure is to provide a secure, strong wound that will heal normally without infection or dehiscence and will form a cosmetically and functionally acceptable scar. Adequate preparation of the patient and surgeon to eliminate skin bacteria will reduce the incidence of wound infection. Good surgical technique is of paramount importance. A minor break, such as a torn glove, changes a clean case to a clean/contaminated case, doubling the risk of wound infection. Choice of the appropriate incision enhances wound healing. A midline incision can withstand three times the force capable of disrupting a paramedian incision. Mass closure of a midline incision has twice the bursting strength of a transverse incision or a linea alba closure.

The techniques used to close a wound depend in part on the type of wound. Most clean incisions and lacerations can be closed primarily; that is, all tissue layers are closed at the time of operation. The wound surface is quickly sealed with a coagulum that is resistant to bacterial penetration. If an abscess has been drained or if the wound is contaminated, the skin should be left open. By delaying closure for about 4 days, the wound is given enough time to develop resistance to infection.

The choice of materials for closing wounds is great and at times may be confusing. Should the RN first assistant staple, or sew, or tape, or glue? When the RN first assistant sews, which suture should be used? Nonabsorbable? 2-0? 4-0? Chapter 10, Suturing Materials and Techniques, provides an in-depth discussion of sutures; here, we discuss only the two major classes: absorbable and nonabsorbable.

ABSORBABLE SUTURES

Absorbable sutures are natural or synthetic products that lose tensile strength in tissues within 60 days. The most traditional absorbable suture, catgut, is made from sheep submucosa. It may be treated with chromium salts to increase tensile strength and to diminish breakdown by collagenolysis. Catgut sutures are degraded by proteolytic enzymes and lose strength rapidly. Wet catgut may lose up to 30% of its strength after 2 hours. Compared to nonabsorbable sutures, it has less knot security, less tensile strength, and less strength retention.

Synthetic absorbable sutures are available; these include polyglycolic acid (Dexon), polydioxanone (PDS), polyglyconate (Maxon), and polyglactin 910 (Vicryl). Synthetic absorbable sutures are degraded by hydrolytic enzymes, producing only mild tissue reaction during absorption. Their tensile strength is retained for varying amounts of time.

NONABSORBABLE SUTURES

Nonabsorbable sutures are either natural (silk, cotton) or synthetic (nylon, dacron, polypropylene [Prolene], wire). As a group, they are characterized by longer retention of tensile strength. Silk rapidly loses it strength after 60 days; the synthetics last longer and are not as irritating to tissue. Nylon loses only 16% of its tensile strength after 70 days, and polypropylene keeps its tensile strength for up to 2 years. Degradation products of both sutures may have some antibacterial properties. Nonabsorbable sutures may be monofilament or braided. Monofilament sutures are harder to handle and to tie. Braided sutures are more irritating to tissue and may trap bacteria, potentiating wound infection.

Clips, staples, tapes, and glue all can be used to close wounds. In the past, metal clips were commonly used to close head and neck incisions. They have the disadvantages of being less elastic and weaker than sutures. Instead of clips, most surgeons now use staples, which can be applied quickly, decreasing operating time. Most disposable appliers are designed to evert and appose skin edges automatically. A variety of stapling devices is available for gastrointestinal resection and anastomosis. Very adherent tapes can be used to close small wounds, particularly of the hands and face. Because they leave no needle tracks or staple puncture wounds, tape closures are the most resistant of all to infection, but most prone to wound disruption. Cyanoacrylate glues have a limited role in clinical surgery because of their carcinogenic potential.

Selection of closure materials should be based on the state of the wound, the healing characteristics of the tissue being closed, the patient's condition, and properties of the closure material. The effects of both local and systemic factors on wound healing and the principle of delayed closure must be considered. In infected or contaminated wounds, the less suture the better. Absorbable sutures dissolve rapidly in infected wounds and should not be used. Monofilament nylon and polypropylene are the best sutures for closing contaminated wounds. Fascia and skin take longer to heal than visceral tissues; for this reason, the sutures of choice for fascial and skin closure are those that maintain their tensile strength. To avoid scarring from suture tracts, skin stitches and staples should be removed within 3 to 5 days. Because the skin wound strength is only 5 to 10% of normal at this time, the fascial and subcutaneous closures must be strong enough to support the wound. Alternatively, skin may be closed with a subcuticular absorbable suture or a pullout, nonabsorbable suture and reinforced with skin tapes.

The most common cause of wound dehiscence is faulty technique. Fascia should be closed with a nonabsorbable suture of appropriate gauge, such as a 0 or 1 nylon, placing each stitch 1.0 cm to 1.5 cm back from the wound edge and 1.0 cm apart. Knots tied too tightly do not allow for the normal 30% postoperative wound expansion, leading to tissue ischemia, suture pull-through, and dehiscence. Including muscle along with fascia in each stitch makes the wound stronger than does closing fascia only. A continuous or running suture closure is as good as interrupted closure and has the advantage of being faster. Too fine a suture (*e.g.*, 4-0 instead of 0 nylon) may not be strong enough to support an abdominal wound. Damaged suture—either frayed nylon or polypropylene that has been fractured by grasping with needle holders—can break, leading to wound disruption. Monofilament sutures of nylon and polypropylene must be tied with multiple knots to prevent slippage.

Incisions in the biliary and genitourinary tracts should be closed with absorbable sutures. Nonabsorbable sutures in the common bile duct or the bladder can be a nidus for stone formation. Bowel anastomoses can be performed "by hand" with one- or two-layer closures using absorbable sutures such as catgut in the mucosal layer and nonabsorbable silk in the outer layer, or with staplers. The end-to-end stapler offers tremendous advantages over a hand anastomosis in the distal sigmoid colon and rectum, allowing the surgeon to save the anus when resecting low-lying tumors. Although the stapled anastomosis is probably no better or worse than a sewn anastomosis, it can be done faster.

The suture of choice in vascular surgery is polypropylene because of its lasting power, smoothness, strength, and especially its memory. Each stitch can be placed under direct vision in small, recessed vessels by leaving big loops of suture. On completion of the anastomosis, the entire suture can be pulled up and tied.

DRAINS

Drains are never a substitute for hemostasis or a replacement for meticulous technique. The drain material should be soft, nonirritating to tissue, firm enough to remain in the intended place, resistant to decomposing, and smooth for easy removal. Careful choice, placement, and care of drains is needed. Superficial wounds ordinarily do not need to be drained. In fact, the drain may provide a route for bacteria to gain access to the subcutaneous tissues. Subcutaneous tissues are particularly vulnerable to infection because fat is relatively avascular. If a drain is needed, one that can be attached to a source of suction in a closed system is preferred to one that drains passively.

Drains within the abdominal cavity are placed either for localized infection, such as an abscess cavity, or to drain raw surfaces that may slowly bleed or leak other types of fluid. Placing multiple drains throughout the abdominal cavity in an attempt to drain generalized peritonitis has been proved to be of little value. The drains quickly become isolated from the peritoneal cavity by the bowel and omentum and thus fail to achieve their goal.

When the RN first assistant is placing a drain, the shortest, most direct route to the skin is selected. The stab wound should be just large enough for unobstructed passage of the drain. Placing the stab wound separate from the main incision prevents its potential contamination. The drain is sutured to the skin at the egress site. When the drain is dressed, gauze is first applied, then the drain is taped in such a way that the tape can be removed without pulling the drain.

DRESSINGS

Surgical wounds may be broadly classified as nondraining and draining. The nondraining wound includes most approximated surgical incision sites. For this type of wound, the RN first assistant should select a dressing that provides an optimal environment for epithelial migration at the wound edges and minimizes the likelihood of wound disruption. Draining wounds, where heavy serosanguineous or enzymatic drainage is present, require a dressing that minimizes tissue maceration.

The primary function of a surgical dressing is to protect the wound surface from exogenous contamination before reepithelialization occurs. Occlusive dressings, traditionally consisting of gauze dressings held in place with tape, are more commonly achieved today by application of a transparent, semipermeable film. More appropriately termed "semiocclusive," this film is waterproof yet allows the skin to "breathe" because the film is permeable to water vapor. With this type of dressing, the RN first assistant can inspect the wound without dressing removal. The film prevents wound dehydration; a "moist" rather than dry environment is more conducive to reepithelialization. Before a semipermeable film dressing is applied, the wound and surrounding skin should be as clean as possible. This may be done by first swabbing the wound, then using a fresh swab with an iodophor for the surrounding area. A 70% alcohol swab can be used to remove excess iodophor solution. When the surface is dry, the dressing is applied. These dressings are intended for long-term application. However, excessive or prolonged accumulation of serum beneath the dressing surface must be avoided. This dressing is not recommended for infected wounds. The moist physiological environment, usually desirable for epidermal regeneration, would provide a growth medium for pathogens in an infected wound.

Highly absorbent, nonocclusive dressings are also used for nondraining wounds. After the wound is cleansed, a nonadhering dressing is applied. If light to medium drainage is anticipated, an impregnated gauze dressing is placed first, followed by general use dressing sponges.

Draining wounds require a dressing that will keep wound exudate from healthy skin. A nonadherent dressing is applied directly to the skin in a single layer, followed by a layer of general use dressing sponges to wick exudate. This may be covered with a secondary layer of dressings, added to absorb and contain drainage.

TRAUMATIC WOUNDS

The RN first assistant who works in collaboration with a physician or group practice may be called to assist with injured patients. Before closing any traumatic wound in an emergency department, several questions must be answered. How long has it been since the time of injury? What was the nature of the wounding implement? Where is the wound located? What is the patient's overall condition? The longer the time between injury and wound closure, the greater the likelihood of bacterial infection. For most clean wounds, primary closure can be done safely 6 to 8 hours after injury. This safe period can be extended several hours by using debridement and prophylactic antibiotics in some wounds. Unfortunately, there are no absolutes in dealing with the safety of wound closure, because the development of wound infection depends more on the total wound bacteria count than on time. Whenever there is any doubt about the safety of primary closure, the wound should be left open to heal by secondary intention.

Scalpel blades produce clean lacerations that can be closed primarily. Blunt trauma, such as that which occurs when the head strikes a dashboard, produces stellate laceration. This type of compression injury breaks the skin open and disrupts surrounding tissues, making them ischemic. Devitalized tissue provides an anaerobic culture medium that inhibits phagocytosis, thereby enhancing bacterial growth. Wounds contaminated with feces, saliva, soil, or clothing particles are more susceptible to infection. Before closing crush wounds or contaminated wounds, all dead tissue must be debrided and all foreign matter removed.

Mechanical cleansing of contaminated wounds can decrease the incidence of infection. Simple flooding of the wound with saline or antibiotic-containing solutions is inadequate. Vigorous scrubbing of the wound with a surgical brush may lead to further damage. High-pressure irrigation that mechanically disrupts bacteria from the tissue surface can decrease bacterial wound counts to safe levels. The pressure exerted by saline squirted from a 35 ml syringe through an 18-gauge needle is sufficient to clean most small wounds. Extensive wound irrigation is more easily accomplished with a pulsating device, such as a Water-Pik. It is not necessary—and in fact may be harmful—to add an antibiotic agent to the cleansing solution. High concentrations of povidone iodine solutions kill human cells as well as bacterial cells. Neomycin, kanamycin, and similar antibiotics can be absorbed in large amounts from the wound, leading to renal and auditory impairment and respiratory depression. A nontoxic surfactant, such as Pluronic F-68, can help loosen bacteria from wound surfaces.

CONCLUSION

The role of the RN first assistant can have a major effect on the outcome of the surgical procedure. By understanding essential principles, the RN first assistant can be of immeasurable help in promoting a favorable result. Wound management, although the direct responsibility of the operating surgeon, is enhanced by the collaboration of a knowledgeable RN first assistant. The collegial relationship between surgeon and assistant is initiated based on shared knowledge and complementary skills. As these are elucidated in patient care activities, mutuality and respect develop. Understanding the rationale for a particular surgical approach, implementing principles of tissue handling, and participating in the selection of a skin closure material are all characteristic activities of an RN first assistant whose contribution to patient care is marked by excellence.

REVIEW QUESTIONS

1. Halsted developed an approach to tissue handling that suggests which of the following (circle all that are correct)?
   a. Sharp dissection is preferred over blunt dissection.
   b. The fewer sutures left in a wound, the more chance for wound disruption.
   c. Small vessels will clot with direct pressure.
   d. The hemostat should clamp the vessel and an adequate margin of surrounding tissue.
   e. Dead space invites infection.
2. In the inflammatory phase of wound healing, the vascular response is
   a. vasoconstriction
   b. vessel retraction
   c. vasospasm
   d. vasodilation
3. During a preoperative nutritional assessment, the RN first assistant will assess the patient's dietary intake of which important nutrient for wound healing?
   a. vitamin K
   b. vitamin E
   c. vitamin C
   d. fiber

Fill in the blanks in the following questions regarding surgical technique.

4. The height of the operating room table should reach the level of the RN first assistant's _______.
5. The desired position of the wrist of an assistant is slight _______.

6. If the operating room table is too high, the extensors are _______ and the flexors are _______, which reduces small muscle control and increases fatigue.
7. In general, lights positioned behind the surgeon or assistant _______ optimum illumination.
8. Lateral and vertical movement of the scalpel is controlled by the _______.
9. To prevent beveled edges, the scalpel blade should be held _______ to the skin.
10. In preparation for the skin incision, the RN first assistant should _______ and _______ the skin.
11. As the skin incision is started, the RN first assistant can _______ traction to assist in opening the developing incision.
12. During scissors dissection, the most natural and controlled cut is achieved when it is made _______ from oneself.
13. Holding a Deaver retractor with the hand under the handle, palm up, keeps the tip of the retractor _______, lessening the need for strong pulling.
14. To remove clotted blood from a wound with a sponge, the RN first assistant presses firmly against the clot with a slight grasping or pinching motion and _______ the clot away.
15. Placing a stab wound for drain insertion should be done _______ from the main incision.
16. _______ dressings are waterproof yet allow the skin to "breathe."
17. Mechanical cleansing of contaminated wounds can _______ the incidence of infection.

Answer the following questions about surgical incisions.

18. The _______ approach is preferable among the pararectus, paramedian, and transrectus, since it avoids nerves entering the rectus along its lateral border.
19. _______ rather than incising muscles causes less damage and reduces postoperative incisional weakness.
20. Following _______ in the abdominal wall assists in preventing injury to the vessels and nerves that run parallel to them.

Answers

1. a,c,e
2. d
3. c
4. elbows
5. extension
6. elongated, shortened
7. interfere with
8. wrist
9. perpendicular
10. stretch, fix
11. increase
12. away
13. toed-in
14. lifts
15. separate

16. semipermeable or semiocclusive
17. decrease
18. paramedian
19. splitting
20. Langer's lines

BIBLIOGRAPHY

Coit DG: Care of the Surgical Wound. *In* Care of The Surgical Patient. New York, Scientific American Medicine, 9-1–9-8, 1992

Davis JH, Foster RS, Gamelli RL: Essentials of Clinical Surgery. St. Louis, Mosby-Year Book, 1991

Edgerton MT: The Art of Surgical Technique. Baltimore, Williams & Wilkins, 1988

Rothrock JC: The RN First Assistant and Care Planning. *In* Perioperative Nursing Care Planning. St. Louis, Mosby-Year Book, pp 506–522, 1990

Vaiden RE, Fox VJ, Rothrock JC: Core Curriculum for the RN First Assistant. Denver, Association of Operating Room Nurses, 1990

Wind GG, Rich NM: Principles of Surgical Technique: The Art of Surgery. Baltimore, Urban & Schwarzenberg, 1987

9 Providing Exposure: Retractors and Retraction

Nancy B. Davis

The Association of Operating Room Nurses' (AORN's) Official Statement on RN First Assistant states that "the RN first assistant to the surgeon during a surgical procedure carries out functions that will assist the surgeon in performing a safe operation with optimal results for the patient."[1] A major function of the RN first assistant is to provide exposure of the operative site.

Exposure is necessary for the surgeon to visualize the tissues that are to be dissected or sutured. Retraction may also be needed to prevent injury of tissues in the operative area. Providing physical safety for the patient during the intraoperative period is essential and must involve all members of the surgical team.

NURSING DIAGNOSIS: PREVENTING INJURY

A judgment made by the nurse related to the patient's problems, potential problems, needs, or health status is stated as a nursing diagnosis. When the RN first assistant determines that retraction will be necessary during the operative procedure, the nursing diagnosis could be stated as "High Risk for Injury (trauma) related to retraction of tissues during the operative procedure." A high risk for injury exists when the patient is at risk for harm because of a perceptual or physiologic deficit, lack of awareness, or maturational age.[2] The risk factor in this nursing diagnosis is situational. The surgery, and its required tissue manipulation, presents an environmental hazard for which nursing intervention is required. In planning and implementing intraoperative care for this patient, the RN first assistant's goal would be to prevent this type of injury. For goal achievement, the RN first assistant must implement appropriate first assistant measures to protect the patient from the known, possible injuries. This goal would relate to Standard IV of AORN's Patient Outcome Standards for Perioperative Nursing, which states that "the patient is free from injury related to positioning, extraneous objects, or chemical, physical, and electrical hazards."[3]

STANDARDS OF CARE

For perioperative patients, there are a number of predicted care regimens indicated in specific situations. When this nursing situation occurs, *standards of care* can be developed that contain detailed guidelines representing the predicted care required. The RN first assistant can participate in developing a set of problems, either actual or high risk, that typically occur during the intraoperative phase of first assisting. The associated standards represent the level of care the RN first assistant is responsible for providing. When they are designed to represent the predicted generic care for all intraoperative patients who receive care from an RN first assistant, the standards can become the perioperative nursing unit's standards of care. Because they apply to all patients receiving care from an RN first assistant during the intraoperative period, they do not need to be written on each patient's care plan. Instead, institutional policy can specify that the generic standard will be implemented for all perioperative patients. The prevention of injury during tissue retraction and the other potential injurious perioperative patient care situations requiring nursing intervention by the RN first assistant should be part of the generic standard of care.

Providing exposure of the operative site is usually the first function that the RN first assistant performs. An experienced assistant makes this activity appear easy. The necessary skill and judgment needed for providing exposure are based on knowledge. The assistant must be knowledgeable regarding the operative procedure and the potential injury to tissues. Proper selection and performance of exposure methods is essential. As the assistant becomes more skilled at providing exposure, the surgeon will provide less direction to the assistant. Protecting the patient from injury becomes the standard of care and part of the quality improvement program.

METHODS OF PROVIDING EXPOSURE

The most common method of providing exposure is by using retraction instruments. Other methods include using grasping instruments, sponges, sutures, tapes, Penrose drains, vessel loops, suctioning, the assistant's hands, or plastic bags.

When choosing the method of providing exposure, the RN first assistant must consider several factors. The major considerations are the operative procedure and the stage of the operation. Physical characteristics of the patient that are considered include the patient's age, height, weight, body build, and any physical deformities or limitations. Also, the type of tissue and the location of vascular or nerve structures, as well as the presence of organs, must always be evaluated in relation to the exposure method used.

Traction of tissues is the mechanism that provides exposure. If traction is inadequate, then the operative site will be poorly exposed, which will impede the surgeon. Excessive traction could result in injury related to lacerations or pressure. The assistant must observe the operative site at all times to ensure effective exposure and prevent unnecessary tissue injury. Knowledge of how to provide the correct amount of traction is acquired through an understanding of surgical anatomy and an appreciation of the fragility of tissue structures.

RETRACTORS

Retractors are instruments designed specifically for holding tissues or organs out of the surgeon's field of vision during the operative procedure. Many retractors are intended for use only on selected operative procedures; other retractors are more versatile and can be used for many different procedures.

Selection of a retractor is based on several factors, including:

the operative procedure
the stage of the operative procedure
the tissues or organs being retracted
the complexity of the operative procedure
the length and depth of the wound
the time necessary to perform the operation
the amount of force (effort) needed to provide exposure.

Retractors are of two basic types: hand-held and self-retaining. Retractors come in several designs and may be sharp or blunt; large or small; flat, round, or curved; wide or narrow; short or long; malleable, hinged, or fixed; straight or angled; and composed of one solid piece or several parts. The assistant must know the types of retractors available, the name of each retractor, and how to use each retractor.

Hand-Held Retractors. As the name implies, hand-held retractors are held continuously by the assistant during use. This is the major disadvantage of this type of retractor, because the assistant's hand or hands are not available to provide other assistance during the operation. In certain operations this may not be a problem, because the surgeon may need a minimal amount of assistance during the procedure. But in more complex operations, if the assistant is holding a retractor, more than one assistant may be needed for safe and efficient execution of the surgical intervention.

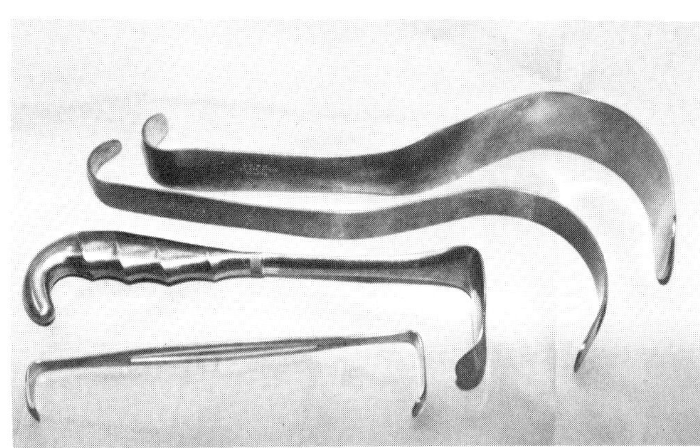

FIGURE 9-1
Examples of hand-held retractors *(Top to bottom)* Two Deavers, Richardson, and Army-Navy.

Nevertheless, the hand-held retractor has several advantages. It can be more quickly positioned, repositioned, and removed. It allows the alert RN first assistant to instinctively vary retractor position to provide more exposure or to let up on the pressure when the harder pull is no longer necessary. The amount of traction placed on the tissues can be altered as necessary, which allows the tissue beneath the retractor to get oxygen and nutrients to its capillary network. For very fragile tissue, the hand-held retractor may be essential to prevent injury. If the accessibility of the tissue needing retracting is difficult, a hand-held retractor may be the retractor of choice.

Hand-held retractors may be designed with or without handles. The handle is designed to provide the assistant with a firmer grip, but many are not designed for comfort. The handle may be round or flat and may have finger notches, rings, or curves (see Figure 9-1). A flat handle is hard to hold for long periods. Retractors without handles usually have straight shafts that may have a different retracting surface at each end (see Figure 9-2). Malleable retractors (ribbons) are flexible and may be bent into various angles. They are available in different lengths and widths (see Figure 9-3). These are versatile retractors;

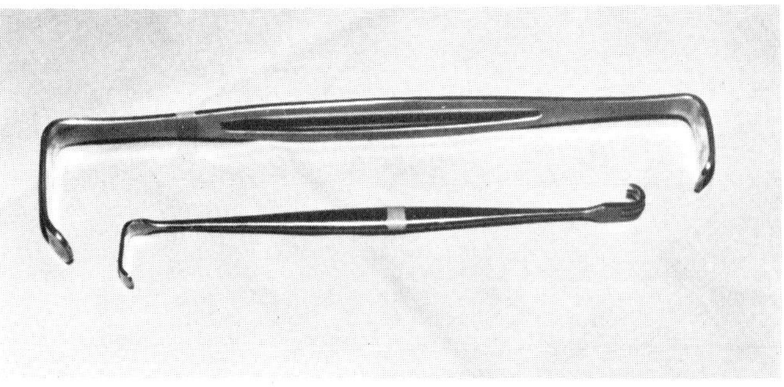

FIGURE 9-2
Hand-held retractors with different retracting surfaces at each end. *(Top)* Army–Navy. *(Bottom)* Senn.

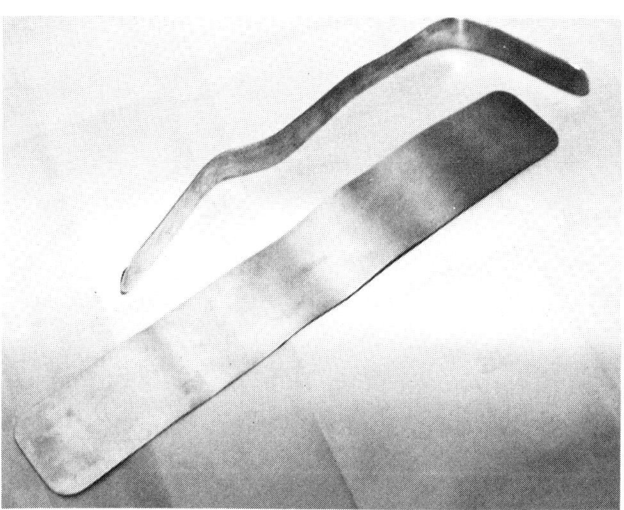

FIGURE 9-3
Malleable retractors. Note bend in narrow retractor.

in addition to retracting where a unique angle is needed, they can help hold in and protect the viscera during abdominal closure.

Retractors designed with prongs are usually used for retraction of shallow tissues, such as the skin or subcutaneous tissue. The prongs may be sharp or dull, and there may be one prong or several (see Figure 9-4). Sharp prongs cause more tissue trauma, but hold better. The assistant must be careful when using the sharp-pronged retractor, as it can easily puncture gloves or tissues, such as the bowel or blood vessels. For this reason, blunt prongs are preferred whenever possible.

When placing the retractor, the assistant must take care not to injure nerves, organs, or vascular structures. Circulation to the tissues should not be compromised. Pinching of tissues or organs can occur if the retractor is placed improperly. Underlying structures should be protected from excessive pressure or tension that could result in tissue damage.

The assistant should hold the retractor in a position that causes the least amount of discomfort, strain, or fatigue. If the assistant is retracting laterally or away from himself/herself, the retractor should rest comfortably in the hand with the palm supine and the arm flexed at the elbow (see Figure 9-5). When retracting toward himself/herself, the assistant is more comfortable holding the retractor with the palm in the prone position or toward himself/herself (see Figure 9-6). The retractor should not be gripped any harder than necessary, because this only increases hand fatigue. It is important that the assistant not lean or rest the arm on the patient, as this could cause pressure injury to soft tissues or even interfere with respirations and circulation. The assistant's hand should not obstruct the surgeon's view.

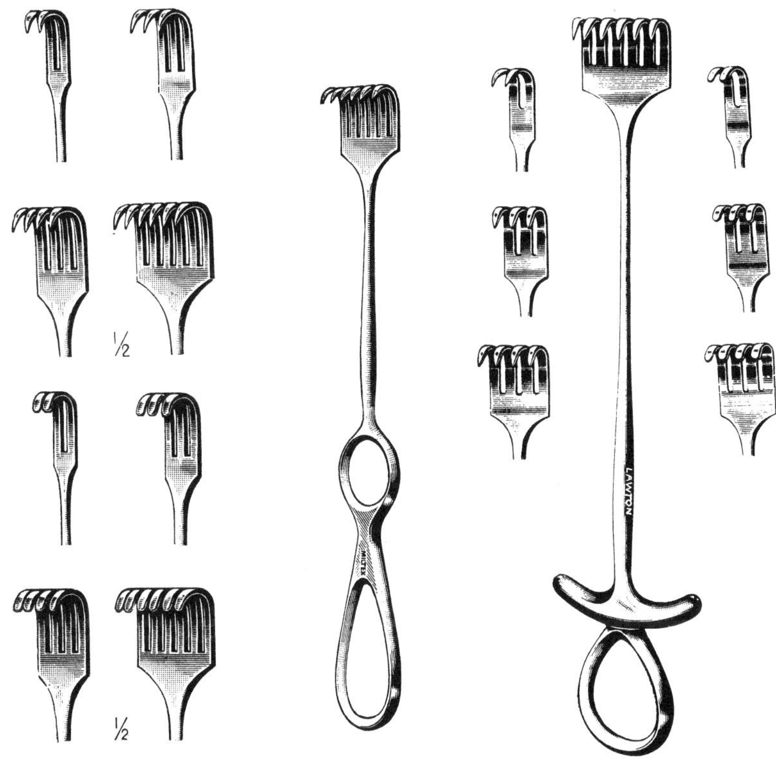

FIGURE 9-4
Rake retractors *(Left)* Volkman retractor. *(Right)* Murphy retractor. *(From Smith EJ, Smith YR: Smiths' Reference and Illustrated Guide to Surgical Instruments, pp 633, 646. Philadelphia, JB Lippincott, 1983)*

The pull on the retractor should provide adequate exposure of the operative field without distorting tissues that are being dissected or sutured by the surgeon. Excessive pulling on the retractor could result in tissue laceration or slipping of the retractor from the incision. Inadequate pulling results in poor exposure and may allow retracted tissues to slip into the field and obstruct the surgeon's visualization. The assistant must observe the effect of the retraction and alert the surgeon if the retractor or tissues are slipping so that the retractor may be readjusted. The assistant tires with long or difficult retracting, and must advise the surgeon when this is occurring.

Self-Retaining Retractors. The self-retaining retractor is designed to provide continuous and unchanging retraction of tissues. Once placed, this retractor does not need to be held, thereby freeing the assistant's hands for other activities. Various self-retaining retractors are available, and the assistant needs to be

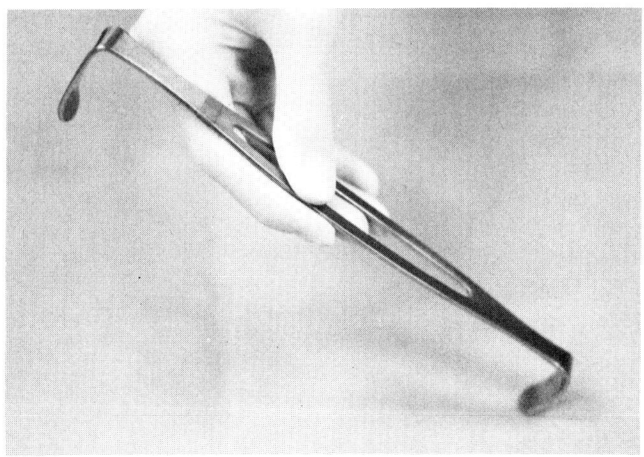

FIGURE 9-5
Position for holding retractor when retracting laterally or away from self.

familiar with the commonly used ones. Some retractors are versatile; others are designed for a specific operative procedure. Self-retaining retractors are especially useful during long operations and are essential when much effort is needed to provide retraction (*e.g.*, during thoracotomy).

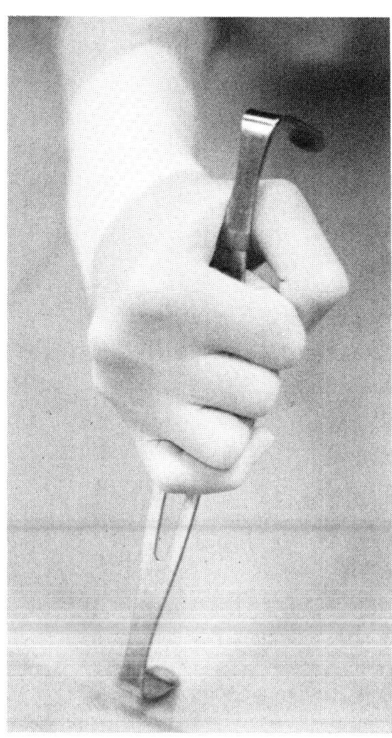

FIGURE 9-6
Position for holding retractor when retracting toward self.

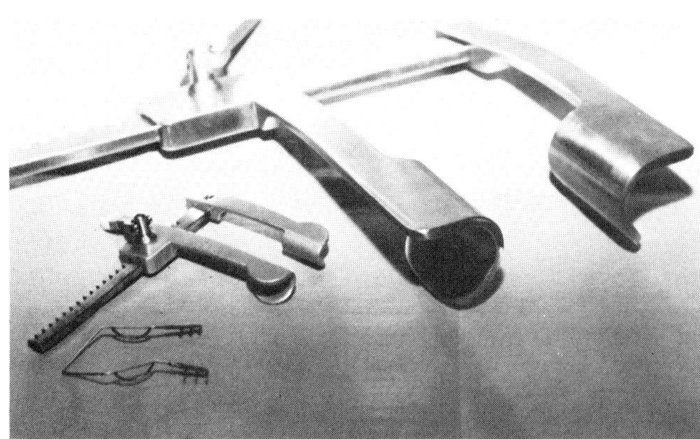

FIGURE 9-7
Examples of self-retaining retractors. *(Left to right)* Parsonnet epicardial retractor, pediatric Cooley sternal retractor, and adult Cooley sternal retractor.

Self-retaining retractors are more complex than hand-held retractors. Such a retractor may be designed as a frame with fixed blades or prongs (see Figure 9-7), or the retracting surfaces may be detachable, with several variations available (see Figure 9-8). The retracting blades or prongs may vary in width, depth, and angulation. The mechanical components of the retractor may include ratchets, springs, cranks, or nuts that open the retractor and hold it in the open position. Any removable parts must be accounted for and included in the formal instrument count.

Good visualization is necessary when placing the retractor. Care must be taken not to injure nerves, vascular structures, organs, or tissues by accidentally pinching them in or under the retracting surfaces or mechanisms. It is often necessary to protect the wound edges from the retractor blades by padding with a sponge. Moistening the sponge can prevent drying of the tissues. The RN first assistant should keep in mind that the greater the exposure and the longer the procedure, the more fluid loss and tissue dessication occur. The need to use moist pads is determined by these factors.

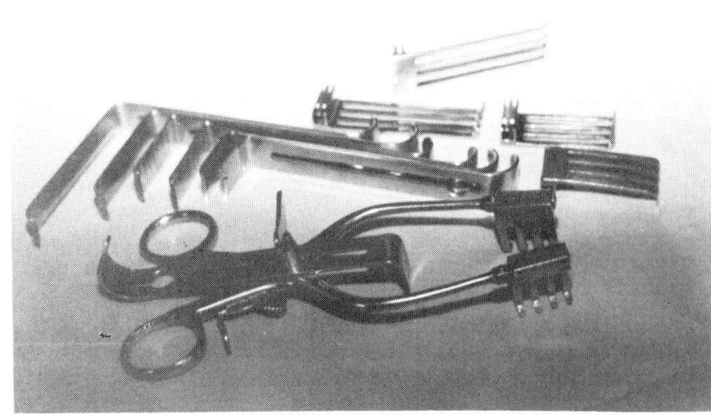

FIGURE 9-8
Henly retractor with various blades for altering depth of retraction.

The retractor should be opened carefully and under direct visualization. It may be necessary to hold the wound edges in the retractor blades while opening the retractor to prevent slipping. With self-retaining abdominal wall retractors, the RN first assistant should keep a hand over each blade to avoid trapping viscera between the blade and the abdominal wall as the retractor is being opened. In operative procedures where retraction requires increased force, the retractor should be opened slowly and possibly in stages. The retractor should not be overexpanded, which will cause excessive pulling on tissues and, possibly, tearing lacerations. For extremely lengthy operations, the self-retaining retractor should be removed periodically to prevent ischemic injury to the wound edges.

GRASPING INSTRUMENTS

Several instruments may be used to provide a secure hold on tissues so that traction can be applied, thereby providing exposure. Grasping instruments will cause varying degrees of tissue damage, depending on the type of tissue grasped, the instrument being used, how the instrument is applied to the tissue, and the amount of traction exerted on the tissue. Judgments made by the assistant when using grasping instruments are based on knowledge and experience.

Tissue Forceps. *Tissue forceps* are instruments that provide an extension of the thumb and fingers for pinching-like action. Forceps are some of the most commonly used surgical instruments, and the assistant must be skilled in using them with either hand. They are quick and easy to use once the skill has been acquired.

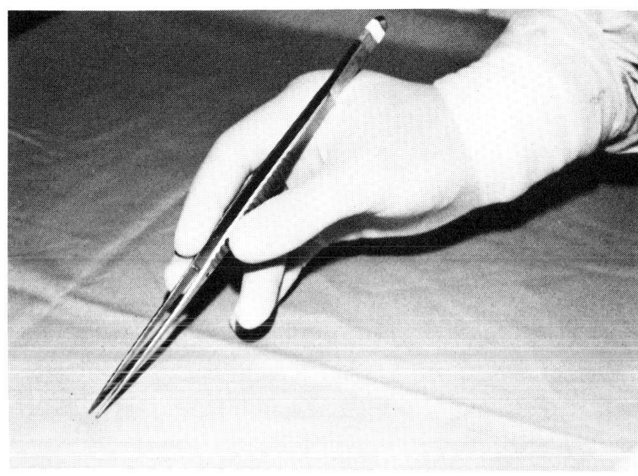

FIGURE 9-9
Position for holding tissue forceps (opened).

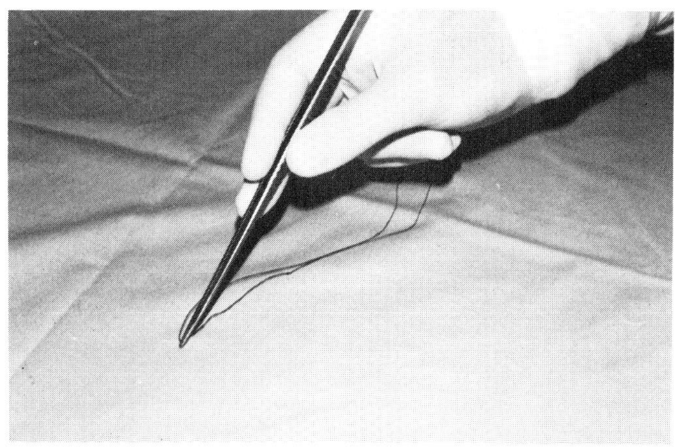

FIGURE 9-10
Tissue forceps closed, grasping suture ligature.

The forceps is held like a pencil (see Figure 9-9), and the tips are forced together by applying pressure with the thumb and fingers (see Figure 9-10). Grasping pressure must be sufficient to provide a secure hold with minimal damage to the tissues. With tissue forceps, pressure can be altered easily and with more precision than with a clamping type of instrument.

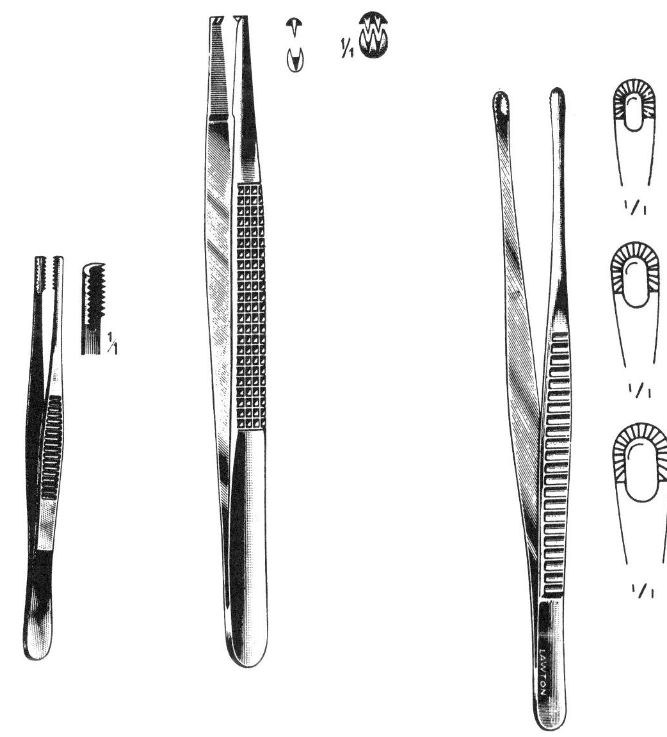

FIGURE 9-11
Examples of toothed tissue forceps. *(Left)* Brown, *(center)* Bonney, *(right)* Russian. *(From Smith EJ, Smith YR: Smiths' Reference and Illustrated Guide to Surgical Instruments, pp 183, 188, 350. Philadelphia, JB Lippincott, 1983)*

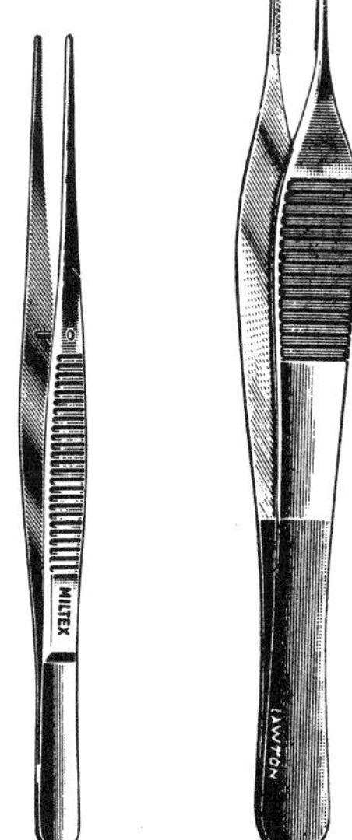

FIGURE 9-12
Examples of smooth forceps *(Left)* Semken. *(Right)* Adson. *(From Smith EJ, Smith YR: Smiths' Reference and Illustrated Guide to Surgical Instruments, pp 365, 417. Philadelphia, JB Lippincott, 1983)*

The tissue forceps is basically two blades joined at one end that spring apart at the other. The blades do not lock. The most commonly used forceps are straight, but they vary in length, width, and tip design. Some forceps are very delicate; others are bulky. Each forceps is designed for use on specific types of tissues, and the assistant must know which forceps is to be used where. Toothed forceps may have one tooth or several teeth at the tip. The teeth may be fine or heavy (see Figure 9-11). Forceps without teeth, called "smooth forceps," are used to grasp tissues that might be easily perforated. Smooth forceps are useful for holding gauze sponges, because the gauze material will not become caught in the tips (see Figure 9-12).

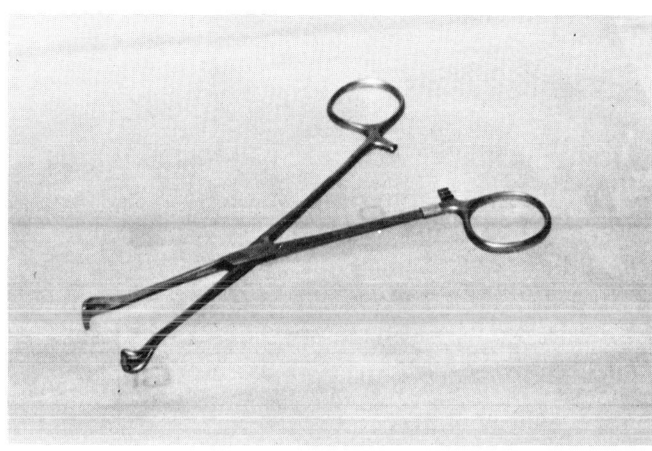

FIGURE 9-13
Babcock clamp. Note smooth grasping surfaces.

When using tissue forceps, tissue should not be held any longer or more firmly than necessary because this increases the damage to the tissues. The amount of traction used when holding tissue with the forceps must be appropriate for the type of tissue. If the traction is too great, the tissue may tear or the forceps may slip. The RN first assistant should carefully inspect the forceps to ensure that the tips meet correctly and that there are no barbs or hooks that could injure tissue.

Clamps. Several types of clamps are used to grasp tissue. These clamps are available in various lengths and may be straight, curved, or angled. They have ringed handles and racheted boxlocks to secure their grasp. Clamp structure varies from delicate to heavy, and the jaws may be smooth or serrated. The tip of the clamp may be fine, pointed, rounded, blunt, or triangular, or it may have interlocking teeth.

Delicate clamps cause less trauma to the tissues and are used for soft or fragile tissue, such as lung or bowel (see Figure 9-13). Delicate clamps must not be used to grasp heavier tissues, because the clamp may slip when traction is applied. Also, the clamp will be damaged if forced to clamp heavy or bulky tissue.

Clamps with teeth are used only on tissues that will not be seriously injured by tooth perforation. The teeth increase the clamp's grasping power, so that greater amounts of traction can be applied (see Figure 9-14). The tips may be very sharp; the assistant must be careful not to perforate gloves or delicate structures like bowel or blood vessels.

Heavy clamps can cause crushing injury to tissues and must be used appropriately. Frequently, just the clamp's tip is used to grasp tissue and apply traction (see Figure 9-15). Excessive traction will cause the clamp to slip or the tissue to tear. The assistant may need to simultaneously hold several

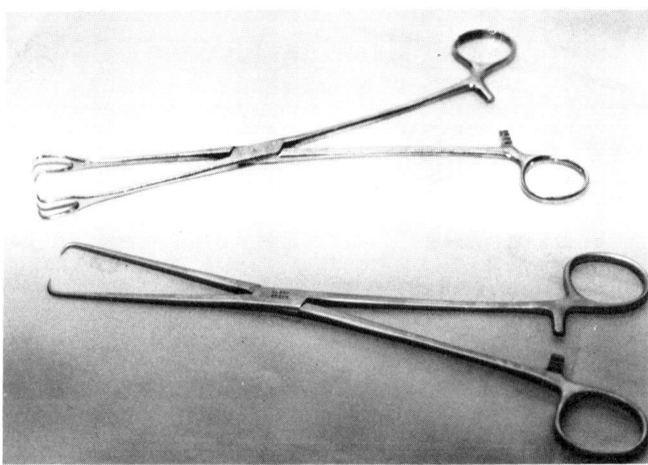

FIGURE 9-14
Tenaculum forceps (single- and double-toothed)

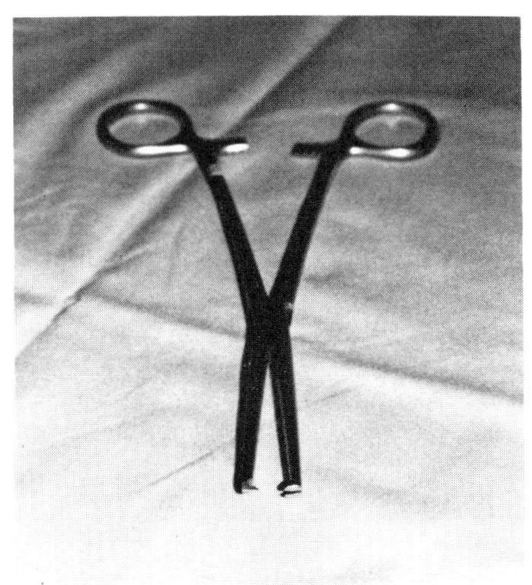

FIGURE 9-15
Ochsner forceps. Note grasping tooth at tip of clamp.

clamps that are providing retraction at different points of a structure. When a clamp is attached to tissue, it should be held by the shaft rather than by the ring handles, because there is less chance of accidentally unlocking the clamp when it is held in this manner (see Figure 9-16).

SPONGES

Sponges are used in different ways to provide exposure. Several types and sizes of sponges are used in the operating room. Laparotomy sponges, gauze

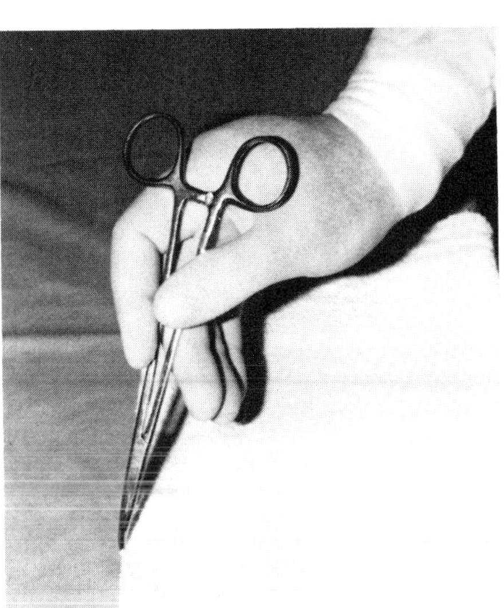

FIGURE 9-16
Position for holding clamp by shaft.

4 x 4 x 8 inches, cottonoid pledgets, and "peanuts" (pills, kitners, pushers, dissectors) are the most frequently used types.

The most common use of the sponge is to absorb fluid or blood that accumulates in the operative site and obstructs the surgeon's field of vision. Sponges are designed to soak up blood and should be used to blot tissues. Rubbing tissue with the sponges is abrasive and can remove clots, increase bleeding, and cause tissue damage.

Sponges may be used with an instrument to remove blood and fluids or as dissectors or retractors to gently push or pull tissues from the operative area. A 4 x 4 inch gauze pad can be folded and clamped into a sponge stick (stick sponge), or a peanut may be clamped in the tip of a curved clamp, such as a peon (see Figure 9-17). It is important that the sponges extend beyond the end of the clamp to protect tissue from injury by the clamp tips. The assistant must be careful to not use excessive pressure with this type of sponge, or else tissue may be perforated or torn. Also, blood supply can be compromised if pressure is applied too firmly or in the incorrect area.

Slippery structures (*i.e.*, bowel or lung) can be held more securely by using a sponge under the fingers. The sponge's coarse fibers will increase the friction and improve traction. Dry sponges provide a better grip than wet ones, but cause more tissue abrasion. This tissue trauma can result in adhesion formation, which could cause postoperative complications, especially with abdominal surgeries. Using a sponge (4 x 4 x 8 inch or lap sponge) under the fingers may also reduce the likelihood of contaminating internal tissues with skin bacteria when retracting skin edges.

Sponges can also be used to stabilize tissues. Organs or tissues that would "fall" into the operative field and obstruct the surgeon's vision can be packed out of the way with sponges. Loose structures, such as bowel, can be better retracted if they are wrapped with moistened laparotomy sponges. Tissues can be protected from retractor blades by using sponges for padding.

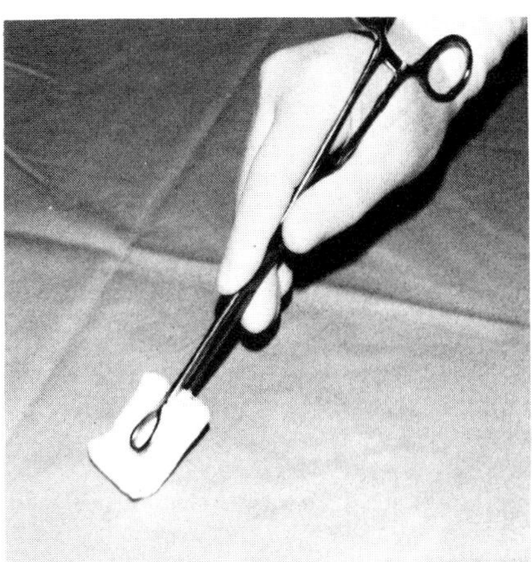

FIGURE 9-17
Sponge stick holding folded gauze sponge.

SUTURES

Sutures are frequently used to provide exposure. They are particularly helpful in everting or fixing small mobile structures, such as the inner surface of the eyelid. They also can be used to stabilize or hold tissues. Skin, pleural, pericardial, dural, peritoneal, and certain other tissue edges are commonly retracted with sutures (see Figure 9-18). Suturing is frequently considered as a retraction method when delicate structures require intermittent release and retraction over an extended period.

The amount of tension or pull that can be exerted on the suture depends on the tissue's fragility and the suture's tensile strength. Sutures must be placed securely in the tissue. Traction on the sutures is applied by the assistant's hand or by clamping/suturing the stitch to the drapes, wound towels, or wound edges. When clamps are placed on the end of a retraction suture, the clamp should not be left unattended. Holding it, or fixing it to a drape, minimizes the risk that someone will mistakenly pick it up without realizing that its jaws are clamped to a suture.

For very fragile tissues, the surgeon may use a pledget of Teflon felt (see Figure 9-19). The felt keeps the suture from cutting into the tissue. When sutures are held with a clamp, the jaws might need to be shod to keep the

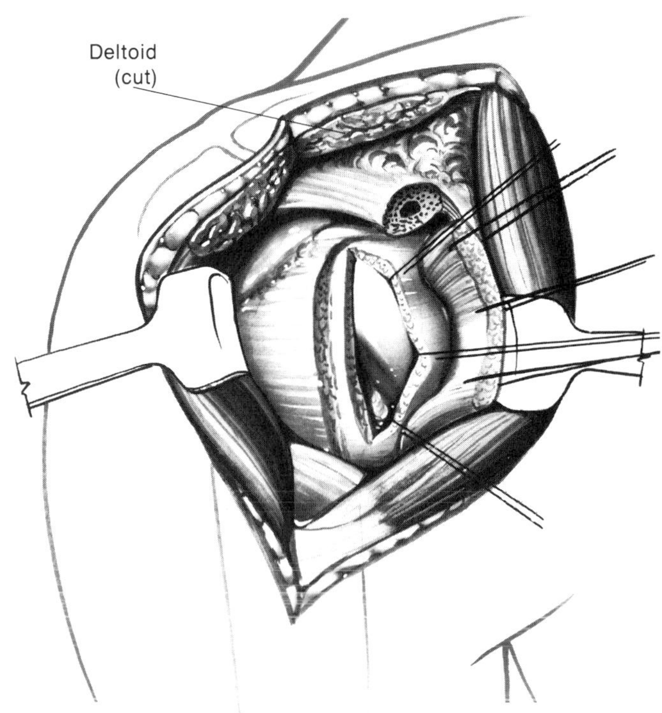

FIGURE 9-18
Use of sutures to retract tissue edges. *(From Hoppenfeld S, deBoer P: Surgical Exposures in Orthopaedics: The Anatomic Approach, p 13. Philadelphia, JB Lippincott, 1984)*

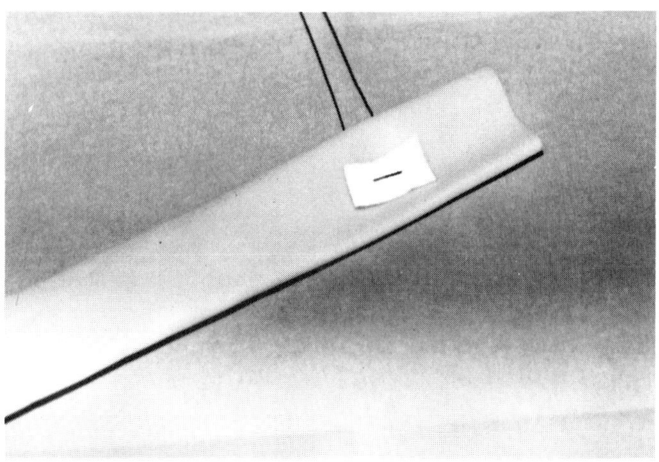

FIGURE 9-19
Illustration of how Teflon felt can be used with a suture for retracting delicate tissues.

suture from being cut. Various prepackaged, sterile shods are available. When the sutures are stitched to drapes or to other structures, tension must be appropriate for the tissue and the sutures, knots must be tied securely, and sutures must be cut close to the knot to prevent other sutures from catching on the knots.

Sutures provide good retraction without the bulk of instruments or retractors. If fastened correctly, they will hold tissue in a continuous position.

Umbilical tapes, *Penrose drains*, and *vessel loops* can also be used to retract blood vessels, nerves, and gastrointestinal structures. These structures are fragile and slippery, which makes them difficult to retract; they also can be easily traumatized, which will result in serious problems.

Once the structure needing retraction is dissected free from surrounding tissues, an angled clamp is used to go under the structure. This clamp must be long enough and have a wide enough angle to slip around the structure easily. Various clamps are available; those used most commonly include kidney pedicle clamps, Semb ligature carriers, Rumel thoracic right-angle forceps, and lower gallbladder forceps.

Once the clamp is passed under the structure, it is opened, and the tape (drain or loop) is inserted into the open jaws; the clamp is then closed and pulled back under the structure (see Figure 9-20). This must be done carefully and gently so that the structure or surrounding tissues are not injured by the clamp. The tape (drain or loop) should be moistened to decrease the friction on the surrounding tissues. The assistant usually uses two hands when placing a tape. One hand holds the clamp or forceps used to hold the end of the tape, while the other hand holds the tape taut. To prevent excessive drag through the tissue, only just enough tape to be grasped securely should be placed in the clamp's jaws.

Once the tape encircles the structure, it is clamped with a hemostat. The assistant can provide traction by pulling on the hemostat, or the hemostat can

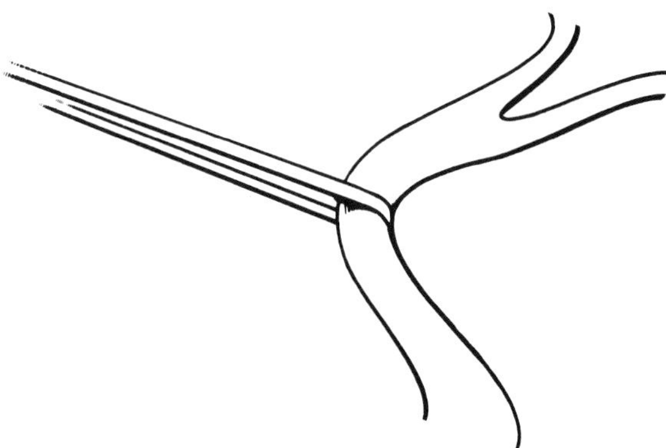

FIGURE 9-20
Vascular structure being retracted with a tape.

be used to clamp the tape, preventing any possibility of injury to the structure itself.

SUCTIONING DEVICES

Suctioning devices remove blood or fluids from the operative area, which is essential for adequate visualization. Suction tips come in various shapes and sizes.

The Frazier suction tip is small and has an opening on the end. It is very useful for small incisional sites with little blood loss. For operative procedures with larger incisions and increased fluid or blood loss, a Yankauer tonsil suction tip or an abdominal suction tip may be used. The Yankauer suction tip's configuration makes it useful in retracting tissue as well as in suctioning blood or fluids.

Aspiration injury of tissue can occur with suction tips that have a single end opening. This can be prevented by protecting the tissue with a sponge so that the suction is not applied directly on the tissue. Should tissue be aspirated, the suction tip should not be pulled away forcibly. Instead, first the suction should be broken by bending off the suction tubing, then the tissue gently removed. Some suction tips have a finger hole. When the hole is covered, the suction force increases; when it is uncovered, suction force decreases.

When using a suction tip, good visualization of the tip is important. Trauma to tissue can occur if the tip is used carelessly; a fine-pointed tip could puncture, tear, or abrade tissue.

The suction tip is used to remove blood or fluids in the area where the surgeon is working. It must never obstruct the surgeon's vision. The RN first assistant may need to use suction frequently and briefly in coordination with the surgeon's activities. The assistant must observe the operative site continuously to anticipate the need for and timing of suctioning.

The assistant also must be alert to the potential for losing removable parts of the suction tip. It is important to have a method of accounting for these parts. For example, the off/on controls may be held in place with screws that can back out and drop into the wound. Occasionally, the surgeon may find it necessary to unscrew the end of the suction tip, which is then given to the scrub nurse for safekeeping until needed again.

RETRACTING WITH THE HANDS

The ideal retractor to provide exposure is frequently the assistant's *hands*. The hand is gently padded, soft, and responsive to the texture of tissue being retracted through tactile sense. Fingers and hands can be repositioned or removed easily and quickly from the operative area. The amount of pressure or traction exerted on tissue can be readily adjusted.

After the initial incision, the assistant uses the fingers to retract the skin edge while the subcutaneous layers are being cut. Fingers are usually used for retracting while the retractor is being positioned. By spreading the fingers, a broad area can be retracted with one hand. The assistant should flatten the hand as much as possible. This causes less obstruction to the operative area and allows for better visualization by the surgeon.

By placing a sponge under the fingers, the assistant can grip the tissue more securely. However, with prolonged retracting, the assistant's fingers and hand may become fatigued. The assistant must inform the surgeon when this is occurring to avoid untimely slipping of the retracted tissues. A brief rest or repositioning the hand will usually relieve the fatigue.

Plastic bags (sterile) have been designed for retracting small intestines during extensive abdominal operations. The bowel must be secured properly within the bag, or else it will slip into the operative area.

CONCLUSION

The effects of the RN first assistant's retracting or providing exposure are apparent during the operative procedure. If exposure is poor, then the assistant must find the first practical moment and method to improve it. By close observation, the assistant can determine the effectiveness of his or her actions. It is not uncommon for the surgeon to situate retractors or determine the method of providing exposure. In some situations, the surgeon determines how and what is retracted. The assistant contributes significantly to the effectiveness, efficiency, and safety of the operative procedure by providing good exposure of the operative site for the surgeon.

Tissue injury resulting from carelessness while providing exposure will usually be apparent at the time of the surgical intervention. However, some injuries—such as nerve injury—may not be noticed until the postoperative period. Postoperative evaluation of the patient's status provides the assistant with information that will be helpful in determining whether any injury related to providing exposure has occurred intraoperatively.

REVIEW QUESTIONS

Fill in the blanks in the following questions.

1. A judgment made by the nurse related to the patient's problems, needs, or health status is stated as a _______.
2. Surgery is the _______ risk factor for the perioperative patient with a high risk for injury.
3. Detailed guidelines for predictable care regimens may be developed as intraoperative _______.
4. A major consideration in selecting the appropriate method of providing exposure is the _______ of the operative procedure.
5. It is easier for the RN first assistant to vary the position of the retractor and force of retraction with _______ retractors.
6. Pronged retractors are usually selected for retraction of _______ tissue.
7. When retracting away from oneself, the retractor should be held in the hand with the palm _______ and the arm flexed at the elbow.
8. The longer the surgical procedure, the more _______ loss and tissue _______. For this reason, moist sponges are used under retractor blades.
9. Overexpansion of a self-retaining retractor can cause excessive pulling on tissue and subsequent _______.
10. Grasping pressure of tissue forceps is controlled by the _______.
11. A clamp with _______ allows more grasping power and tissue traction.
12. When a clamp is attached to tissue, it should be held by the _______ to prevent accidental unlocking.
13. When a sponge is used to absorb blood in the field, a _______ motion prevents tissue damage.
14. A gauze dissector should be inserted into a clamp with the end of the dissector _______ the end of the clamp.
15. A particularly useful way to fix a small, mobile structure is to use a _______ as a retraction method.
16. To keep a suture from cutting into fragile tissue, a _______ may be used with the suture.
17. If tissue is aspirated into the end of a suction tip, the assistant should first _______, then gently remove the tissue.
18. The _______ is often the best retractor; it is softly padded and responsive through tactile sense.
19. Before repositioning any retracting device, the RN first assistant should _______________.
20. During surgery, the best way to determine the effectiveness of retraction is by _______________.

Answers

1. nursing diagnosis
2. situational
3. standards of care
4. stage
5. hand-held
6. shallow/subcutaneous
7. supine
8. fluid/dessication
9. tearing/laceration
10. thumb and fingers
11. teeth
12. shaft
13. blotting
14. beyond
15. suture
16. pledget of felt
17. break the suction
18. hand
19. inform the surgeon
20. observation

REFERENCES

1. Association of Operating Room Nurses: AORN official statement on RN first assistants. AORN J 39:404–405, 1984
2. Carpenito LJ: Nursing Diagnosis: Application to Clinical Practice. Philadelphia, JB Lippincott, 1992
3. Association of Operating Room Nurses: Standards and Recommended Practices for Perioperative Nursing. Denver, Association of Operating Room Nurses, II:7-2 1992

BIBLIOGRAPHY

Anderson R, Romfh R: Technique in the Use of Surgical Tools. New York, Appleton-Century-Crofts, 1980

Cardiovascular, Thoracic, General Surgical Pilling Instruments. Fort Washington, PA, Narco Scientific, 1980

Davis JH, Foster RS, Gamelli RL: Essentials of Clinical Surgery. St Louis, Mosby–Year Book, 1991

Groah L: Operating Room Nursing, Perioperative Practice. Norwalk, CT, Appleton & Lange, 1990

Kneedler J, Dodge G: Perioperative Patient Care. Boston, Blackwell Scientific, 1987

Meeker M, Rothrock, J: Alexander's Care of the Patient in Surgery. St Louis, Mosby–Year Book, 1991

Rothrock JC: Perioperative Nursing Care Planning. St. Louis, CV Mosby, 1990

Swartz S, Shires GT, Spencer F, Storer E: Principles of Surgery, 4th ed. San Francisco, McGraw-Hill, 1984

Vaiden RE, Fox VJ, Rothrock JC: Core Curriculum for the RN First Assistant. Denver, Association of Operating Room Nurses, 1990

10 Suturing Materials and Techniques

Nancy B. Davis

Suturing skills are required by the RN functioning as a first assistant during operative procedures. Suturing is one of the unique nursing behaviors identified for RN first assistants in the Association of Operating Room Nurses' (AORN's) Official Statement on RN First Assistants (see Appendix 1). The use of the term "suturing" is broad; variations in practice environments and state nurse practice acts may further quantify and define parameters for what types of structures may be sutured. Like all skill acquisition, learning and performing the techniques of suturing progress from basic competency to excellence in skill performance.

Preparation and handling of suture materials, needles, and needleholders are basic functions of a scrub nurse. The nurse learns about the types of sutures and how and when they are used. By observing the surgeon, the scrub nurse becomes familiar with suturing techniques. These experiences as a scrub nurse are most helpful to the RN first assistant when learning to suture.

Learning to suture should first be undertaken in a simulated setting. Such laboratory experience facilitates educational assumptions about psychomotor skill learning. Skills are learned first by imitation; the skill is demonstrated, and the learner follows the example of the demonstrator. As the learner practices, skill in manipulation follows; the technique can be carried out without constant demonstration. As the RN first assistant learns to manipulate hand and arm movements in suturing, precision in the technique follows. Eventually, the skill becomes naturalized; it is done with smooth, fluid motions, and the correct technique is selected for each application. Laboratory practice is especially helpful when learning more complex suturing techniques, such as microsurgery. Following practice and initial skill evaluation, suturing skills are refined in the operating room under the direction and supervision of the surgeon.

Although the choice of suture materials and techniques is often determined by the operating surgeon, the RN first assistant must consider the influence of the patient's condition, age, presence of infection, and type of tissue being sutured. Preoperative patient assessment provides data about the patient from which the RN first assistant identifies potential complications. Suture materials are foreign substances; in selecting the type of suture and suturing technique, the RN first assistant must consider patient risk factors and the potential for such problems as wound infection, inadequate wound healing, wound dehiscence, and excessive scarring. Taking these factors into consideration, the goal is to leave minimal foreign material in the wound. This is achieved, in part, by selecting the suture with the highest tensile strength and the smallest diameter and that holds knots well, requiring fewer turns and throws during tying.

USES AND SELECTION OF SUTURES

The three common uses for sutures during operative procedures are as follows:

1. Strands of suture are used as ligatures to "tie off" blood vessels and control bleeding.
2. Sutures are used to sew tissue together (reapproximate) and to hold the tissue securely until they are healed.
3. By applying tension to sutures placed through tissue, that tissue can be retracted, facilitating exposure of the operative site for the surgeon.

Sutures are considered to be medical devices and as such must meet certain standards established by the federal Food and Drug Administration (FDA). Since 1937, government regulations have established criteria for ensuring the safety and effectiveness of sutures. Sterility, tensile strength, size, dyes, needle attachments, coating or impregnation of suture material with other substances, packaging, and labeling are some of the areas addressed in these regulations.

A primary factor to consider when selecting a suture is the tissue being sutured. The suture must be as strong as the tissue it is holding, and the strength of the suture must last until the tissue is healed. Thus the rate of suture absorption should correspond to the rate of healing. Tissues heal at different rates; healing can be affected by such factors as infection, obesity, fever, debilitation, chronic disease, and age. The smallest diameter of suture is used to minimize tissue reaction and injury. The suture material should be pliable, strong, and hold knots securely; suture security depends on its intrinsic tensile strength and ability to hold a knot. Other considerations include location and length of the incision, desired cosmetic results, personal experiences, cost, and availability.

CLASSIFICATION OF SUTURES

Sutures are classified according to the effects of tissue enzymes and body fluids. A suture is a foreign body; the body reacts to it by attempting to dissolve or digest it. If this is possible, then the suture is *absorbed*. *Nonabsorbable sutures*, in contrast, cannot be dissolved or digested; rather, they become encapsulated by the body tissues.

Sutures are also classified according to the number of strands of material used. A suture with two or more strands of suture material twisted or braided together is termed a *multifilament suture*. Although the multifilament suture's higher coefficient of friction helps it hold knots, the multiple strands make it harder to drag through tissue, thus increasing tissue trauma and tissue reaction. This type of suture has a capillarity (transfer of body fluids along the suture strand) due to the interstices in the braided or twisted strands; capillary action can be reduced by coating the suture with silicone or paraffin. A *monofilament suture* consists of one strand of suture material that is noncapillary and causes very little tissue reaction.

ABSORBABLE SUTURES

Absorbable sutures are temporary; they will be digested or dissolved. Tensile strength, retention, and absorption rate vary among the absorbable sutures, and these factors must be considered separately. For example, a suture may lose its strength quickly and be absorbed slowly. These sutures can be treated to delay the absorption rate or coated with agents that have an antimicrobial action. Absorbable sutures vary in texture, structure, size, and color (see Table 10-1).

Surgical Gut. Surgical gut (catgut) is used less frequently since the introduction of synthetic absorbable sutures. Gut is made from the submucosal layer of sheep intestine or the serosa layer of beef intestine; it is a highly purified collagen. Gut is processed by electronically spinning and polishing the strands into various sizes. The suture can be left "plain," or it may be dipped in chromium salt solution. "Chromicizing" the suture increases its resistance to the digestive action of the tissue enzymes, which delays suture absorption. This treated suture is called "chromic." *Plain* suture loses its tensile strength in 7 to 10 days and is absorbed in 70 days. *Chromic* suture's tensile strength lasts 10 to 14 days; it is usually not absorbed before 90 days. Chromic suture causes less tissue reaction than does plain suture, which may elicit a marked foreign-body response.

Surgical gut suture must be handled as little as possible, because handling may cause the suture to fray. The suture material loses its pliability if allowed to dry. Pliability can be restored by moistening the suture with sterile water or saline. The suture must not be soaked any longer than a few seconds, because soaking decreases tensile strength and knot security.

Synthetic Absorbable Sutures. Polymers made from polyglycolic acid, polyglactin 910, polyglyconate, or polydioxanone, synthetic absorbable sutures are prepared as monofilament or multifilament sutures. Tissue reactions are mild and are decreased further when the monofilament suture is used. This type of suture is stronger than surgical gut, and the tensile strength lasts longer. After 14 days, 60% or more of the suture's tensile strength remains. Absorption occurs through hydrolysis, and the suture will not be totally absorbed for 60 to 90 days. The polydioxanone suture will not be absorbed until after 90 days, and absorption may take as long as 180 days.

The braided polymers handle like silk sutures; because of their higher coefficient of friction, knot security is good. However, the monofilament or the coated sutures (polyglactin 910 and calcium stearate coating) are smoother and slicker, so they will require additional throws for knot security.

NONABSORBABLE SUTURES

Nonabsorbable sutures are not digested by tissue enzymes or hydrolyzed by body fluids. They are considered permanent sutures. Nonabsorbable sutures are used when the suture strength needs to be retained longer than 2 to 3 weeks. They are often used when it is necessary to minimize the tissue reaction or trauma that can occur with the absorbable sutures (see Table 10-2).

With the exception of wire sutures, nonabsorbable sutures should not be used in the presence of infection. The suture itself could become a site for the infection, perhaps necessitating suture removal.

Surgical Silk. In the past, surgical silk was the most commonly used nonabsorbable suture because of its easy handling, its tensile strength, and the security of its knots with a minimal amount of throws. All other sutures are compared with silk in relation to these handling properties. However, silk does cause a higher degree of tissue reaction than do the other nonabsorbable sutures. Silk is made from the silk of silkworms. After the silk filaments are processed, the strands are braided or twisted, treated to decrease capillary action, and usually dyed black. Silk loses up to 20% of its strength if moistened; therefore, it is used dry. The tensile strength of silk decreases after 90 to 120 days, and the silk usually is absorbed after 2 years. It is not a true nonabsorbable suture, but is classified as such because of the time that it remains in the tissues. Strict aseptic technique is necessary when using silk, and silk is never used in an infected wound.

Virgin Silk. Virgin silk is processed differently than other silk. The sericin gum normally present on the silk filaments is not removed but rather is left on to hold the fine filaments together. The suture is very fine (8-0 or 9-0) and is used primarily for ophthalmic procedures.

Surgical Cotton. Surgical cotton is made from natural cellulose cotton fibers. The fibers are twisted into strands, processed, and coated to provide a smoother

(text continues on page 193)

TABLE 10-1

Absorbable Sutures Commonly Used in Surgery

Suture	Types	Frequent Uses	Tissue Reaction	Contraindications	Warnings	Tensile Strength Retention *in vivo*	Absorption Rate
Surgical gut	Plain	Ligate superficial vessels; suture subcutaneous and other tissues that heal rapidly; sometimes used in presence of infection, as opposed to a braided nonabsorbable suture Ophthalmology	Moderate	Should not be used in tissues that heal slowly and require support	Absorbs relatively quickly	Lost within 7–10 days (Individual patient characteristics can affect rate of tensile strength loss)	Digested by body enzymes within 70 days
Surgical gut	Chromic	One of the most versatile of all materials; may be used in presence of infection; used in tissues that heal relatively slowly but intended for use as absorbable suture or ligature Ophthalmology	Moderate, but less than plain surgical gut	Being absorbable, should not be used where prolonged approximation of tissues under stress is required	Protein-based absorbable sutures have a tendency to fray when tied	Lost within 21–28 days (Individual patient characteristics can affect rate of tensile strength loss)	Digested by body enzymes within 90 days

Polyglactin 910 Polyglycolic acid suture	Braided	Ligate or suture tissues where an absorbable suture is desirable except where approximation under stress is required	Mild	Being absorbable, should not be used where prolonged approximation of tissues under stress is required	Safety and effectiveness in neural and cardiovascular tissue have not been established	Approximately 60% remains at two weeks; approximately 30% remains at three weeks	Minimal until about 40th day; essentially complete between 60–90 days; absorbed by slow hydrolysis
Polydioxanone	Monofilament	Abdominal and thoracic closure, subcutaneous tissue, colon and rectal surgery; can use in presence of infection Orthopaedic, plastic	Slight	Being absorbable, should not be used where prolonged approximation of tissues under stress is required	Safety and effectiveness in neural and cardiovascular tissue have not been established	Approximately 70% remains at 2 weeks; approximately 50% remains at 4 weeks; approximately 25% remains at 6 weeks	Minimal until about 90th day; essentially complete within 210 days; absorbed by slow hydrolysis

Adapted from Ethicon: Wound Closure Manual, pp 24–25. Somerville, NJ, ETHICON, Inc, a Johnson & Johnson Company, 1985.

TABLE 10-2

Nonabsorbable Sutures Commonly Used in Surgery

Suture	Types	Frequent Uses	Tissue Reaction	Contraindications	Warnings	Tensile Strength Retention *in vivo*	Absorption Rate
Surgical silk	Braided	Most body tissues for ligating and suturing; general surgery, ophthalmology and plastic surgery	Moderate	Should not be used for placement of vascular prostheses and artificial heart valves	Slowly absorbs	Loses most or all in about 1 year	Usually cannot be found after 2 years
Surgical cotton	Twisted	Most body tissues for ligating and suturing	Minimal	None	None	Loses 50% in 6 months; has 30%–40% at end of 2 years	Nonabsorbable; remains encapsulated in body tissues
Surgical steel	Monofilament Multifilament	Abdominal wall and skin closure, sternal closure, retention, tendon repair, orthopaedic and neurosurgery	Low	Should not be used when a prosthesis of another alloy is implanted	May corrode and break at points of bending, twisting, or knotting	Indefinite	Nonabsorbable; remains encapsulated in body tissues
Nylon	Monofilament	Skin closure, retention; plastic surgery, ophthalmology, and microsurgery	Extremely low	None	None	Indefinite	Nonabsorbable; remains encapsulated in body tissues
	Braided	Most body tissues for ligating and suturing; general closure, neurosurgery					
Polyester fiber	Braided	Cardiovascular, general, and plastic surgery retention; ophthalmology	Minimal	None	None	Loses 15%–20% per year	Degrades at a rate of about 15%–20% per year
Polypropylene	Monofilament	General, plastic, cardiovascular surgery and skin closure; ophthalmology	Minimal transient acute inflammatory reaction	None	None	Indefinite	Nonabsorbable; remains encapsulated in body tissues

Adapted from Ethicon: Wound Closure Manual, pp 24–25. Somerville, NJ, ETHICON, Inc, a Johnson & Johnson Company, 1985.

surface. The weakest nonabsorbable suture, surgical cotton is used less frequently than silk. Cotton's tensile strength is increased 10% by moistening the suture immediately before use. Although 50% of tensile strength is lost in 6 months, 30% to 40% of tensile strength may remain after 2 years.

Linen. Rarely used, linen is made from twisted flax fibers. The tensile strength of linen is inferior to that of the other nonabsorbable sutures.

Stainless Steel. Surgical stainless steel wire sutures are made from a strong, flexible, and uniform steel alloy and can be used with stainless steel hardware or prostheses. (They should not be used in the presence of another alloy, because electrolytic reactions could occur.) Stainless steel wire is strong, minimally tissue reactive, and one of the most secure suture materials available. The suture is prepared as a monofilament wire or as braided multifilament wire. The monofilament wire kinks easily, but both types can be held securely in place by twisting or knotting the suture. However, knot security may be compromised when wire suture is twisted rather than tied. The major disadvantage is related to handling the suture; gloves can be punctured or tissue injured by the sharp ends of the wire. Wire's tensile strength is very high, and tissue reaction is very low. Wire cutters must be used, because the wire will damage suture scissors.

Nonabsorbable Synthetics. *Nylon* is made from a synthetic polyamide polymer. Its tensile strength is high, and tissue reaction is extremely low. This monofilament suture is noncapillary and is easy to handle. It does require additional throws for knot security, however. Moistening nylon suture makes it easier to handle and more pliable. Multifilament nylon is braided very tightly and treated for noncapillarity. It handles like silk but causes much less tissue reaction. Nylon suture loses 15% to 20% of its tensile strength per year in tissue and will not provide indefinite support.

Polyesters are made from polyethylene terephthalate fibers braided together. This suture is strong, and very little tissue reaction occurs. However, the uncoated polyesters can cause tissue trauma by friction as they are pulled through the tissues. They may be coated or impregnated with Teflon, polybutilate, or silicone to reduce the amount of friction produced when passing through tissue; but then additional throws are needed for knot security.

Polybutester is a monofilament that is more flexible and elastic than some of the other nonabsorbable monofilament sutures. Another new nonabsorbable suture, expanded *polytetrafluoroethylene* (PTFE) is strong relative to other monofilaments and has pliability and comparable knot security.

Polypropylene is made from a polyolefin of polymeric linear hydrocarbons. It is formed into a strong, smooth monofilament suture that does not weaken in tissues and causes very little tissue reaction. It is easy to handle, slides through tissue easily, and holds knots securely.

Polyethylene is a synthetic made from thermoplastic resins formed into

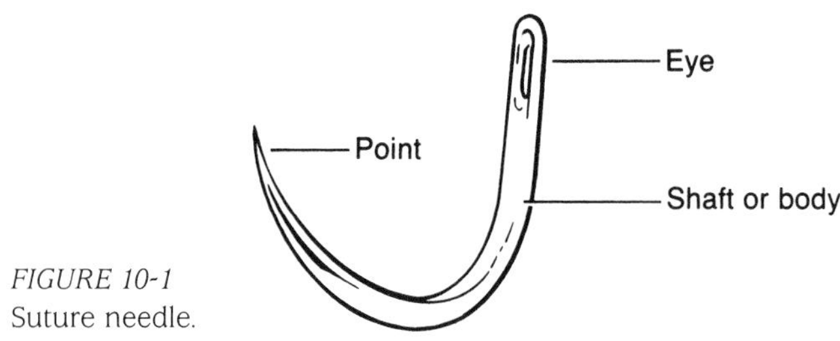

FIGURE 10-1
Suture needle.

monofilament sutures. It is easy to handle, passes smoothly through tissue, causes minimal tissue reaction, ties easily, and holds knots securely.

SURGICAL NEEDLES

The surgical needle transports the suture through the tissues during surgical operations with the least amount of trauma to the tissues. High-quality steel alloy is used in manufacturing surgical needles. The different sizes of needles are made from wire of various thicknesses. The wire is heat treated and tempered to provide the necessary strength and flexibility. A needle must be strong enough to penetrate the tissue without bending or becoming deformed. Because it is flexible, the needle can bend slightly without breaking. Bending alerts the user that the tissue is too tough for the needle.

Needles are carefully sharpened, finely polished, and smoothed for ease in tissue penetration. Silicone coatings are occasionally used. Because needles are noncorrosive, flaking of foreign material from needles into the surgical wound cannot occur. Before using, needles should be carefully inspected for any barbs, hooks, or rough areas.

NEEDLE DESIGNS

Basically, needles have three components: the eye, the shaft or body, and the point (see Figure 10-1).

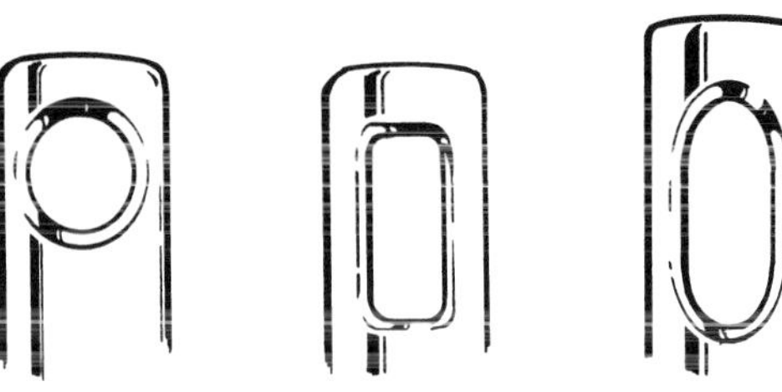

FIGURE 10-2
Closed-eye needles.

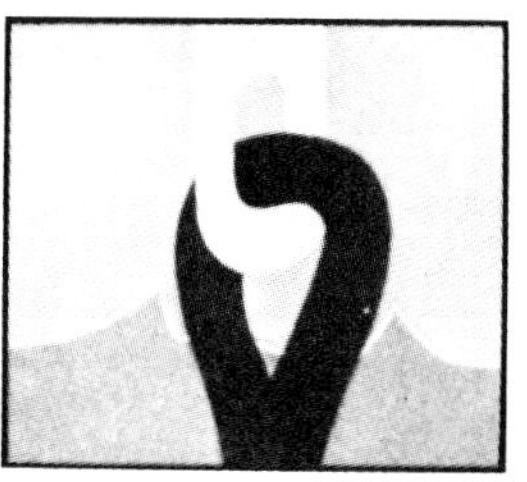
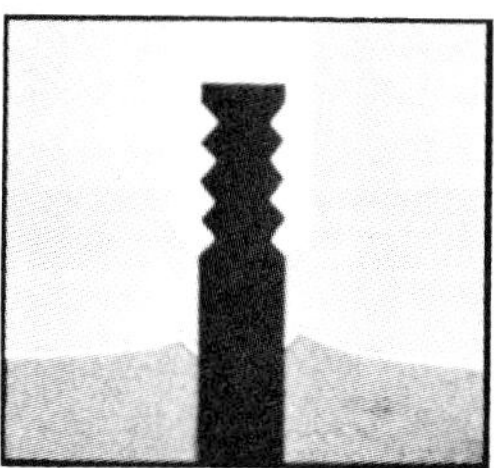

FIGURE 10-3
(Left) Tissue disruption caused by double suture strand with eyed needle. *(Right)* Tissue disruption minimized by single suture strand swaged to needle. *(From Wound Closure Manual, 1985. Courtesy of ETHICON, Inc., a Johnson & Johnson Company, Somerville, NJ)*

Eye. The eye of the needle is located at the end of the needle where the suture is attached. The three types of needle eyes are closed, French or split, and swaged.

The *closed-eye needle* has a round, square, or oblong hole through which the suture is threaded (see Figure 10-2). The eye must be smooth to avoid cutting the suture. Eyed needles may be reusable or disposable.

Although eyed needles may be economical, the eye must be larger than the suture; the additional bulk of a double suture causes increased damage to the tissue that the needle penetrates (see Figure 10-3).

The *French-* or *split-eye needle* has a spring opening (see Figure 10-4) allowing the suture and the needle to be almost the same size, which decreases tissue trauma. The double suture still must be pulled through the tissue, however. French-eye needles are quicker to thread but are usually finer needles that have limited use.

The *swaged* or *atraumatic needle* is actually an eyeless needle. The suture is attached to the end of the needle and is only as large as the needle itself. This type of needle provides the least amount of tissue trauma. Although expensive, swaged sutures are easier, quicker, and in some situations necessary to use. Many of the fine, synthetic nonabsorbable sutures are used for delicate surgery, such as microsurgery or vascular surgery. This type of surgery necessitates minimal tissue injury, as results from using a swaged needle. Optimum sharpness is ensured because the swaged needle is used only with that suture and then discarded. Sutures are now available with swaged needles that can be removed from the suture with a slight tug. Generically called "pop-off" or "break-away" sutures, "control release" is the trade name for this type of suture, manufactured by Ethicon. These are used

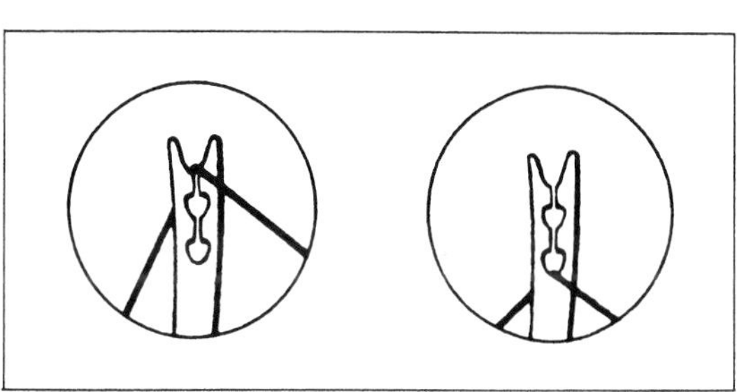

FIGURE 10-4
French-eyed (split-eye) needle. *(From Wound Closure Manual, 1985. Courtesy of ETHICON, Inc., a Johnson & Johnson Company, Somerville, NJ)*

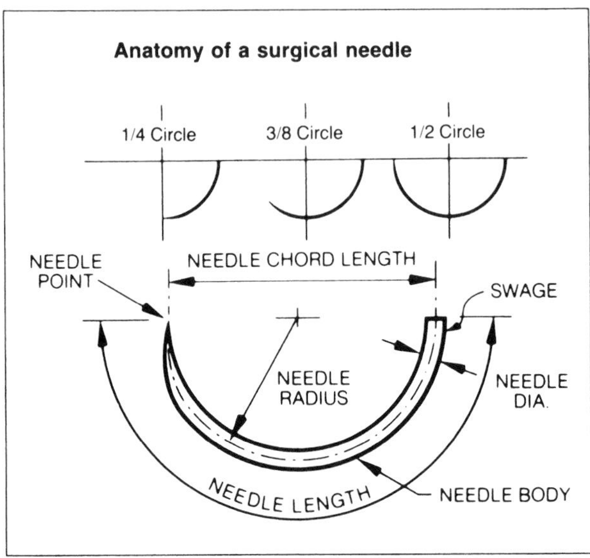

FIGURE 10-5
Methods of measuring the size of a suture needle. *(From Wound Closure Manual, 1985. Courtesy of ETHICON, Inc., a Johnson & Johnson Company, Somerville, NJ)*

for interrupted suturing techniques in which several sutures can be placed rapidly.

The choice of *needle eye* is based on the location and type of tissue being sutured, the size of the suture being used, the availability of various needles, and considerations related to decreasing surgery time. The assistant must be familiar with the surgeon's preferences in all operative procedures with which he/she assists.

Shaft. The shaft, or body, determines the needle's shape, size, and diameter. This area of the needle is grasped or held while being placed through tissue. The body may be straight, curved, or partially curved. The various needle sizes are determined by measuring the chord length, needle length, and needle radius (see Figure 10-5).

A needle may be oval, round, triangular, side-flattened rectangular, or trapezoidal in design. Some needles are flat and ribbed in the area where grasped by the needleholder. This reduces slippage of the needle in the needleholder while suturing.

Needle shape, size, and thickness must all be considered when selecting a needle. The shape and size depend on the location and accessibility of the tissue being sutured. The thickness is determined by the type of tissue and size of the suture being used. The needle must be strong enough to penetrate the tissue without bending or breaking and be as close to the diameter of the suture as possible (see Figure 10-6).

Point. The needle point is the end that first penetrates the tissue being sutured. The design of the point varies according to the type of tissue to be penetrated (see Figure 10-7). The basic point types are cutting, taper, and blunt. Cutting needles are designed to penetrate tough tissue like skin, tendons, fibrous or calcified tissue, and sternal bone. The variations in the cutting edges alter the direction of cutting and promote ease in tissue penetration.

Taper needles, usually called "round" needles, cause the least trauma but must be used on tissue that they can penetrate easily.

The blunt needle does not have a sharp point; it basically dissects the tissue as it is pushed through it. It can be used on very fragile tissue.

SUTURING

The RN first assistant needs skill in suturing. The application of this skill varies depending on the practice setting and legal constraints that may exist. Commonly, the RN first assistant will suture subcutaneous and skin tissue during wound closure.

In the scrub nurse role, the perioperative nurse has had the opportunity to observe suturing. Through this observation, and by active inquiry, the nurse can learn how to handle tissues when suturing, principles for reapproximating tissues, different suturing techniques, and the criteria for selecting suture materials and suture needles. Practicing suturing techniques should first be done in a laboratory setting; skill refinement occurs during the operative procedure, under the direction of the surgeon.

ASSISTING DURING SUTURING

The RN first assistant can perform essential nursing behaviors to facilitate suturing. One of the first requirements is to know ahead of time the surgeon's preferences for suturing materials and techniques. As wound closure approaches, the field should be cleared of sponges and extraneous instruments to prepare for counts. The wound should be inspected for bleeders, and any found should be controlled. Overhead lights may need to be adjusted and retractors repositioned for better visibility. The RN first assistant and surgeon should have a synchronized plan for who will tie knots and who will cut sutures. When tying a suture that is being used only once, the RN first assistant will take the needle and its suture, tie the first knot with the correct tension, then rapidly throw on the additional knots. Both ends of the suture are then presented for cutting, the needle and remaining suture are returned to the scrub nurse, and the assistant gets ready as the surgeon places the first bite of the next suture. When several stitches will be made with the same suture, the assistant needs to grasp enough of the short end to tie rapidly and accurately; while the knot is being tied, the surgeon will be repositioning the needle on the needleholder for the next stitch. The suture is cut, the short end discarded, and the long end retained as the process continues. When the suture becomes too short for convenient tying, another is requested.

(text continues on page 202)

Shape	Typical Applications	
Straight	Gastrointestinal tract Nasal cavity Nerve Oral cavity	Pharynx Skin Tendon Vessels
Half-curved	Skin, rarely used	
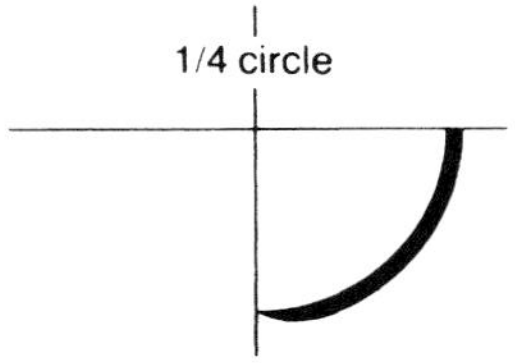 1/4 circle	Eye, primary application	Microsurgical procedures

FIGURE 10-6
Needle shapes and uses. *(From Wound Closure Manual, 1985. Courtesy of ETHICON, Inc., a Johnson & Johnson Company, Somerville, NJ)*

(continued)

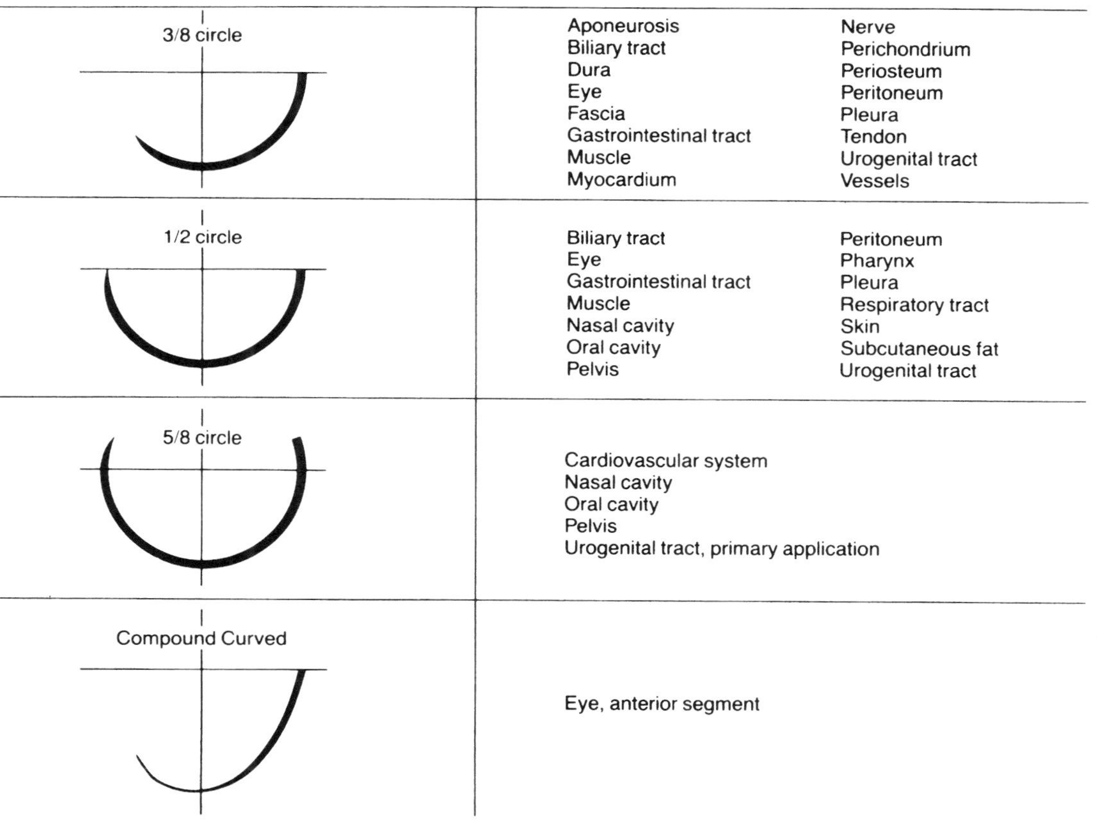

Needle shape	Applications	
3/8 circle	Aponeurosis Biliary tract Dura Eye Fascia Gastrointestinal tract Muscle Myocardium	Nerve Perichondrium Periosteum Peritoneum Pleura Tendon Urogenital tract Vessels
1/2 circle	Biliary tract Eye Gastrointestinal tract Muscle Nasal cavity Oral cavity Pelvis	Peritoneum Pharynx Pleura Respiratory tract Skin Subcutaneous fat Urogenital tract
5/8 circle	Cardiovascular system Nasal cavity Oral cavity Pelvis Urogenital tract, primary application	
Compound Curved	Eye, anterior segment	

FIGURE 10-6 *(continued)*

Needle Point and Body Shape	Typical Application
Conventional Cutting POINT BODY	Ligament Nasal cavity Oral cavity Pharynx Skin Tendon
Reverse Cutting POINT BODY	Fascia Ligament Nasal cavity Oral mucosa Skin Tendon sheath
MICRO-POINT* Reverse Cutting Needle POINT BODY	Eye
Precision Point Cutting POINT BODY POINT BODY	Plastic or cosmetic procedures Skin

FIGURE 10-7
Suture needle points and shapes. *(From Wound Closure Manual, 1985. Courtesy of ETHICON, Inc., a Johnson & Johnson Company, Somerville, NJ)*

(continued)

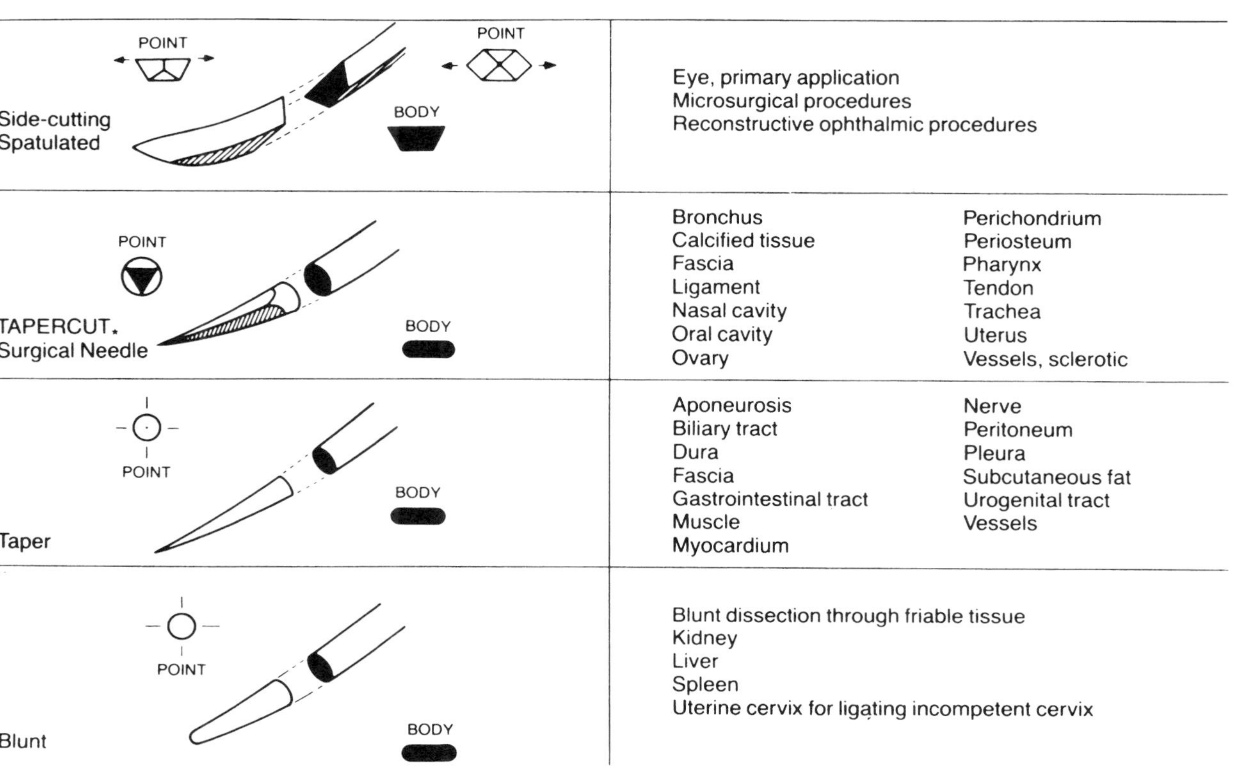

Side-cutting
Spatulated
POINT
POINT
BODY
Eye, primary application
Microsurgical procedures
Reconstructive ophthalmic procedures
TAPERCUT.
Surgical Needle
POINT
BODY
Bronchus
Calcified tissue
Fascia
Ligament
Nasal cavity
Oral cavity
Ovary
Perichondrium
Periosteum
Pharynx
Tendon
Trachea
Uterus
Vessels, sclerotic
Taper
POINT
BODY
Aponeurosis
Biliary tract
Dura
Fascia
Gastrointestinal tract
Muscle
Myocardium
Nerve
Peritoneum
Pleura
Subcutaneous fat
Urogenital tract
Vessels
Blunt
POINT
BODY
Blunt dissection through friable tissue
Kidney
Liver
Spleen
Uterine cervix for ligating incompetent cervix

FIGURE 10-7 *(continued)*

At times, the RN first assistant may be required to assist in grasping a needle as it exits tissue. The assistant may first use the tip of the unopened needleholder to provide a downward counterforce on the tissue (usually skin) where the needle is exiting. As the needle exits and the surgeon pauses to readjust, the assistant should grasp the needle with the needleholder behind the point of the needle, rotating the needle 90 degrees through a natural curve. This will bring most of the needle above the skin surface. Some of the needle should remain below the skin surface; this provides a position of stability for the surgeon to regrasp it. As the surgeon pulls the needle through, the assistant reaches for the suture as it emerges behind the needle and begins the first throw of the knot. This is referred to as the "needle fixation and presentation" technique.[1]

SUTURING TOOLS

Needleholders and tissue forceps are the basic instruments required for suturing. Through years of experience, the perioperative nurse is familiar with the various needleholders and tissue forceps and their uses. Functioning in the scrub nurse role is an excellent method of learning how and when these instruments are used during operative procedures. However, actual use of instruments necessitates mastery of new technical skills.

Needleholders. *Needleholders* are similar to hemostats. Most needleholders are designed with ring handles and ratchet locks. Some of the delicate needleholders are designed like tissue forceps and have spring locks (see Figure 10-8). The tips of needleholders are usually short and blunt, but some are designed with very fine, pointed tips. Needleholders are available in various lengths and sizes (see Figure 10-9).

Selection of a needleholder is based on the depth of the area where the sutures will be placed and on the size of the suture needle. Using a light, fine needleholder on a heavy suture needle could damage the instrument by springing the jaws or damaging the jaw inserts. Individual preference is another factor, understandable considering the numerous needleholders available.

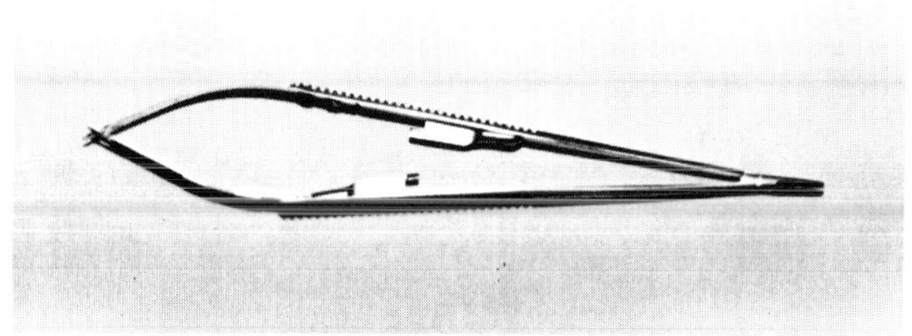

FIGURE 10-8
Castroviejo needle holder with spring lock.

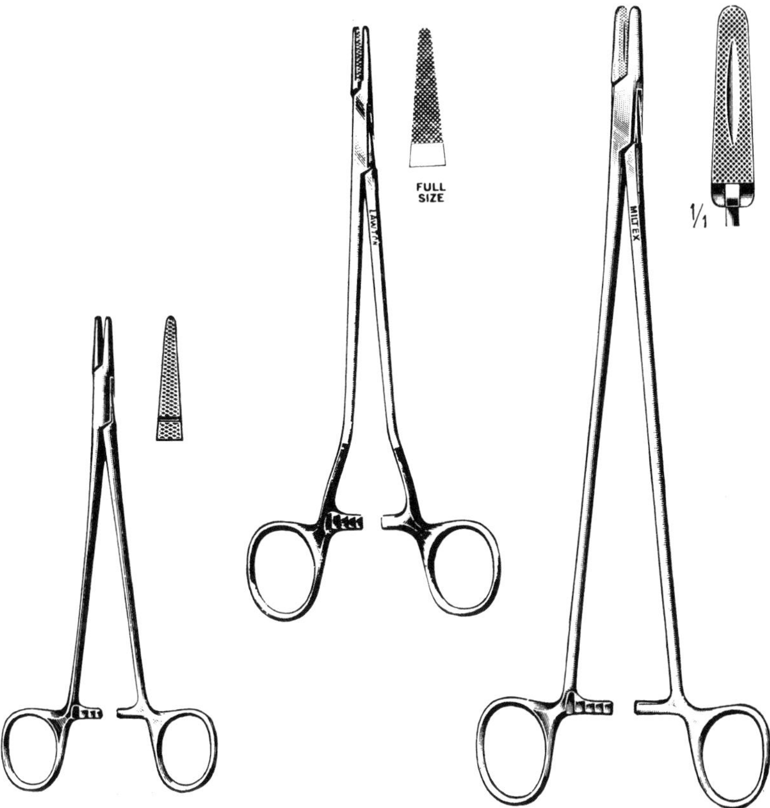

FIGURE 10-9
Examples of needleholders. *(Left)* Crile-Wood, *(center)* Sarot, *(right)* Masson. *(From Smith EJ, Smith YR: Smiths' Reference and Illustrated Guide to Surgical Instruments, pp 510, 517, 541. Philadelphia, JB Lippincott, 1983)*

Needleholders must be inspected to ensure that they function correctly. The jaws must hold the needle securely so that it will not slip as it is passed through the tissue. The jaw insert should be inspected for worn areas, and the security of the needle should be tested by gently attempting to move it with the fingers. The needleholder must open and close easily; resistance might result in inadvertent needle displacement in the tissue.

Placement of the suture needle in the needleholder is important. The needle is grasped at a point approximately one-quarter to one-half of the distance from the eye end (or swaged end). If the needle is grasped too close to the eye, it may bend as it is placed in the tissue. The needle may be placed at a right angle to the needleholder or at a slight angle. The needle is grasped in the tip of the needleholder jaws, and the needleholder is ratcheted one or two

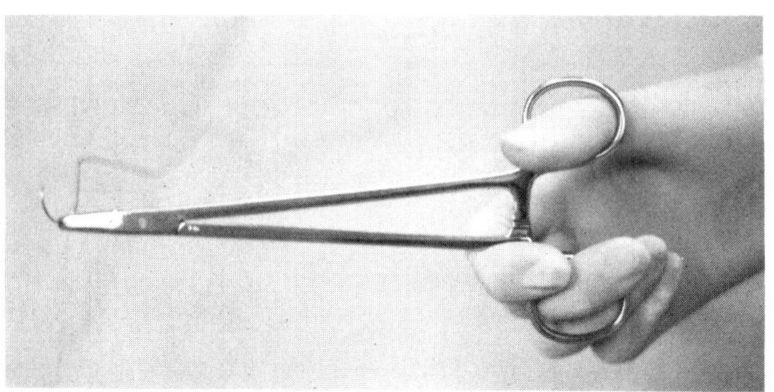

FIGURE 10-10
Needleholder with needle in correct position.

ratchets (see Figure 10-10). If the needleholder tips are allowed to extend beyond the secured needle, they can interfere with suturing by pushing into tissue (see Figure 10-11). The needle can be damaged, notched, or bent if it is clamped too tightly in the jaws of the needleholder. If the needle is placed in the holder in the direction of use, it will not have to be repositioned.

Needleholder Grips. The grip used on a needleholder depends on the amount of exertion required, the amount of control needed (*i.e.*, delicate), the location of the tissue being sutured, and the ease of suturing encountered.

The palmed grip is used when suturing very dense tissue that is difficult to penetrate (*i.e.*, sternum). The needleholder is held in the palm of the hand and gripped on the shaft, close to the tip (see Figure 10-12). This very secure grip is necessary when exerting a great deal of force on the needle. The direction of the needle is easily altered by rotating the needleholder in the hand. It is necessary to reposition the hand to release and reposition the needle.

The *thenar* grip is used for rapid, easy suturing. Precision is less exacting with this technique. The needleholder is grasped without inserting the thumb into the ring handle. The ball of the thumb (its metacarpal joint) is pressed against the thumb ring of the needleholder for control. This position puts the

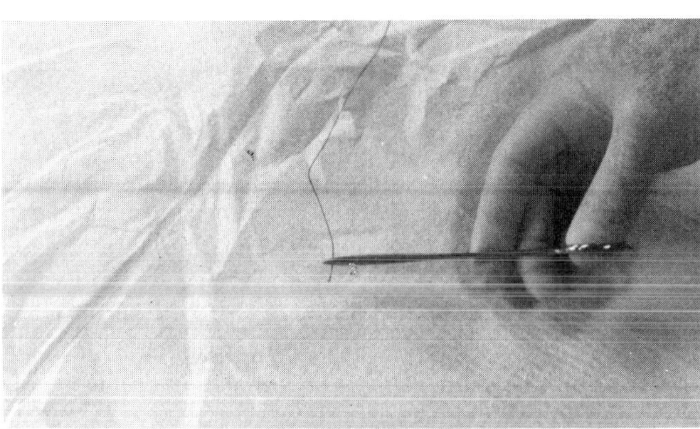

FIGURE 10-11
Needleholder with needle too far back in jaws.

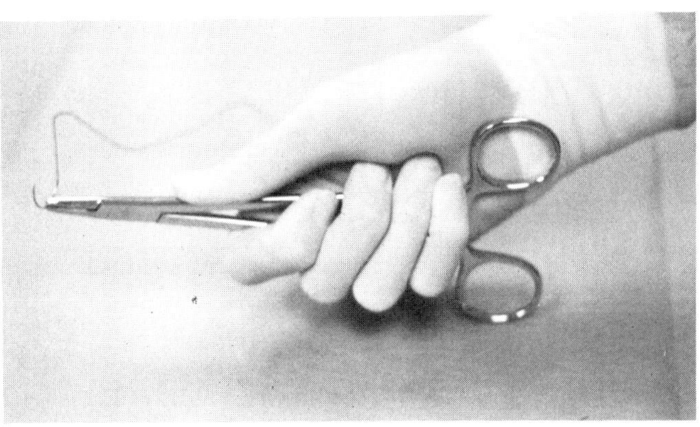

FIGURE 10-12
Palmed grip of needleholder.

needleholder in a direct line with the axis of the forearm; the motion of rotating the needleholder is simple and natural. It also provides the necessary leverage for opening and closing the needleholder (see Figure 10-13). However, the sudden opening of the needleholder can cause movement of the suture needle, a potential problem that must be considered when using this technique.

The *thumb-ring finger* grip is the most traditional method of using the needleholder. This technique is more precise and affords easier control of the needle. Hand position does not have to be changed when opening and closing the needleholder (see Figure 10-14).

The *pencil grip* is used for very fine, delicate needleholders that operate with a spring latch or are latchless. The spring latch can be closed and released with finger pressure. The needleholder is controlled by rotating it between the index finger and the thumb (see Figure 10-15). However, rotation of the needleholder on its axis may require more complex movement of the hand, wrist, and forearm.

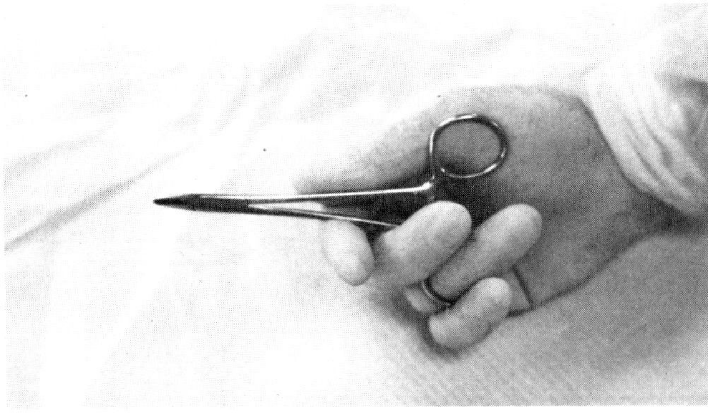

FIGURE 10-13
Thenar grip of needleholder.

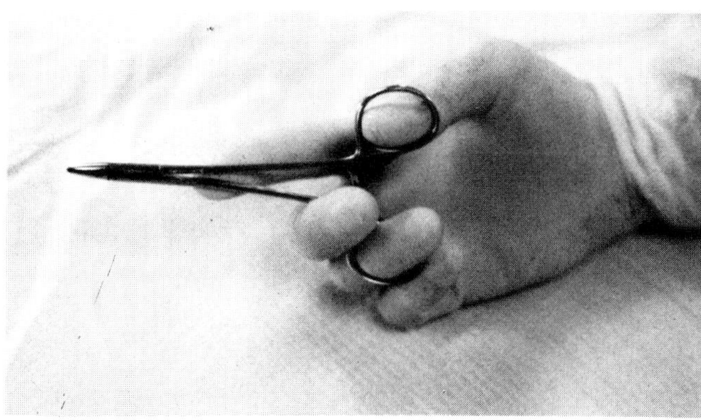

FIGURE 10-14
Thumb-ring finger grip of needleholder.

Suture Scissors. *Suture scissors* vary in length and size and may be straight or curved. The scissors is held in a position that provides stability and control. The "tripod" position provides the best control. The thumb and ringfinger are placed in the ring handles, and the index finger is extended along the shaft of the scissors. The palm of the hand faces down; the position can be easily changed by rotating the wrist (see Figure 10-16).

Good visualization is essential when cutting sutures. The suture knot can be easily seen and the cutting distance estimated by looking through the opened scissor blades. Cutting with the tips of the scissors prevents inadvertent cutting of surrounding structures. Generally the suture is cut as close to the knot as possible, but the length of the suture "tail" that is left is determined by the type of suture. Cutting the knot too short may decrease knot security. If cutting sutures when there is motion, additional support can be provided by resting the scissor hand against the other hand. The suture is held taut as it is cut.

Suture scissors must open and close smoothly. The blades should be sharp; dull or rough blades could snag the suture and cause it to be pulled loose or possibly tear the tissue being sutured.

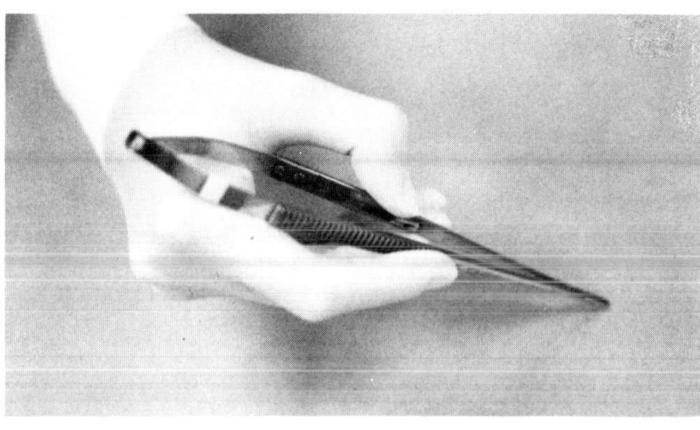

FIGURE 10-15
Pencil grip of needleholder.

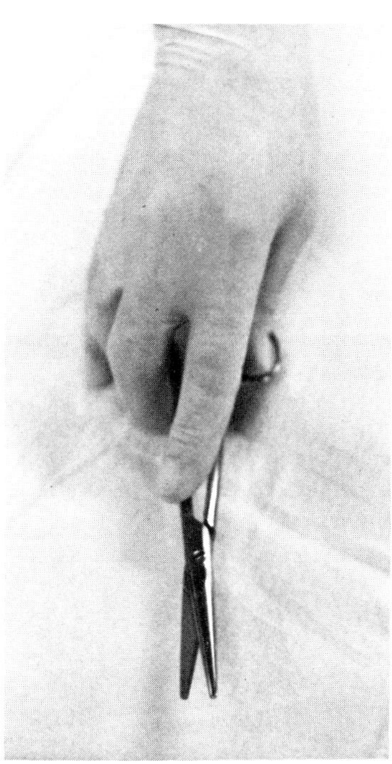

FIGURE 10-16
Position for using suture scissors.

By anticipating the need to cut sutures, the RN first assistant can contribute to the efficiency of the operation. The assistant should have the scissors ready and close to the area where the suture is being tied. By observing and counting the number of throws the surgeon has placed, the assistant can know when the suture is to be cut.

Tissue Forceps. Tissue forceps are used in conjunction with the needleholder. (For more information on forceps and their use, see Chapter 9, Providing Exposure: Retractors and Retraction, and Chapter 12, Using Grasping Instruments.) Using the forceps in the opposite hand allows the tissue to be stabilized and exposure to be provided before the suture needle penetrates the tissue. Tissue must be handled gently to avoid unnecessary injury or trauma that may interfere with healing. The forceps brace the skin as the tip of the needle emerges on the exit side of the incision during closure. The teeth of the forceps should be set into the tissue only when necessary to avoid slipping. The tissue forceps can also be used to grasp and remove the suture needle after it has passed through the tissue. The forceps are then used to hold the needle while it is repositioned on the needleholder.

SUTURING TECHNIQUES

Suturing is the method of reapproximating tissues that have been cut during the operative procedure. The cut tissues should be sutured to resume as near-

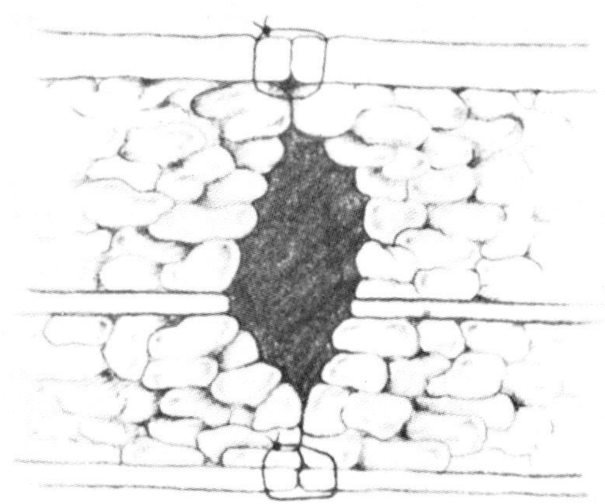

FIGURE 10-17
Dead space in subcutaneous fat. *(From Wound Closure Manual, 1985. Courtesy of ETHICON, Inc., a Johnson & Johnson Company, Somerville, NJ)*

normal a position as possible. It is important to correctly identify the different tissue layers being sutured to properly reposition them. The width and depth of the stitch will depend on the type of tissue being sutured. Suturing provides support to tissues while they heal, so that "gaps" or "dead space" will not delay healing (see Figure 10-17). Dead space not only weakens the suture line; it also is a potential site of bleeding or infection.

Whenever possible, the RN first assistant should sew toward himself/herself (see Figure 10-18). This position is more comfortable and maximizes visi-

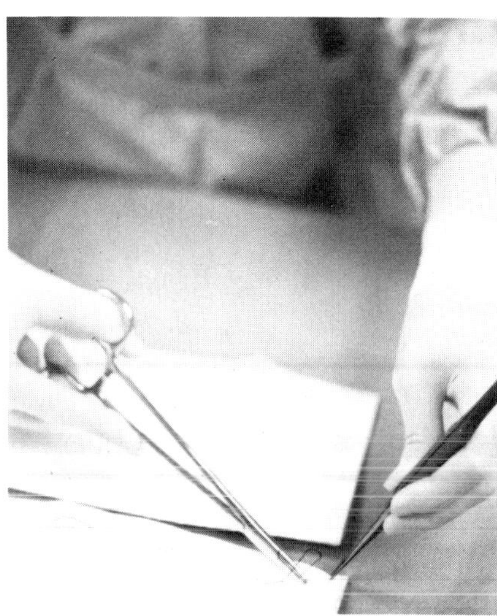

FIGURE 10-18
Suturing toward self.

bility. To begin suturing, the tissue is grasped with the forceps and, with the hand in the prone position, the needle tip is inserted. The needle should enter a structure at right angles to its surface. The hand is rotated at the wrist so that the needle is arched through the tissue. The tip of the needle should be readily accessible after it goes through the tissue. To withdraw the tip of a curved needle, the hand starts in a pronated position. The needle tip is withdrawn with the forceps or the needleholder and pulled through the tissue in a small arc that follows its curve. While doing this, the hand turns 180 degrees to supination; this is a natural movement that involves only the forearm. Damage to the needle tip is avoided by grasping the needle on the body rather than on the tip itself. If the needle does not reach through the tissue, a larger needle is needed. The assistant should not attempt to force the needle through, because it may break. If the tissue layers are close together, both sides may be sutured with one placement of the needle. In many instances the suture needle is passed through one side and then through the opposing side (see Figure 10-19).

INTERRUPTED SUTURES

Interrupted sutures may be used for bowel and fascial tissues or when sutures will be under increased tension. Although this technique is somewhat slower than a continuous suture, it is safer if there is potential of suture breaking due to tension or tissue fragility. Interrupted sutures also enable more precise approximation of tissues and thus are frequently used for plastic surgery, where minimal scarring is desired. When suturing with interrupted sutures, care must be taken to leave an adequate amount of suture on both sides for tying.

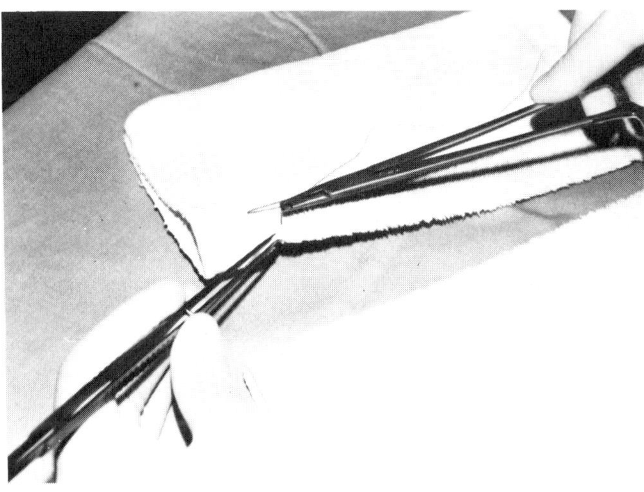

FIGURE 10-19
Placing suture in one side.

CONTINUOUS SUTURES

In this faster suturing method, the suture is pulled through the tissue in one continuous motion after the needle has been passed through both sides of the wound (see Figure 10-20). Care must be taken not to pull the suture too tightly; this will either strangulate tissue and cause possible necrosis or cause the suture to cut through the tissue.

FOLLOWING A SUTURE

Following the suture for the surgeon using a continuous suture must be done carefully and correctly if it is to be effective. The assistant holds adequate tension to keep the tissue layers together without distorting or strangulating the tissues. Whenever possible, the suture is held from the exited side of the wound, because there is less chance of tearing the tissue with the suture (see Figure 10-20). The suture should be held close enough to the wound to avoid shortening the suture length, but not so close as to obstruct the placement of the needleholder and sutures. When releasing the suture, it should not be allowed to become entangled in drapes, instruments, or other sutures. Timing between the assistant and the surgeon is important in relation to releasing and grasping the suture. If tension is released prematurely, the suture line may loosen, resulting in poor approximation of the tissues, or the remaining suture may fall onto the suture site and obscure the surgeon's view before he moves the needle to reload it.

It may be necessary to grasp the suture with a forceps rather than with the fingers, as when the suture is too short to grasp with the fingers or when the operative site is deep or restricted. When grasping the suture with a for-

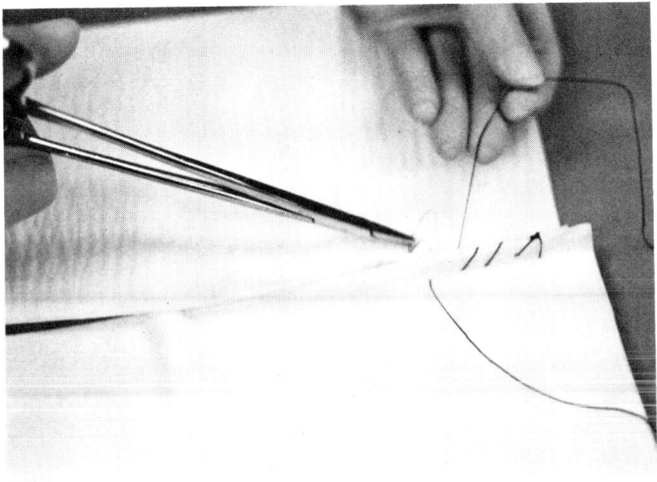

FIGURE 10-20
Technique for placing continuous sutures.

ceps, the assistant must be careful not to grasp too tightly or use a crushing type of forceps; damage to the suture could cause the suture to break immediately or could weaken the suture, causing it to break later.

If necessary, it is possible to follow one's own suture when suturing. To do so, the suture is grasped with the little finger in the hand holding the tissue forceps (see Figure 10-21). This technique can be most useful and is easily learned.

SUBCUTANEOUS SUTURES

Subcutaneous tissue suturing is often done by the RN first assistant. The suture is usually an absorbable type. Sutures are used in this type of tissue to provide tissue approximation and eliminate dead space. It is not done to provide strength to the wound, because the tissue is fragile and soft. Sutures are placed vertically through the tissue from one side of the wound to the other. Horizontal sutures should not be used; they can compromise the blood supply to the skin. Sutures must be placed close enough together to eliminate any "gaps" in the suture line. Tension on the sutures must be adequate to hold the tissue together but must not be excessive, or else the suture may pull through the tissue or strangulate the tissue itself. The suture needle must not be placed too deep into the tissue, because it is possible to inadvertently penetrate the skin, exposing the suture to the skin surface and providing a potential route of wound infection.

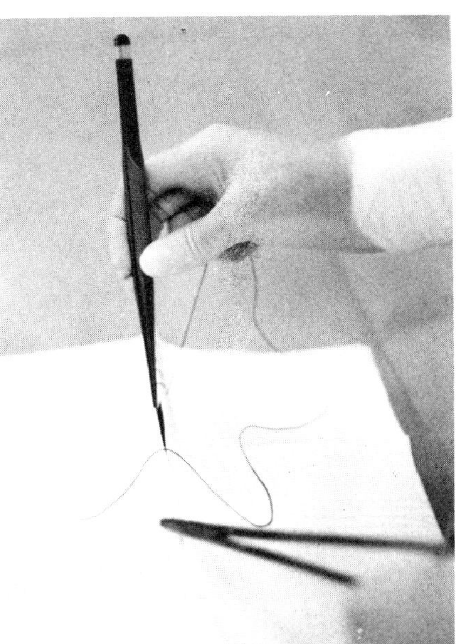

FIGURE 10-21
Following own suture. Note that suture is grasped by little finger.

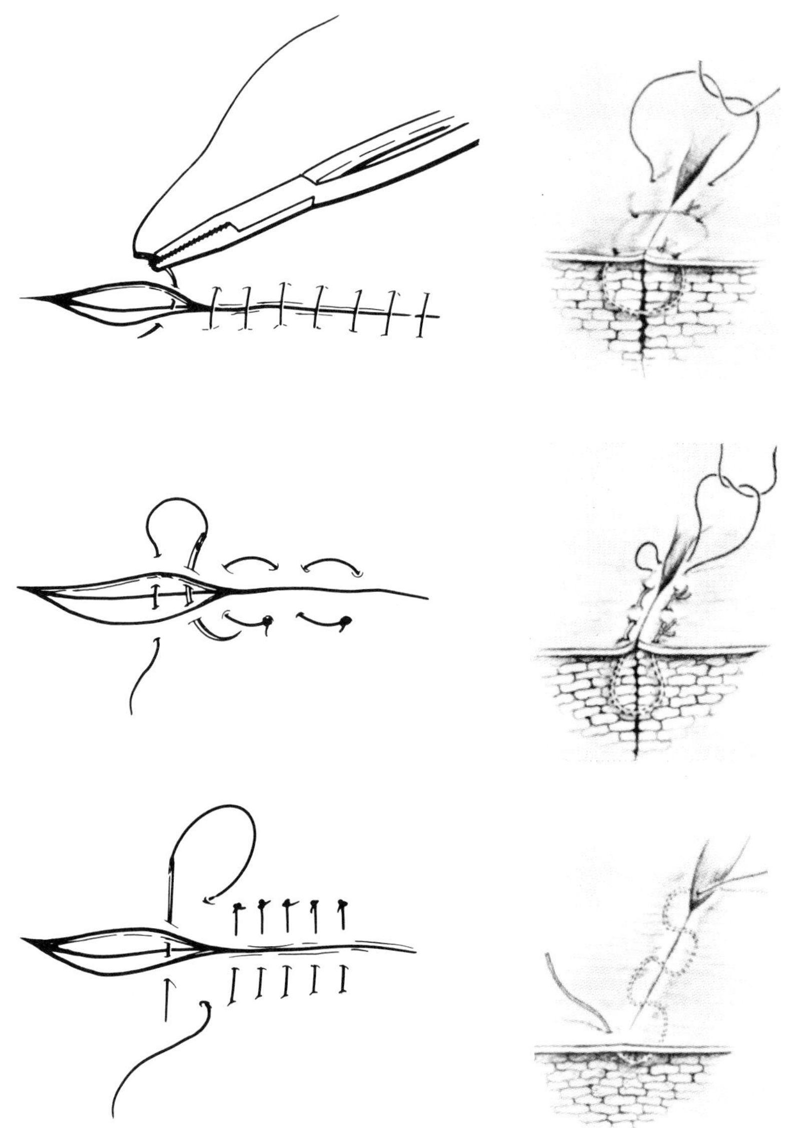

FIGURE 10-22
Examples of interrupted skin sutures. *(Top)* Simple interrupted suture. *(Center)* Interrupted horizontal mattress suture. *(Bottom)* Interrupted vertical mattress suture. *(From Wound Closure Manual, 1985. Courtesy of ETHICON, Inc., a Johnson & Johnson Company, Somerville, NJ)*

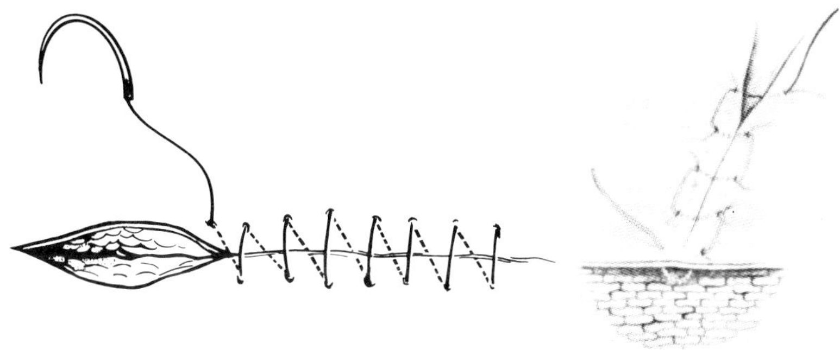

FIGURE 10-23
Examples of continuous skin suturing technique. *(Left)* Continuous over-and-over suture. *(Right)* Continuous horizontal mattress suture. *(From Wound Closure Manual, 1985. Courtesy of ETHICON, Inc., a Johnson & Johnson Company, Somerville, NJ)*

SKIN SUTURES

Skin suturing technique depends on the type of incision, its location, the patient's condition, the desired result, and the surgeon's preference. RN first assistants commonly do this type of suturing.

Suture materials used for the skin are nonabsorbable and must be removed postoperatively. Monofilament sutures are more commonly used because they are less traumatic to the tissue. This type of suture is smooth and easier to remove. Braided materials may harbor infectious organisms and potentially cause superficial wound infection. More tissue reaction will occur with the braided sutures. The suture selected should be as fine a gauge as possible, while still providing the necessary support to the skin edges as they are reapproximated.

Interrupted sutures provide a better cosmetic result as the wound heals. The "simple" interrupted suture is frequently used. Simple interrupted sutures are placed by entering the skin on one side of the wound edge and exiting on the other side. The entry and exit points are usually only a few millimeters from the incision site and should be approximately the same distance from the skin edges on each side, to avoid distortion of the incision line. After the suture is tied, the knot is pulled to one side of the wound, close to the skin. This technique will adjust the tension and equalize the skin edges. The result of the simple suture is a square-shaped suture that encloses an equal area of dermis on both sides and avoids inverting skin edges.

"Interrupted mattress" sutures may be needed in instances where increased accuracy is necessary. Mattress sutures also provide more support to the suture line; this may be needed in situations where there is increased strain on the suture line itself (see Figure 10-22). The horizontal mattress is

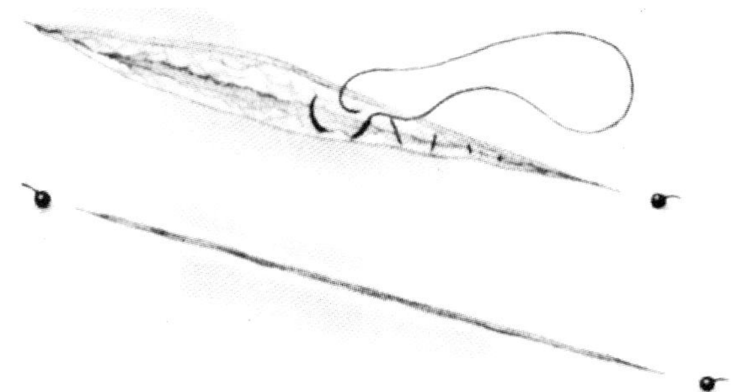

FIGURE 10-24
Continuous subcuticular closure anchored with lead shot. *(From Wound Closure Manual, 1985. Courtesy of ETHICON, Inc., a Johnson & Johnson Company, Somerville, NJ)*

more commonly used in fascia than on skin. The interrupted mattress is placed by entering and exiting the skin edges at a slightly greater distance than with the simple interrupted stitch. Once the first stitch is placed, the needle is passed back through the skin very close to the edges (approximately 2 mm to 3 mm) and then tied in place. Again, gentle, loose tying approximation allows for the slight edema that occurs during wound healing.

Continuous suturing is frequently used on the skin because it can be done quickly, but the cosmetic result is not as good as with the interrupted techniques. To place the sutures, the assistant begins on one side of the incision and exits on the other side at approximately the same distance from the skin edges on each side. The suture is tied, and the short end of the suture is cut. The suture is then used in a "running" fashion or in an "over and over" looping fashion until the wound is closed. A continuous mattress suturing technique can be used if needed (see Figure 10-23).

A subcuticular suture technique gives the best cosmetic result, with a scar that is very fine. The RN first assistant will find that subcuticular sutures are most valuable for skin closure in parts of the body with a thick dermal layer or where skin is firmly attached to strong subdermal fascia. If the dermis is thin, subcuticular closure should be avoided. An absorbable suture is usually used; however, a nonabsorbable suture can be used and removed later. To remove the nonabsorbable suture, it is necessary to secure the ends of the

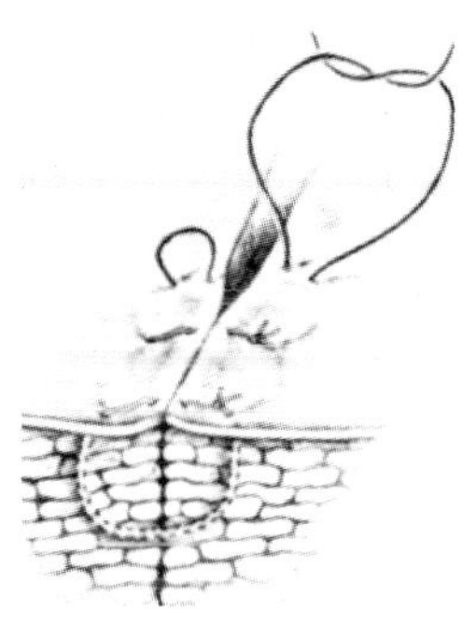

FIGURE 10-25
Continuous subcuticular suturing technique. *(From Wound Closure Manual, 1985. Courtesy of ETHICON, Inc., a Johnson & Johnson Company, Somerville, NJ)*

PROXIMATE* skin staplers

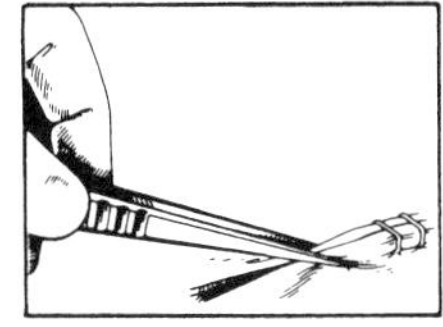

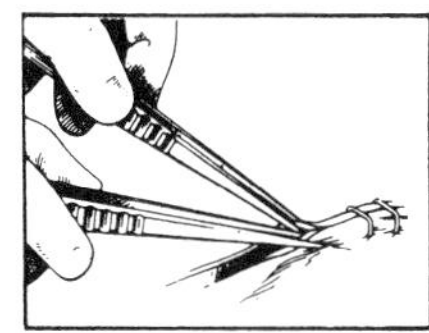

1. Evert and approximate skin edges as desired with one or two tissue forceps.

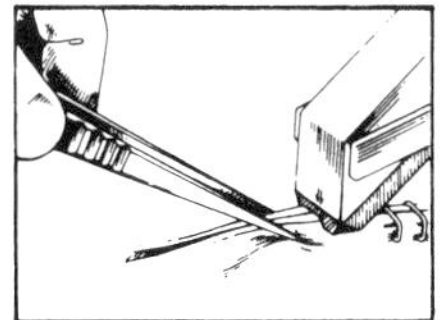

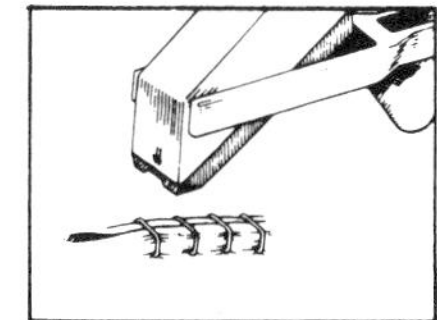

2. Position stapler very lightly over everted skin edges and squeeze trigger.

3. Back stapler off the staple.

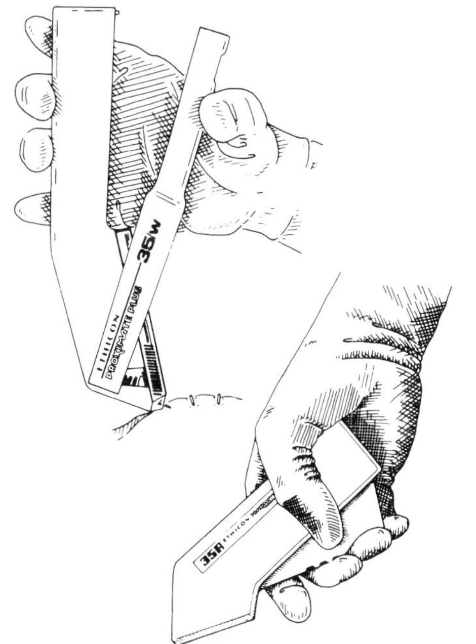

4. Both stapler configurations can be fired from any angle.

FIGURE 10-26
Skin stapling device. *(From Wound Closure Manual, 1985. Courtesy of ETHICON, Inc., a Johnson & Johnson Company, Somerville, NJ)*

suture at the skin level, where they can be easily grasped to remove (see Figure 10-24). Subcuticular stitches are placed in the lower part of the dermis layer. The first stitch is placed into the corner of the incision just below the dermal–epidermal junction. The stitches are placed in a horizontal fashion and alternated from one side to the other, with each stitch taking small epidermal bites. The stitches must be placed at the same depth on each side; if not, the wound will be uneven (see Figure 10-25). When the suture line is completed, the suture is tightened by pulling the ends, and an instrument tie completed on each end at skin level.

Skin staples are being used with increasing frequency and are very versatile. The skin edges are everted and approximated with one or two tissue forceps as the staple is applied (see Figure 10-26). Staples cause minimal tissue trauma or compression, and provide a superior cosmetic result to that produced by continuous or interrupted skin sutures.

Regardless of the type of skin suturing technique used, some basic principles must be followed. Bleeding in the subcutaneous layer and skin layer should be controlled before suturing these layers. Bleeding can distort the wound, disrupt the suture line, and create hematomas that could result in a potential site for infection. When the first bite of the needle is made, the wrist should be presupinated to cock the hand in a position that gives strength to drive the needle through the skin. Sutures are placed with as little trauma as possible. Tissue is handled carefully and gently, and crushing injury is avoided. Sutures are never pulled tightly, because tissue can become strangulated and the blood supply compromised. Sutures should be made only just tight enough to hold the opposing tissues together. Tissue edema in the postoperative period can increase the pressure of tissue against the sutures, resulting in "hatchmark" scarring; this can be avoided by leaving sutures slightly loose when placed. To achieve this technique, the assistant notes when the skin edges first make contact approximation during a closing stitch. The skin at the site rises just slightly above the surrounding skin surface. This is usually an indication of the right amount of tension at the suture line; the knot can then be set. Skin edges are slightly everted as they are reapproximated, which results in better healing and a better appearing scar. The skin edges are aligned as closely as possible to their original appearance.

CONCLUSION

Regardless of the suturing material and method used, the RN first assistant's goal during any suturing activity is to achieve a wound that heals without complications. To achieve this goal, the RN first assistant makes educated choices about the type of suture material, suturing instrument, and suturing technique. Coupled with these cognitive abilities, the RN first assistant must be proficient in the manipulative skills involved in suturing. The result will be effective and efficient patient care.

REVIEW QUESTIONS

1. One of the RN first assistant's goals during suturing is to leave minimal foreign material in the wound. To achieve this, suture should be selected that has
   a. a low coefficient of friction
   b. antimicrobial impregnated in it
   c. high tensile strength and small diameter
   d. tightly braided fibers with negligible interstices
2. The rate of suture absorption should correspond to the
   a. tensile strength of the tissue
   b. rate of healing of the tissue
   c. USP designation as type A or B
   d. suture diameter
3. Suture security depends both on knot-holding ability and
   a. suture diameter
   b. incision location and length
   c. intrinsic pliability
   d. suture tensile strength
4. An advantage of multifilament suture is its
   a. ability to drag through tissue
   b. decreased tissue trauma
   c. knot-holding ability
   d. capillarity
5. The most tissue reactive absorbable suture is
   a. plain catgut
   b. chromic catgut
   c. polydiaxanone
   d. polybutester
6. In general, a monofilament suture requires ______ knot throws for security than a multifilament.
   a. fewer
   b. more
   c. the same number of
   d. more, but only if it is coated with a lubricant
7. The major disadvantage of wire suture is its
   a. inertness
   b. need to be twisted for knot security
   c. high tensile strength
   d. handling characteristics
8. When assisting during wound closure with a suture that will be used for several interrupted stitches, the RN first assistant who is tying first grasps
   a. the short end of the suture
   b. the needle
   c. the long end of the suture
   d. a pair of forceps

9. To assist in grasping a needle as it exits tissue during skin closure, the RN first assistant grasps the needle with a needleholder and
   a. brings most of the needle above the skin surface
   b. brings all of the needle out in a 90-degree arc
10. A needle that is grasped in a needleholder too close to the eye may
    a. break
    b. notch
    c. bend
    d. slip
11. When suturing very dense tissue, the RN first assistant may select the _______ grip.
    a. palmed
    b. thenar
    c. thumb-ring finger
    d. pencil
12. The most traditional needleholder grip, and one that yields both precision and needle control, is the _______ grip.
    a. palmed
    b. thenar
    c. thumb-ring finger
    d. pencil
13. When using a very fine needleholder, the _______ grip is used.
    a. palmed
    b. thenar
    c. thumb-ring finger
    d. pencil
14. Although precision is less exacting with the _______ grip, it is used for rapid, easy suturing.
    a. palmed
    b. thenar
    c. thumb-ring finger
    d. pencil
15. When suturing, the hand begins in what position?
    a. supine
    b. prone
    c. semi-supine
    d. right-angled
16. When following a suture for a surgeon, it is more desirable to hold the suture from which side of the wound?
    a. exit
    b. entry
17. During subcutaneous closure, _______ sutures should not be used because they can compromise blood supply to the skin.
    a. vertical
    b. horizontal

18. During skin closure, the RN first assistant uses a technique that _______ skin edges.
    a. everts
    b. inverts
19. During subcuticular closure, each stitch takes small _______ bites.
    a. dermal
    b. epidermal
20. The right amount of tension at the suture line takes into consideration the potential for
    a. dehiscence
    b. suture sinus tract infection
    c. hematoma formation
    d. postoperative swelling

Answers

1. c	8. a	15. b
2. b	9. a	16. a
3. d	10. c	17. b
4. c	11. a	18. a
5. a	12. c	19. b
6. b	13. d	20. d
7. d	14. b	

REFERENCES

1. Edgerton MT: The Art of Surgical Technique, pp 149–153. Baltimore, Williams & Wilkins, 1988

BIBLIOGRAPHY

Cardiovascular, Thoracic, General Surgical Pilling Instruments. Fort Washington, PA, Narco Scientific, 1980

McShane R, Perry A: Skin lacerations: Suturing and caring for the wound. Clinical Nurse Practitioner, 2(2):8–10, 1984

Swartz S, Shires GT, Spencer F, Storer E: Principles of Surgery, 4th ed. San Francisco, McGraw-Hill, 1984

Wind GG, Rich NM: Principles of Surgical Technique: The Art of Surgery. Baltimore, Urban & Schwarzenberg, 1987

Wound Closure Manual. Somerville, NJ, ETHICON, 1985

11 Wound Healing

*Jane C. Rothrock**

Wound healing focuses on the reestablishment of normal tissue physiology. This is a normal reaction to injury and is the keystone in the foundation of surgical principles. The surgeon and RN first assistant collaborate to augment the forces of repair and resistance to infection. Surgical wound management is based on knowledge of the physiology of wound healing and interference with the body's natural mechanism of self-repair. Though it is beyond the scope of this chapter to discuss in entirety the complex mechanisms of wound healing, fundamental principles of this process are shared by all types of wounds found in surgery. Understanding these principles is germane to the quality of wound care provided by the RN first assistant and the type of results obtained. This chapter focuses on the biology of wound healing in the subcutaneous tissues along with those considerations involved in daily preoperative, intraoperative, and postoperative wound management encountered in perioperative patients.

TYPES OF WOUNDS

Wounds may be classified by etiology as either surgical or traumatic and further subdivided on the basis of tissue loss as either closed or open. A closed wound heals by *primary intention*; it is a sharply made wound that is accurately reapproximated within hours of the incision and heals with minimal space between its edges (see Fig. 11-1). An open wound heals by *secondary intention*; the tissue defect decreases in size by contraction and is filled by the

* *In the first edition, this chapter was written by Leonard T. Yu.*

formation of large amounts of new connective tissue, vessels, and epithelium. The new tissue regenerated in this process is known as granulation tissue. Open wounds are usually external, but healing by secondary intention is also seen in the healing of a closed space created after a pneumonectomy or a serum collection under a skin flap after mastectomy.

PHYSIOLOGY OF WOUND HEALING

Several biologic properties are shared by both closed and open wounds. This discussion of wound healing examines the physiology of closed and open wounds and then focuses on events that are unique to wound healing.

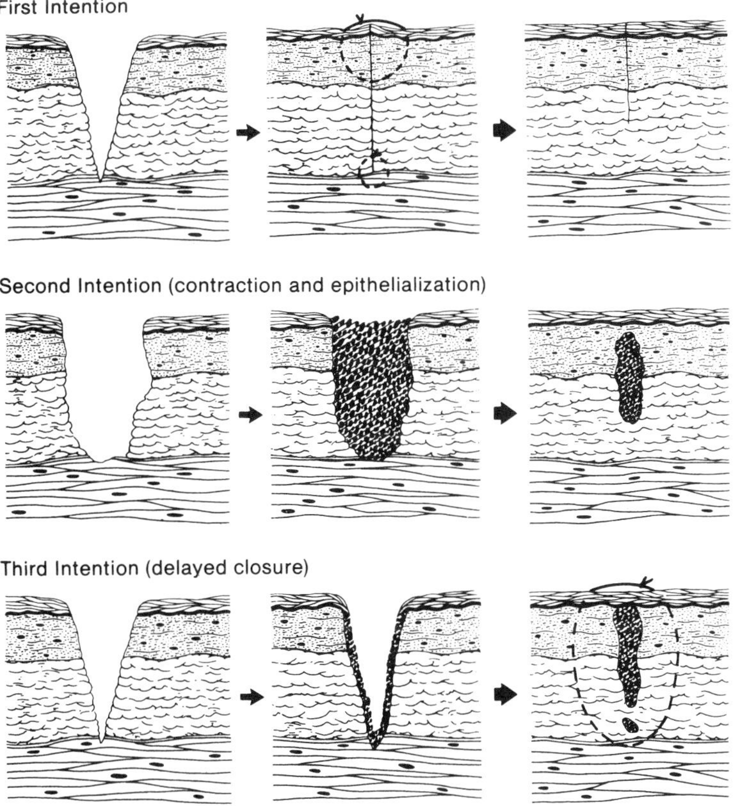

FIGURE 11-1
Classification of wound healing. *First intention*—A clean incision is made with primary closure; there is minimal scarring. *Second intention* (contraction and epithelialization)—The wound is left open to granulate in with resultant large scab and abnormal dermal-epidermal junction. *Third intention* (delayed closure)—The wound is left open and closed secondarily when there is no evidence of infection. *(Hardy JD Hardy's Textbook of Surgery, 2nd ed. Philadelphia, JB Lippincott, 1988, p 107.)*

CLOSED WOUNDS

Healing of closed wounds involves several phases. Although they are discussed as separate entities, the phases frequently overlap chronologically and may occur simultaneously. Following tissue injury, an *inflammatory phase* is initiated; vascular and cellular responses occur immediately when tissue is cut or injured. The length of the inflammatory phase is related to the degree of wound contamination; it may extend from several days to several weeks. The less contaminated the wound, the faster it will heal. In clean wounds, those created aseptically in surgery, few inflammatory cells are seen after 5–7 days.

Injury disrupts tissue integrity; blood vessels are damaged, cells are broken, and the complement cascade is initiated. Transient vasoconstriction occurs, followed by blood vessel dilation. Capillaries become permeable to plasma proteins and plasma that leaks into the site of injury. White blood cells stick to vascular endothelial surfaces and then move through vessel walls into the adjacent tissue. Within hours after the initial insult, the wound fills with a cellular inflammatory exudate containing white blood cells, red blood cells, plasma proteins, and fibrin. The duration and intensity of this phase depends on the amount of local tissue damage. Extensive injury or the presence of foreign material in the wound can prolong this phase for months. In the usual clean surgical incision, inflammation lasts several days.

The white blood cells are the key cells in the inflammatory response. Acting as the digestive tract of the wound, they engulf and remove injured tissue and cellular debris. Injured tissue and bacteria are believed to release chemotactic substances (chemoattractants) to draw leukocytes and other macrophages into the wound. This stimulates fibroblast activity and neovascularization in the wound space.

The *migratory* phase (also referred to as the epithelial phase) evolves from the inflammatory phase. Neutrophils, the predominant inflammatory cells, are gradually replaced by macrophages. These cells engulf damaged tissue and bacteria, digesting them in lysosomes. If wound contamination is excessive, then the white blood cells are overwhelmed; as these cells die, they release lysosomal enzymes such as proteases and collagenases, which contribute to tissue damage and prolong the inflammatory response.

Many substances attract fibroblasts and other mesenchymal cells into the wound during the migratory phase. A protein known as platelet-derived growth factor (PDGF) seems to initiate the healing cascade by recruiting infection-fighting cells. Fibroblast growth factor (FGF) promotes growth of new blood vessels that supply local cells with nutrients. These natural proteins are currently the foci of research studies seeking to speed postsurgical healing of immunosuppressed patients.[1,2]

The epidermis adjacent to the wound edge thickens as early as 24 hours after injury. Basal cells enlarge, undergo mitosis, and migrate across the surface of the wound defect, but these epithelial cells migrate only over viable tissue. They are stopped by contact inhibition. By 48 hours, the wound surface may be completely re-epithelialized. After the wound is bridged, a layering of the epithelium is reestablished and keratinization proceeds.

The *proliferative* (also referred to as the cellular or fibroblastic) phase of wound healing begins at this time and may last for several weeks. By 2 or 3 days following injury, fibroblasts derived from locally injured or stimulated mesenchymal (perivascular) tissues invade the wound; these predominate by day 10. Fibroblasts are responsible for the synthesis and secretion of collagen, elastin, and the proteoglycons of ground substance. The fibrin strands that had filled the wound earlier now act as scaffolding for fibroblast movement. Collagen fibers subsequently appear soon after this cellular invasion.

Rapid capillary proliferation by budding of existing venules promotes neovascularization as the nutritional needs of the healing wound increase and a new vascular network is generated. New vessels develop from existing vessels as capillaries. Capillaries grow from the wound edges toward areas of inadequate perfusion. When they meet other developing capillaries, they join and establish new blood vessels. The lymphatic system is also reestablished at this time, facilitating local drainage of interstitial fluid.

A phase characterized by fibroplasia becomes evident by 4–5 weeks, when the fibroblasts decrease in number and collagen fibers fill the wound. These fibers initially appear as early as 4–5 days after injury in randomly oriented bundles. They gradually enlarge and produce a massive, dense, collagenous structure (the scar), which binds the severed tissues together. A phase of *scar remodeling* then ensues. During this phase, the collagen fibers in the scar are altered (cross-linked) and rewoven into different architectural patterns that affect the gross appearance of the "healed" wound. In reality, it is more accurate to think of scar physiology as a continuous dynamic process rather than an event that ceases at a given time. This process may last many years and is the reason an "old wound" may be affected by later events in particular patients.

Collagen. The body's principal structural protein, collagen is the major constituent of skin, tendons, ligaments, bones, cartilage, fascia, and the septa of various organs. It is composed of a group of glycoproteins, which are synthesized initially as a gel in the healing wound. The rate of collagen synthesis normally peaks 5–7 days after injury, which coincidentally is the time when the wound experiences its most rapid increase in tensile strength. Paradoxically, collagen also undergoes lysis or enzymatic modification of its fibers while synthesis takes place. The breakdown of old collagen at the same rate as synthesis of new collagen is known as scar maturation; it serves to orient and weave the collagen fibers along lines of stress. The resulting architectural patterns determine the mechanical properties of the scar. Although the cross-links between the collagen strands increase during the remodeling phase, scar tissue never reaches the tensile strength of unwounded tissue.

OPEN WOUNDS

Open wounds share many of the basic healing processes discussed for closed wounds; however, the need to repair a tissue defect in these injuries also involves wound contraction and granulation tissue formation. Following the loss of tissue, an inflammatory exudate collects on the surface of the wound.

Cellular mitosis and migration from adjacent tissues give this wound bed a finely "granular" appearance. After a delay of 2–3 days, the wound undergoes contraction during the healing process. The wound margins move toward each other, stretching surrounding skin to make the surface defect smaller. Contraction is most rapid by 5–10 days and slows by 2 weeks. The cells responsible for this phenomenon are known as myofibroblasts. In areas of loose, mobile skin, little deformity and acceptable cosmetic results may be obtained by wound contraction. Regions of the body with poor skin mobility (*e.g.*, face, anterior lower leg, hands, neck, breasts) cannot be healed by this mechanism, and severe contraction deformity, a nonhealing ulcer, or healing by epithelialization alone may result.

Epithelialization occurs beneath whatever nonliving covering (*e.g.*, scab eschar) is on the wound. Epithelial cells migrate from the wound margins over the collagenous granulation tissue at the base of the wound bed. They usually cannot migrate more than a few centimeters from the wound edges, and the resulting junction of epithelium and underlying scar tissue is relatively weak. It is a poor substitute for skin, because minor shearing forces can disrupt this layer. It frequently deteriorates after traumatization. Epithelialization and contraction may be minimized by a combination of immediate skin coverage of the open wound and mechanical splinting of the adjacent tissues.

Examination of these wounds shows that heavily contaminated open wounds display markedly decreased bacterial counts during the 3–6 days after injury. Consequently, many of these wounds can safely be left open for healing by secondary intention or closed after several days with markedly decreased rates of wound infection. This latter technique is known as *delayed primary closure* (DPC) (see Figure 11-1).

SKIN GRAFTS

If a wound can be directly approximated without excessive tension or distortion, then this is most often the method of choice. Wounds deficient in surface covering may require closure by a skin graft or flap if secondary or delayed primary closure cannot be done. The skin graft is a segment of dermis and epidermis that has been separated from its blood supply and site of origin (donor site) before being transplanted to another area of the body (recipient site). It may consist of the epidermis and a portion of the dermis (split thickness) or the epidermis and all of the dermis (full thickness). It is usually used as a permanent wound covering and may be used to close any wound with a sufficient blood supply to produce granulation tissue.

A skin graft is placed in contact with its recipient bed, from which it initially absorbs a plasma-like fluid. A fibrin network forms between the graft and the bed, holding the graft in place. Vascular buds grow into this network and then into the graft during the first 48 hours after grafting. Lymphatics are also restored, so that drainage from the graft is established by the fourth or fifth postoperative day. The capillary buds that grow into the graft race to vascularize the graft before its cells undergo autolysis and death, as the plasmatic flow from the bed into the graft is insufficient to support indefinite survival. Improper tension on the graft, fluid (blood or serum) beneath the graft, and movement of the graft on its bed will delay or prevent revascularization and may result in graft failure. For these reasons, the RN first assistant will need to consider a patient care regimen that includes skin graft immobilization during the first 5–7 days after placement; compression dressings may help with this. The risk of seromas and hematomas can be limited by elevating the part, if possible. In patients with flaps, the blood supply must not be impaired by pressure from a dressing, poor patient positioning, or hematoma formation; drains are frequently placed to encourage tissue approximation, as well as to prevent the collection of blood and serum under the flap.[3]

PHYSICAL EVENTS

Wounds begin to gain strength immediately after repair, irrespective of the type of closure. Initially, only relatively weak intercellular forces—that is, protein adhesion and fibrin polymerization—are responsible. After collagen fibers begin to appear, near the third day after injury, wound strength increases rapidly. The healing wound has its greatest mass approximately 3 weeks after injury, but the gain in strength continues at a rapid, constant rate for close to 4 months. After this the rate slows, but the wound continues to gain strength for about 1 year, reflecting prolonged collagen turnover. Wounds rarely if ever regain the strength and resilience of uninjured tissue; normal elasticity is lost in scars, which become relatively inelastic and brittle.

The scar undergoes a progressive change in its appearance during this period of remodeling or maturation. It usually demonstrates a gradual loss of redness and firmness, becoming white, soft, and nonadherent to underlying structures. The healed wound may appear narrow or wide, raised or depressed, and delicate or thick. These varied end results reflect a combination of surgical technique, the activity of collagenase (which causes collagen turnover), and physical forces that act on the healing wound. Fibroblasts and collagen fibers tend to align along lines of tension; even minor stresses on the healing wound affect their activity. Incisions crossing lines of changing dimension (joints) produce large hypertrophic scars. Incisions within normal skin creases where tension is minimal tend to produce small, well-healed scars. For unknown reasons, scars exhibit more rapid wound maturation in older patients than in children.

SECONDARY HEALING

A wound reopened within a week of primary repair will heal more rapidly than the original wound. This phenomenon, called *secondary healing*, is believed to be related to an immediate onset of fibroplasia without the usual 4- to 6-day lag period after injury. These wounds do not demonstrate increased rates of wound healing, and the ultimate strength of the healed wounds is the same as that of wounds that underwent primary repair. The sole difference is the absence of a lag phase in secondary healing wounds; the healing process already under way simply continues without alteration or delay.

Reopening an old, mature wound starts a different set of events than those that occurred when previously uninjured skin was incised. The scar that results from a second wound is different than the initial scar in both physical characteristics and appearance. The final secondary scar usually has less collagen and appears less hypertrophic than the initial scar.

METABOLIC REQUIREMENTS OF WOUND HEALING

All the steps involved in wound healing require numerous synthetic and energy-consuming reactions. The inflammatory response and the delicate balance between collagen synthesis and lysis are particularly dependent on the patient's metabolic status. The wound makes a nutritional demand; unless this demand is met by dietary sources, the body is forced to turn on itself, catabolizing certain of its own tissues to acquire the metabolites needed for repair. It should be noted, however, that patients undergoing major elective surgery who have no nutritional disturbances before the surgery are not apt to develop wound healing problems secondary to metabolic alterations induced by the operation unless a complication, such as serious shock, infection, renal failure, or liver failure, develops.

Proteins and amino acids must be available for cell multiplication and synthesis of the enzymes and substrates critically involved in the healing process. Protein deficiency—particularly deficits or imbalances in essential amino acids such as methionine, cystine, and lysine—delay almost all aspects of healing, including neovascularization, fibroblast proliferation, collagen synthesis, and wound remodeling. If protein deficiency is prolonged or liver function is severely impaired, serum albumin levels decrease, resulting in excessive edema that may impair wound healing. Resistance to infection is seriously lowered in protein-deficient patients, which can further complicate repair.

Glucose is the body's major metabolic fuel. Short-term deficits may be supplemented by gluconeogenesis. Fibroblasts and leukocytes metabolize glucose, and glucose availability is vital during the first few days after injury. Glucose is of little value if a lack of insulin prevents its utilization, as in diabetes. Furthermore, hyperosmolarity resulting from hyperglycemia, another consequence of diabetes, also interferes with wound repair.

Certain unsaturated fatty acids (arachidonic, linoleic, and linolenic) are considered to be essential and must be supplied exogenously. They are important for the production of prostaglandins, which regulate cellular metabolism, inflammation, and circulation.

Vitamin A aids the entrance of macrophages into wounds. It is vital to the initiation of repair and may accelerate wound healing. Vitamin C (ascorbic acid) is involved in collagen turnover and can alter the balance of collagen metabolism. A deficiency of vitamin C (scurvy) causes new wounds to heal poorly and old wounds to reopen. Vitamin K is required for synthesis of clotting factors. Lack of this vitamin may lead to clotting abnormalities and excessive bleeding into wounds.

Several minerals, particularly magnesium, are involved in many energy-producing cycles and protein synthesis. Of the trace elements necessary for wound repair, zinc (deficient in burned or highly stressed patients) affects epithelialization, wound strength, and collagen protein production. Iron is needed for the hydroxylation of collagen; copper and manganese are important in the enzyme systems required for collagen cross-linking.

Patients with wounds healing by secondary intention are usually discharged from care before the wound is closed. A study of the adequacy of overall calorie, protein, Vitamin C, and zinc intake in a small group of such patients indicated that most of the patients had inadequate caloric and zinc intake, over half had inadequate protein intake, and a third had inadequate vitamin C intake. This study suggests that RN first assistants should pay serious attention to patient education and postdischarge follow-up of nutritional intake with patients whose wounds are healing by secondary intention.[4]

WOUND MANAGEMENT

With the advent of modern wound management, the devastating consequences of wound infections, and their significant mortality, has decreased. In early attempts to control wound infections, the perioperative team's effort was primarily directed towards controlling infecting organisms through antiseptic and aseptic surgical technique. The epidemiology of wound infections has changed as the perioperative team has worked to control sources of bacterial contamination. The 1990s has brought an increased focus on the host defense mechanisms as the effort to provide improved results of wound healing continues.

PREOPERATIVE CONSIDERATIONS

Optimal wound healing requires careful attention to the details of preoperative, intraoperative, and postoperative management. The chief preoperative concern for all types of wounds is reducing factors that may lead to postoperative wound infection. For elective surgery, this includes skin antisepsis and judicious antibiotic administration so that an adequate tissue level of the appropriate antibiotic is attained before the operative procedure. (See Chapter 4, Microbiologic Basis of Asepsis, for more information.) For traumatic wounds, major considerations include length of time between injury and treatment and the strength and type of foreign inoculum in the wound. An absolutely "safe" number of hours between injury and treatment that permits closure of traumatic wounds without the risk of subsequent wound infection does not exist. Rather, the decision to primarily close a traumatic wound depends on the injury's clinical appearance, its location on the body, method of injury, and ultimately the surgeon's judgment.

In many cases, contaminated wounds may be converted to clean ones for closure soon after inoculation. This frequently requires anesthesia of the involved area to permit adequate surgical debridement of nonviable tissue and foreign material. But although local anesthetics containing vasoconstrictors may prolong the duration of anesthesia, they may damage wound defenses in contaminated wounds by restricting local blood flow. Antibiotics have limited usefulness in preventing wound infection in most traumatic injuries; a fibrinous coagulum frequently surrounds bacteria in these wounds and serves to isolate them from contact with the antibiotic. Tetanus prophylaxis should not be neglected in these patients.

INTRAOPERATIVE FACTORS

The determinants of an infectious process are the infecting organism, the environment in which the infection occurs, and the host defense mechanisms. Controlling sources of infecting organisms—in surgery, most often bacteria— is vital. Endogenous bacteria play a significant role in wound infection. Remote infections, even those of the urinary tract, should be treated before elective surgery. The skin is a primary source of infection following clean operations (see Table 11-1). The perioperative team and the environment are other potential sources of exogenous contamination. Basic principles of asepsis are predominant, controllable factors by the RN first assistant. Less controllable is expected duration of the surgical procedure. During lengthy procedures, the sources of bacteria represent increased time at risk for contamination. Abdominal surgery is another risk factor; because major concentrations of endogenous bacteria are located in the abdomen, these operations are more likely to involve bacterial contamination. In all surgical procedures, the RN first assistant should work closely with the surgeon to carry out a procedure with minimal blood loss, avoidance of shock, and maintenance of blood volume, tissue perfusion, and tissue oxygenation. All of these efforts combine to minimize trauma and the secondary, unintended immunologic effects of major surgery.[5]

The many intraoperative factors that affect wound healing are discussed in detail in other chapters of this book. The driving force in the prevention of wound infection is knowledge and expertise in the fundamentals of aseptic

TABLE 11-1
Classification of Surgical Wounds

Classification	Description
Clean	Nontraumatic No inflammation No break in technique Respiratory, GI, GU tracts not entered Primary closure Drainage by closed system
Clean-contaminated	Respiratory, GI, GU tracts entered under control (no spillage)
Contaminated	Fresh, traumatic wound Gross spillage
Dirty/infected	Acute inflammation Traumatic wound with retained, devitalized tissue Perforated viscera

technique. An understanding of the microbiological principles of asepsis (see Chapter 4, Microbiologic Basis of Asepsis) assists the RN first assistant in breaking the chain of infection. The importance of preoperative skin antisepsis and the use of microbial barriers in creating and maintaining the sterile field (see Chapter 6, Perioperative Patient Preparation) guides the RN first assistant in initiating preventive patient care measures. Ensuring proper tissue handling (see Chapter 8, Principles of Tissue Handling), providing adequate exposure (see Chapter 9, Providing Exposure: Retractors and Retraction), judiciously selecting suture materials and suturing techniques (see Chapter 10, Suturing Materials and Techniques), skillfully handling clamps (see Chapter 12, Using Grasping Instruments), and achieving meticulous hemostasis (see Chapter 13, Providing Hemostasis) are all intraoperative maneuvers with which the RN first assistant is intimately involved. The critical role played by the RN first assistant during the intraoperative period contributes significantly to satisfactory patient outcomes related to wound healing. For this reason, much of this book explores in detail these critical elements of RN first assistant functions. Table 11-2 provides a brief, but not inclusive, review of important RN first assistant nursing behaviors to facilitate wound healing.

POSTOPERATIVE WOUND CARE

Initially applied under sterile conditions in the operating room, dressings prevent wound and suture line contamination, protect wounds from additional trauma, and immobilize surrounding skin. A wound's susceptibility to surface contamination is greatest during the first postoperative day. After this period a coagulum seals the wound, and the wound rapidly gains resistance to infection. Consequently, the dressings on elective surgical wounds are generally

TABLE 11-2

Nursing Diagnosis: High Risk for Infection

Definition: Patient at risk to be invaded by opportunistic or pathogenic agent from external source.

Risk Factors: Depend on endogenous and exogenous factors

Endogenous: Remote sites of infection; skin flora; nature and site of operation

Exogenous: Perioperative team and environment related

Related Factors: Chronic, concomitant diseases; immunosuppression or deficiency; impaired circulation, tissue perfusion; diabetes; obesity; medications (steroids, immunosuppressants, antimicrobials); surgery, especially abdominal; presence of invasive lines; trauma, presence of foreign body; malnutrition; age-extremes (newborn/elderly)

RNFA Care Regimen

1. Assess for risk and related factors.
2. Use nursing diagnosis, High Risk for Infection, when one or more factors is present.
3. Initiate preventive strategies:
   a. Collaborate in treatment of remote infection site
   b. Implement preoperative patient education (prepare patient and family/significant other for postoperative routines/care regimens):
      - early ambulation
      - techniques to promote coughing and deep breathing
      - nutrition
      - wound care
      - reportable signs and symptoms; how to contact RN first assistant/surgeon
      - medication regimen (postoperative, as appropriate)
      - home care referral, as necessary.
   c. Collaborate in:
      - preoperative skin preparation
      - selection of appropriate surgical barriers (gowns/drapes)
      - controlling perioperative environment
      - initiating principles of surgical technique to facilitate wound healing (duration of operation; cautious tissue handling; judicious use of electrosurgery, sutures, drains; careful hemostasis; maintenance of tissue perfusion; correct use of instruments; meticulous attention to surgical asepsis).

left intact until the wound is inspected 1–2 days after surgery. Exceptions may be made for dressings that become saturated with blood or serous drainage and thus effectively disrupt the sterile barrier created by the dressing. Traumatic wounds are at higher risk for wound infection and are generally examined within 24 hours after treatment.

Many skin irritations are mistakenly attributed to a problem with a wound or to an allergic reaction to tape. They may be caused by taping techniques or tape effects on skin. Tape should be applied without tension. It should be applied from the center of the incision outward, with gentle rubbing of the ends to improve adherence.[6] In a small study of the effects of paper-backed and plastic-backed adhesive tapes, skin irritation scores and skin stripping scores were lower for patients with paper-backed tape.[7] Stripping the skin of its superficial layer interferes with the skin's ability to control water metabolism and can interfere with wound healing.

Sutures and clips in skin are usually removed when their purpose has been achieved. Too early removal invites wound dehiscence and scar widening; on the other hand, leaving them in place too long leads to the development of epithelial-lined suture tracts, infection, and unsightly scars. As healing rates vary according to the patient's age and overall condition and the type of wound, an absolute rule for removing all types of sutures does not exist. Generally, in an uncomplicated wound, skin sutures are removed 5–15 days postoperatively. Retention sutures in the abdomen are usually removed after the third postoperative week.[8] Nonetheless, the RN first assistant should understand that such factors as the amount of tension on the wound edges, the presence of any risk factors that would prolong wound healing, and cosmetic concerns are better guidelines than postoperative day counts for the timing of suture or clip removal.

Wound drains and tubes are generally removed before the risk of induced infection or interference with healing outweighs their benefit—usually within 5 days, because most fluid collections will have been decompressed by that time. Changing wound wicks and packing daily helps keep wounds clean by gentle debridement and removal of wound debris and also facilitates delayed primary closure; most of these wounds may be closed safely 5 days after surgery.

Skin graft survival requires adequate continuous contact with the recipient bed. Grafts are usually immobilized with stents or splints to prevent shearing when the patient moves. These wounds are usually inspected 2–3 days postoperatively for fluid collection beneath the graft. Such collection frequently gives the overlying area of the graft a translucent appearance and can prevent successful grafting. Needle aspiration or an incision in the graft can evacuate the fluid while the graft is still viable and prevent potentially devastating complications. Skin grafts on extremities (particularly the lower extremities) are elevated after surgery to decrease dependent edema in the wound until adequate lymphatic drainage is restored.

EARLY WOUND COMPLICATIONS

Problems encountered in healing wounds may be broadly classified into those that occur early in the postoperative period and those that develop late. Infection, the most frequent complication, usually presents several days after surgery. Local signs may be occult, but patients often develop systemic signs of distress with fever, tachycardia, and elevated white blood cell counts that suggest an ongoing infectious process.

INFECTIONS

The nature, diagnosis, and treatment of wound infections is a multifaceted process. Subcutaneous abscesses, cellulitis, necrotizing soft tissue infection, and intrabdominal and retroperitoneal infections, as well as their etiologic agents, must be diagnosed correctly and treated quickly. Wound surveillance, close patient assessment and evaluation, laboratory confirmation, and balancing the risks and inherent benefits of antibiotic therapy are all major considerations in infection control.

Cellulitis. A bacterial infection spreading in tissue planes, cellulitis usually causes intense inflammation manifested locally as tenderness, pain, swelling, erythema, and warmth. The responsible organism is frequently streptococcus. Treatment involves adequate rest to decrease muscle contractions that may force bacteria into lymphatics and veins. Elevation of limbs reduces dependent edema, and heat enhances local blood flow in the affected area. Drainage is rarely used and is indicated only to relieve pressure-induced ischemia. Appropriate systemic antibiotics are indicated.

Abscess. Localized bacterial infection marked by a circumscribed area of pus (necrotic tissue, bacteria, and white blood cells) constitutes an abscess. Abscesses tend to develop point tenderness and fluctuate on palpation. They are often under high pressure and tend to seed bacteria, causing bacteremia or sepsis by invasion of vascular spaces, or cellulitis from involvement of adjacent tissues. They should be surgically drained or excised with the resulting wound packed open to prevent recurrence of a closed-space infection. Rest, heat, and elevation are helpful, but antibiotics may not be indicated unless regional or systemic involvement is evident.

Lymphangitis. Bacterial spread through the lymphatic system, usually arising from a local area of cellulitis or abscess, is known as lymphangitis. Antibiotics, local heat, and rest, along with proper treatment of the infectious source, are appropriate therapy.

Tetanus. A complication of traumatic wounds rarely seen today, tetanus is caused by a toxin from *Clostridium tetani* bacteria that usually manifests itself after an incubation period of 7–10 days after inoculation. Tetanus should be suspected in a patient with insomnia, irritability, tremors, spasms, and rigidity of muscles adjacent to a traumatic wound. Treatment involves tetanus immune globulin administration and sedation. Occasionally, mechanical ventilation and surgical debridement of necrotic tissues with wide excision of the affected area are indicated.

Gas Gangrene. Clostridial myositis, also known as gas or invasive gangrene, is a rapidly progressive infection that causes extensive local and regional tissue destruction and systemic toxemia. It arises from injuries associated with devitalized muscle and decreased local oxygen tension. Swelling and pain present early (within 24 hours) after injury and may be associated with crepitus from gas formation in the muscles. Often, the wound produces a thin, watery, brown, foul-smelling discharge that may contain gas bubbles and bacteria. Skin overlying the affected area may appear bronze-colored and dusky; dark red muscle may protrude through the wound. The patient rapidly develops systemic signs of pallor, weakness, apathy, profuse diaphoresis, dyspnea, and tachycardia that seems out of proportion to the low-grade fever. Such a patient faces impending septic shock. Treatment consists of immediate surgical exploration of the wound with decompression of the involved muscle compartment, wide excision and muscle debridement, antibiotics (usually penicillin), hyperbaric oxygen, and supportive therapy.

Meleney's Ulcer. Progressive bacterial synergistic gangrene, also called Meleney's ulcer, is a necrotic process involving large areas of skin that may ulcerate 1–2 weeks after the placement of stay sutures or drainage of abdominal or thoracic abscesses. It may also follow operative procedures in poorly vascularized tissues. The lesions are caused by a mixed infection from *Staphylococcus aureus* and a streptococcus. They are characterized by a tender, centrally brown, shaggy area of necrosis and ulceration surrounded by a purple zone and a red cutaneous flare. These wounds are treated by radical excision and antibiotics.

Actinomycosis. Actinomyces is frequently responsible for chronic suppurative infections with multiple draining cutaneous sinuses complicating recent wounds. The purulent exudate characteristically contains yellow sulfur granules. In addition, local granulomatous tissue proliferates, forming parallel cutaneous ridges in the wound. Treatment consists of incision and drainage with prolonged antibiotic therapy.

Dehiscence. The breakdown and separation of tissue layers in a wound, dehiscence usually occurs 5–8 days postoperatively. Although half of all cases are associated with infection, dehiscence may also occur in many patients who did not demonstrate a cutaneous "healing ridge" of tissue in their incisions. Poorly managed ischemic wounds and wound closure under extreme tension are other common causes of dehiscence. If dehiscence is noted within 6 hours and is caused by premature suture removal, the wound is immediately resutured. Otherwise, the wound is usually managed with open packing and secondary or delayed primary closure. When there is serosanguineous drainage from an abdominal wound 5–8 days after surgery and the healing ridge is absent, then the wound should be explored to define the extent of facial dehiscence. If facial dehiscence is significant, it may lead to evisceration. If immediate operative reclosure is not possible, then evisceration is prevented with abdominal binders and bedrest.[9]

Serum or Blood Collections. Seromas frequently complicate wounds involving undermined tissues, such as mastectomy flaps or large incisions in obese patients. Although these collections are initially sterile and resistant to infection, they quickly become susceptible to contamination and should be drained. Hemorrhage within a wound may be related to hypertension, coagulopathy, or excessive postsurgical motion. However, most wound hematomas are the result of surgically controllable bleeding, such as an unligated vessel; these should be evacuated under sterile conditions, as they predispose wounds to infection and may take months to organize and resorb. They can be resutured unless infection or ongoing bleeding is present. If a seroma develops after a drain is removed, it should be aspirated intermittently. If it does not resolve, then the closed suction drains should be reinserted or the wound allowed to heal by secondary intention. Antibiotics and graded compression dressings may be indicated.

Nonhealing Wound. This phenomenon is usually the manifestation of a local complication in the wound healing process, such as undue tension on tissue edges with ischemia and necrosis of tissues, hematoma, infection, or retention of foreign material. Occasionally, other etiologies or underlying systemic diseases may need to be ruled out (see Table 11-3).

LATE WOUND COMPLICATIONS

Certain wound complications have catastrophic implications. One often focuses on such factors as wound dehiscence, its related factors, prevention, and nursing intervention. Yet in the broad sense of potential morbidity of wound complications, the RN first assistant must consider an array of complicating events that are not as emergent as dehiscence but nonetheless are consequential to the patient.

TABLE 11-3

Causes of Nonhealing Wounds

Cancer	Drug therapy
Basal cell carcinoma	Infections
Leukemia	Nutrition
Melanoma	Starvation (protein depletion)
Squamous cell carcinoma	Inflammatory bowel disease (malabsorption)
Chronic trauma	Radiation
Factitious ulcer	Locally irradiated tissues
Hyperactivity	Radiation enteritis
Peripheral neuropathy	Vascular disorders
Poor hygiene	Arterial ischemia and atherosclerosis
Proximal nerve injury	Diabetes
Pruritus	Pressure sores

INCISIONAL HERNIA

Incisional hernia is considered to be iatrogenic in origin. It usually occurs after abdominal wounds and is rare in chest or flank incisions. These hernias are frequently multiple and represent a failure of healing. The most common cause of incisional hernia is wound infection, but technical errors in closing wounds, severe obesity, and prior dehiscence all predispose to this complication.

EPITHELIAL CYST

Cysts are occasionally seen along suture lines. The needle and suture used to approximate skin edges create a microwound that epithelial cells migrate into and line when sutures are left in skin for an excessive time. Cysts may be prevented by properly timed skin suture removal (usually within 5 days).

SUTURE SINUS

Developing from small abscesses in or near a wound associated with localized infection around a suture, suture sinuses persist as long as the suture remains in the tissue and may resolve spontaneously after several weeks as the suture is ejected from the wound. Suture sinuses occur most frequently with silk, cotton, or heavy multifilament plastic sutures.

HYPERTROPHIC SCARS AND KELOIDS

Large, firm masses of scarlike collagenous tissue may arise in healing wounds for unknown reasons. Certain races (blacks and Orientals) and younger patients may be more susceptible to these lesions; however, the lesions also may be seen in patients with normal scar formation and may even occur interspersed between areas of normal scar formation in the same healing wound. Hypertrophic scars usually stay within the boundary of the wound and tend to occur around joints, where areas of varying motion and tension exist. Keloids characteristically grow beyond the original incision. The management of these lesions is extremely varied and beyond the scope of this discussion.

CONTRACTURE

This is occasionally an end result of wound contraction involving shortening of skin and soft tissues adjacent to an area of injury. Motion around joints may be severely limited, and distortion of adjoining tissue structures may result.

WOUND PAIN

Irritating nonabsorbable sutures or traumatic neuromas are frequent etiologies for late postoperative wound pain. Although most of these complaints usually resolve spontaneously, some may require surgical intervention. Hyperesthesia around a wound is usually due to local sensory nerve injury and frequently diminishes or becomes well tolerated.

CANCER

Any chronic ulcer in a wound that has not healed after several months should be investigated for malignant changes. Ulcerated keloids and chronic sinus tracts may be prone to malignancy. Squamous cell carcinomas have been known to develop in old burn wounds (Marjolin's ulcer).

HIGH-RISK PATIENTS

Experience has shown that certain groups of patients are predisposed to developing wound complications postoperatively. Patients at high risk for these problems usually have local or systemic conditions that make them more susceptible to wound infections, affect the inflammatory response to injury, or alter collagen synthesis and maturation.

LOCAL FACTORS

A wound's general condition significantly influences its final result. Well-made and well-tended wounds resist infection, whereas ischemic tissues dessicated by electrosurgery, strangulated by haphazardly placed ligatures, approximated by excessive tension, or sustaining prolonged exposure to air all heal poorly. Grossly contaminated wounds that have been inadequately debrided or closed primarily tend to become infected.

Previous therapy at the injury site will also affect tissue repair. Radiation to a wound site frequently leaves a wasteland of relatively hypoxic and poorly vascularized tissues. The replication of vascular endothelial cells is often suppressed and contraction is retarded, but these are usually more deleterious to open wounds healing by secondary intention.

SYSTEMIC FACTORS

Malnutrition has been demonstrated to cause poor wound healing through both delayed repair and increased susceptibility to infection. Patients who present as significantly malnourished, such as from ethanol abuse, starvation, chronic illness, or malabsorption, should have their nutritional abnormalities corrected before major surgery is performed. Healthy patients will generally not encounter these problems if they are allowed to resume nutritional intake within 1 week. If a patient cannot be expected to begin adequate nourishment by oral or nasogastric tube routes after this time, then total parenteral nutrition (TPN) should be instituted.

Victims of multiple trauma are included in the high-risk group. Massive injury alters the body's metabolic "steady state" markedly by increased heat production and gluconeogenesis; negative nitrogen, potassium, sulfur, and phosphorus balances; early hyperglycemia; and altered carbohydrate utilization. The body's reaction to acute injury or illness appears to involve almost all its metabolic pathways. At no time are the body's nutritional demands as great as they are following serious injury, especially when complicated by infection. Wound repair is influenced by the nutritional disorders stemming from altered metabolic processes associated with severe injury, as well as by the patient's previous nutritional status. Persistent imbalances, frequently seen after major multiple injury, can produce serious malnutrition and impair wound healing. Superimposed on these disturbances are problems posed by contaminating microorganisms, foreign bodies, and compromised blood supply to the injured tissues.

Poor nutrient and oxygen delivery to wounds related to anemia or hypotension retards repair. Oxygen is essential to white blood cell and fibroblast functions, which are depressed by hypoxia. Oxygen is also needed for energy production in the healing wound through hydroxylation and oxidative metabolism. Both functioning systems are required for collagen synthesis.

Several diseases are associated with poor wound healing. Patients with Cushing's syndrome exhibit delayed repair secondary to a glucocorticoid excess, which can depress the inflammatory response. Diabetic patients are highly susceptible to local wound infections secondary to dysfunctional white blood cells. In addition, these patients frequently manifest microvascular disease, which creates local wound hypoxia. Peripheral neuropathy in this illness may lead to repeated accidental trauma to a healing wound. Vasculitis and atherosclerosis also have been implicated in delayed healing due to poor circulation. Disorders of the immune system, especially in leukopenic patients, may lead to a decrease in the natural immunity of the wound and higher infection rates.

Extreme age and obesity have been associated with higher incidence of wound complications. Both elderly and obese patients tend to heal poorly, suffer infection, and experience dehiscence more often than do their younger and leaner counterparts.

Concomitant drug therapy has been proven deleterious to wound repair in several instances (see Table 11-4). In general, any agent that interferes with the inflammatory process or cell proliferation retards healing. Corticosteroids and other anti-inflammatory agents are notorious for this side effect. They suppress repair if administered within 2–3 days after injury; healing will continue, but very slowly. The inflammatory response is decreased, fibroblastic proliferation and collagen synthesis are depressed, epithelial migration is hindered, and wound contraction is limited. Open wounds, by their dependence on all these factors, are particularly vulnerable to these effects. Several chemotherapeutic agents are cytotoxic (*e.g.*, methotrexate and nitrogen mustard) or antimitotic (*e.g.*, vinblastine). Their activity against cell division does not differentiate between malignant cells or those involved in wound healing. Occasionally, these drugs are combined with corticosteroids and may be dev-

TABLE 11-4
Drugs That Delay Wound Repair

Anticoagulants	Methysergide
Hematoma formation	Causes excess scarring
Anti-inflammatory agents	Penicillin
Suppress inflammation	Liberates penicillamine
Suppress protein synthesis	Pentazocine
Suppress contraction	May cause extreme fibrosis
Suppress epithelialization	Radiation
Chemotherapeutic agents	Suppresses cell replication
Arrest cell replication	Destroys blood supply by endarteritis
Suppress inflammation	
Suppress protein synthesis	
Colchicine	
Arrests cell replication	
Suppresses collagen transport	
Diphenylhydantoin	
Causes hypertrophic scars	

astating to wound repair. Anticoagulant therapy (coumadin and heparin) may lead to wound complication from excessive bleeding into wounds.

CONCLUSION

RN first assistants are involved in all phases of wound healing, from perioperative patient assessment through intraoperative dimensions of tissue handling and suturing to postoperative wound evaluation. It should be evident from this abbreviated discussion that wound healing is a complex process involving many facets of human physiology. Because all patients are to some degree individual and variable in biologic behavior, one cannot impose rigid guidelines for their care. Rather, one may only hope to optimize the conditions for the repair of injury based on sound surgical experience and knowledgeable attention to details of proper treatment tailored to each particular situation and patient. Successful wound management relies on this understanding by the RN first assistant and all members of the patient care team.

REVIEW QUESTIONS

1. Sharply made wounds that are reapproximated and heal with minimal space between their edges are classified as
   a. open wounds
   b. closed wounds
   c. aseptic wounds
   d. primary wounds

2. When a tissue defect decreases in size by wound contraction, it is designated as healing by

   a. primary intention
   b. secondary intention
   c. tertiary intention
   d. delayed intention

3. Following tissue injury, the initial vascular and cellular response is the

   a. inflammatory phase
   b. phagocytic phase
   c. injury phase
   d. epithelial phase

4. This initial phase lasts

   a. a few days
   b. 24 hours
   c. 5–7 days
   d. a few days to a few weeks

5. Key to the effectiveness of the cellular response is the activity of

   a. vasoconstriction
   b. chemotaxis
   c. leukocytes
   d. fibroblasts

6. During the migratory phase of wound healing, epithelial cells travel over viable tissue to bridge the wound; they cease migration through

   a. the effects of fibroblast growth factor
   b. mitosis
   c. the healing cascade
   d. contact inhibition

7. What cells are responsible for the synthesis and secretion of collagen and elastin?

   a. proteoglycons
   b. ground substance
   c. fibroblasts
   d. collagenases and elastinases

8. Scar remodeling is the effect of

   a. plastic surgery
   b. collagen reweaving
   c. capillary cross-links
   d. lymphatic drainage of interstitial fluid

9. If a skin flap is required to cover a tissue defect, the RN first assistant will most likely assist in

   a. drain insertion
   b. splint application
   c. compression dressing changes
   d. seroma evacuation

10. One reason that diabetic patients may have compromised wound healing is the presence of
    a. protein deficiency
    b. amino acid deficits
    c. hyperglycemia
    d. impaired serum albumin
11. Dietary sources of _______ are important for collagen turnover and metabolism in healing wounds.
    a. vitamin A
    b. vitamin C
    c. calories
    d. lysine
12. Preoperative patient considerations in preventing wound complications are focused on
    a. providing antimicrobial prophylaxis
    b. assessing and treating risk factors
    c. performing wound classification
    d. correcting host defenses
13. When taping dressings in place, the RN first assistant applies tape without tension, working from
    a. the center of the incision outward
    b. the edge of the incision toward the center
14. Nursing research indicates that skin irritation and skin stripping may be lower when _______ is used.
    a. plastic-backed adhesive tape
    b. paper-backed adhesive tape
15. Cellulitis may be treated by
    a. needle aspiration
    b. heat and elevation
    c. surgical debridement
    d. drain insertion
16. When palpating an area that may be an abscess, the RN first assistant will note that the area usually _______ on palpation.
    a. has crepitus
    b. sounds hollow
    c. fluctuates
    d. resonates
17. Gas gangrene, a rapidly progressive infection, is accompanied by swelling, pain, and
    a. high fever
    b. low-grade fever
    c. septic shock
    d. dark, red muscle

18. A wound that is closed under extreme tension may exhibit what wound complication?
    a. dehiscence
    b. myositis
    c. cutaneous healing ridges
    d. shaggy necrosis
19. Locally irradiated tissue may cause
    a. Meleney's ulcer
    b. draining cutaneous sinuses
    c. nonhealing wounds
    d. pruritus
20. Among those patients classified as at high risk for wound infection are those with
    a. alcoholism
    b. diabetes
    c. hypoxia
    d. hypoglycemia

Answers

1. b	8. b	15. b
2. b	9. a	16. c
3. a	10. c	17. b
4. d	11. b	18. a
5. c	12. b	19. c
6. d	13. a	20. b
7. c	14. b	

REFERENCES

1. Erickson D: Growth factors may help heal stubborn wounds. Scientific American, 265(6):141, 1991
2. Falango V, Zitelli JA, Eaglstein WH: Wound healing. J Amer Acad Derm, 19:559–562, 1988.
3. Lawrence WT, Bevin AG, Sheldon GF: Acute wound care. Care of the Surgical Patient, Vol I, 8-1–8-15. Scientific American, New York 1990
4. Stotts NA, Whitney JD: Nutritional intake and status of clients in the home with open surgical wounds. Research Review: Studies for Nursing Practice, 7(2):1, 1990
5. Meakins JL: Guidelines for prevention of wound infection. Care of the Surgical Patient, Vol I, 5-1–5-10. Scientific American, New York 1990
6. Weber BB: Timely tips on adhesive tape. Nursing 91, 21(10):52–53, 1991
7. Weber BB, Speer M, Swartz D, Rupp S, O'Linn W, Stone KS: Irritation and stripping effects of adhesive tapes on skin layers of coronary artery bypass graft patients. Research Review: Studies for Nursing Practice, 4(4):1, 1988
8. Coit DG, Sclafani L: Care of the surgical wound. Care of the Surgical Patient, Vol I, 7-1–7-10. Scientific American, New York 1990
9. Ibid, p 7-2

12 Using Grasping Instruments

Sergius Pechin

Grasping instruments may be defined as those used for clamping tissues for hemostasis, for retraction, and for dissection. Grasping instruments are also used in tissue approximation. This chapter will not attempt to catalog all the numerous types of grasping instruments. The operating surgeon will obviously have an individual preference based on personal experience and technique. The RN first assistant should have no difficulty in adapting to a particular technique when the fundamental principles are understood.

Both the American Nurses' Association (ANA) Standards of Clinical Nursing Practice and the Association of Operating Room Nurse (AORN) Standards of Professional Performance address the expectation that a nurse will acquire and maintain current nursing practice knowledge and evaluate her or his own nursing practice. Such an expectation extends to the RN first assistant in many of her or his nursing behaviors. It becomes necessary, then, for the RN first assistant to actively identify self-learning needs, including critical thinking, interpersonal, and technical skills.[1] Constructive feedback, peer review, and self-evaluation should be part of the RN first assistant's regular performance appraisal to establish areas for practice development.[2]

HEMOSTASIS

Hemostasis is temporarily provided with application of the hemostat, after which the vessel may be secured either with a tie or with the use of a desiccating current by touching the instrument with the active electrode of an electrosurgical unit. Because one of the RN first assistant's primary roles is to provide a dry field, and because one way of attaining this is with the hemostat, complete familiarity with this instrument is mandatory. Superficial bleeding provides little potential for difficulty, and the well-educated and skilled RN first assistant may clamp with impunity. However, control of deep bleeders and large amounts of bleeding must be left to the expert RN first assistant, inasmuch as blindly grasping at brisk bleeding lying in a large pool of blood invites disaster.

HEMOSTATS

Small, short hemostats are used for superficial vessels. Deeper bleeders may need a hemostat designed for specific requirements. These may be long and curved or long and straight. The curve may be gentle or sharply angulated, with each design providing, by its length and contour, the best aid for each particular anatomic circumstance.

HEMOSTAT TECHNIQUE

The RN first assistant should develop a definite technique in handling and using the hemostat. Such a technique is described and illustrated in Figure 12-1. As the assistant develops this technique, certain important general principles become part of her or his skill repertoire in all instrument handling techniques. The RN first assistant should first become familiar and comfortable with the feel of the hemostat and its balance in the hand. As this familiarity is established, the instrument gradually becomes an extension of the assistant's hand. As awkwardness lessens, the hemostat becomes easy to position naturally and comfortably. Soon, the need to grasp it tightly disappears, and the RN first assistant becomes adept at holding it with just enough of a grip to allow the best feel of the tissue to which the hemostat is applied.

Securing a bleeding vessel with a hemostat can be accomplished with either the tip or jaw technique. The tip technique has the principle objective of grasping only the open vessel, with a minimum of surrounding tissue. This minimizes tissue devitalization. In the tip technique, the hemostat tip is pointed toward the vessel. In contrast, the jaw technique grasps the vessel in the greater curvature; the tip points away from the vessel. This technique allows the hemostat tip to extend beyond the exposed vessel, trapping a ligature more easily as it is passed during tying. However, with this technique, more tissue is included in the hemostat jaw, and therefore more tissue is devitalized. The RN first assistant may be tempted to use the jaw technique during vessel occlusion to save time; this desire for speed should be a result of perfection of technique, not a goal for its own sake. The jaw technique should be selected when it is most useful; for example, when clamping across uncut tissue before transection. In this case, the jaw technique is superior. When transecting vascular pedicles, omentum, or other structures between clamps, knot tying is easier if the clamp jaws are applied with tips pointed toward the intended cut (and away from the vessel).

FIGURE 12-1A
Hemostat technique. (1) In grasping a bleeder, the method shown in **A** is obviously the most sure. Only the very tip of the instrument is used to capture the smallest amount of tissue containing the bleeder. Consequently, the smallest amount of tissue is devitalized by ligature or electrical current.

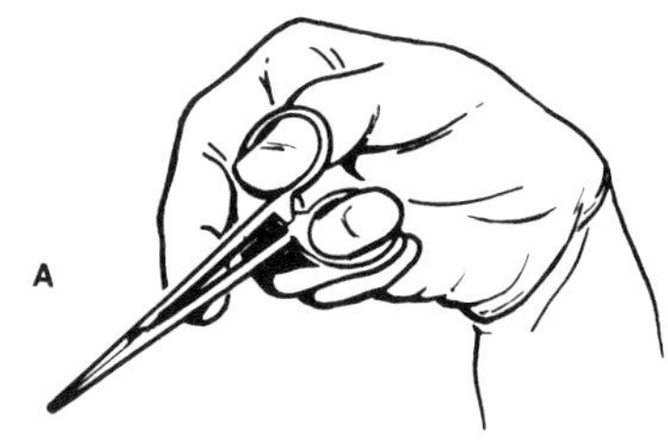

FIGURE 12-1B
Once the hemostat is placed, however, the fingers should be withdrawn from the rings, and the hemostat should be grasped as in **B**. The ring closest to the assistant is grasped between thumb and middle finger; the index finger is kept mobile enough to release the ratchet of the instrument by pressure against the ring. In this maneuver, the whole instrument is firmly stabilized with the ring that is contained between the thumb and third finger. If this technique is developed, it allows the assistant to manipulate the point of the instrument through an almost 360-degree arc, which would not be possible if the fingers were still incorporated in the rings as shown in the original position, shown in **A**. Performing the recommended technique will require practice and expertise to develop smooth manual dexterity.

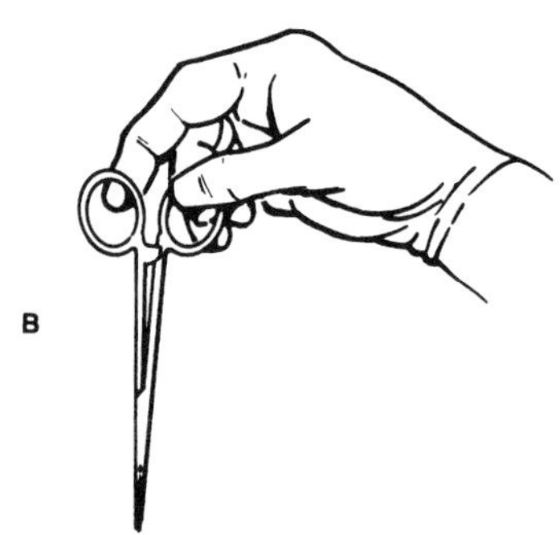

FIGURE 12-1C
Once the hemostat has performed its function, it may be carried for immediate reuse as indicated in **C**. The lower ring is hooked by the distal end of the fourth finger, and the body of the instrument is then held to the palm of the hand by the fifth finger. This allows the thumb, middle, and third fingers to be mobile. The assistant's ability to continue to assist is not limited, inasmuch as an entire operative procedure can be expertly handled with just these three digits. Any time the hemostat is to be used again, it can be flipped out to the attitude shown in A and then returned to the position shown in C again when its duty is accomplished. It might be added that this maneuver need not be limited to just the use of the hemostat. It can be used with scissors or any comparable ringed instrument that is not too long.

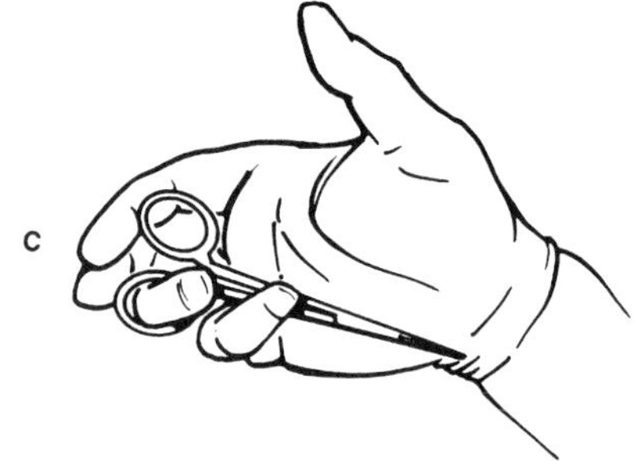

When hemostasis is achieved and it is time to proceed with vessel ligation, the RN first assistant should hold the hemostat without fingers in the finger rings. This permits optimal rotation for tie placement without twisting the vessel. The handles of the hemostat are held away from the wound to facilitate placement of the hands of the person tying the knot. Once the first loop of the ligature is placed, the handles are depressed and the hemostat tip is elevated and exposed without pulling. As the first knot throw is secured, the hemostat is gradually removed. In situations permitting easy access to the wound, such as with superficial layers, the fingers do not need to be in the rings for clamp removal. The finger ring on the left is grasped by the thumb. The ring is pinched between the thumb and the ring finger, and the lock is disengaged by pressing the index finger on the finger ring. Then the clamp is gently removed and discarded.

During critical situations, the RN first assistant will select the three-point grasp, with the thumb and index fingers in the instrument rings to facilitate controlled release of the clamp. To release the hemostat from this grip, the tip is rested on a firm surface as the index finger presses on the closed shanks, "pushing" the clamp from the hand.

RETRACTION

Grasping instruments may be used for retraction, either to facilitate visibility or to help with dissection by providing tension on the appropriate tissue. Here, instrument application must be done carefully and deliberately to obviate trauma to tissue not adapted to this technique. Specific types of retracting instruments have been devised; the most common of these are described in the following sections.

KOCHER INSTRUMENT

The Kocher instrument is used mainly where retraction is necessary; for example, in the dissection of heavily scarred or fibrotic areas, such as the reopening of an old incision. The clamp is a better tissue holder for these cases than a tissue forceps; the static use of the forceps would cause fatigue. During dissection and separation of adhesions, the Kocher is well-suited to lift and hold peritoneum as underlying surfaces are exposed. It is also useful during midline closure of the abdomen; the dense fascia can be grasped and stabilized with a Kocher immediately adjacent to the site where the stitch will be placed. This instrument is toothed, and care must be taken not to mistake it for the smooth hemostat. A curved Kocher can be mistaken for a curved Kelly, in which case its inadvertent use could inflict damage.

The Kocher is considered to be a "crushing" instrument; its small jaws apply great pressure to a small area. When a Kocher is used during transection of an area, such as bowel, a cuff of tissue should be left distal to the clamp. Tissue is less likely to slip between the jaws this way.

ALLIS CLAMP

The fine-toothed Allis clamp is used for retracting more delicate tissue. It has been used at times on cut bowel edge. The numbers and fineness of the teeth of an Allis clamp vary, in part delineating the type of tissue that it might grasp. Like a Kocher, this clamp also applies great pressure to a small area. This enables the RN first assistant to hold it with minimal pressure, knowing that the jaws will not slip.

BABCOCK CLAMP

This broad but thin-bladed, untoothed clamp is used primarily to lift and retract bowel and other delicate structures. Considered one of the nontraumatic clamps in the surgical armamentarium, the Babcock is commonly used to encircle tubular structures and gently hold soft tissue. The ratchet on the Babcock should be tightened only enough to hold the tissue.

TENACULUM

A more heavily toothed instrument than the Allis, the tenaculum is used particularly for retracting heavier tissue. A prime example is the tenaculum forceps used for retraction in thyroid gland dissection.

It might seem appropriate to declare that smooth instruments are designed for bowel and delicate tissue and that toothed instruments are theoretically designed for tougher, firmer tissue. However, it has not really been determined that this is true. Smooth instruments can crush tissue, and toothed instruments sometimes can cause less trauma, because less metal comes in contact with tissue and less pressure needs to be exerted to lift tissue when gently biting. Suffice it to say that gentle handling of tissues with any instrument is the prime consideration.

THUMB FORCEPS

The thumb forceps provides an extension of the surgeon's and RN first assistant's fingers to allow for more precise handling of tissue. Forceps are commonly used by the nondominant hand to assist maneuvers undertaken by the dominant hand. Thus, they are commonly used as an adjunct to the needle holder to stabilize tissue while suturing; to the scalpel and scissors to hold tissue while cutting; and to the hemostat to retract tissue for exposure before clamping. Forceps are also used to grasp vessels for electrosurgical coagulation, to pack sponges, to grasp objects for extraction, and to grasp the end of needles. Their versatility requires that a large variety of thumb forceps be available, each adapted to a particular situation.

Here, as with other grasping instruments, the question of plain as opposed to toothed instruments is to be decided. The RN first assistant will likely be asked to provide countertraction in dissection, so the choice of forceps must be based on knowledge of tissue type and requirement of the traction. In general, fibrotic, scar-type tissue warrants the use of a toothed forceps, such as the broad-toothed Russian forceps. Bowel and peritoneum, on the other hand, require a nonpuncturing forceps. Anatomic proximity of tissue guides the RN first assistant in selecting a long forceps or a shorter forceps, such as the Adson. This small-toothed forceps has variation with longitudinal rows of teeth, which distribute the force and allow firm fixation without trauma. An Adson is well-suited to moderately dense tissue such as the skin. The fine points on the teeth give more holding power by concentrating force in a small area; they cause less tissue destruction than smooth forceps when holding skin.

It is this type of experiential knowledge, gained from scrub nurse function, that makes the RN first assistant such a valuable asset to the surgeon. However, understanding the proper use of an instrument such as a tissue forceps must be translated into clinical skill in actual instrument use. Consider the following simple routine in using tissue forceps to lift the peritoneum during abdominal surgery. The surgeon first picks up peritoneum with tissue forceps; the RN first assistant remains still during this move. The surgeon then remains still while the assistant picks up peritoneum a few millimeters away. The assistant gently holds the tissue forceps while the surgeon readjusts the forceps to ensure that only a single layer of peritoneum is within its jaws. Once this is ensured, both the surgeon and assistant hold the forceps still while the peritoneum is opened between the two sets of forceps. It is this kind of clinical skill, knowing how to and when to, that sets the RN first assistant apart. It is a feeling and knowledge of move-countermove that is smoothly synchronized between surgeon and RN first assistant, producing a flowing, dynamic continuity throughout the surgical intervention.

Tissue forceps should be held so that one blade acts as an extension of the thumb and the other acts as an extension of the opposing fingers. The grip should be gentle and balanced; if hard squeezing is needed to hold the tissue, then either the wrong forceps are being used or a clamp is needed. The most maneuverability is obtained from holding the forceps in the pencil position, or in a modified pencil grip. When not in active use, the forceps may be palmed and supported by extending the ring and little finger; the unflexed middle finger thus is still free for use. Palming an unused instrument, when alternately grasping with forceps and fingers, saves time. If the little finger and ring finger are required for use, as when completing a one-handed tie, the forceps can be temporarily pinched in the web between the thumb and index finger. To move forceps back to a position of use, the palm is turned down and the thumb and index finger are used to grasp the forceps in the desired place.

CONCLUSION

This basic understanding of gentleness in handling tissue, experience founded on good training in manual skills, knowledge of anatomy and procedural aspects of the intervention, and familiarity with instruments are the fundamental prerequisites necessary to provide good surgical assistance. Perioperative nurses, functioning in the expanded role of intraoperative first assistant, are in an ideal position to elaborate their knowledge of surgical interventions and augment role function as they continue to provide quality patient care.

REVIEW QUESTIONS

Indicate whether each of the following statements is true (T) or false (F):

_____ 1. The ANA's standards of professional performance require that the nurse systematically evaluate the quality and effectiveness of medical practice.

_____ 2. Hemostasis can be secured with a clamp either by applying the tip to the bleeding vessel or by trapping the bleeding vessel in the convexity of the clamp's jaws.

_____ 3. Crushing clamps, such as a Kocher, used during transection are more secure from having tissue slip between their jaws if a cuff of tissue is left distal to the clamp.

_____ 4. The objective of the jaw technique of applying a curved hemostat is to include a minimum of surrounding tissue.

_____ 5. Tip clamping makes it easier to pass a ligature around a vessel.

_____ 6. Speed should be the primary goal of surgical technique.

_____ 7. An accurate and secure hemostat grip is the "tripod," where the thumb and ring finger are inserted in the instrument rings and the index finger is placed on the shaft.

_____ 8. To manipulate a hemostat during vessel ligation, the hemostat should be held for encirclement by the ligature with the fingers in the rings.

_____ 9. In a deep wound, the RN first assistant should trap the ligature beneath the tip by gently pressing the clamp deeper in the wound and rotating the tip away from the person tying the knot.

_____ 10. While the knot tier tightens the first half-hitch, the RN first assistant should quickly snap the hemostat off the wound.

_____ 11. The three-point grasp is the more secure and accurate grip for a clamp in a critical situation.

_____ 12. A left-handed assistant removes a clamp by grasping the left ring between the thumb and index finger and disengaging the lock by pressure of the middle, ring, and little fingers on the right finger ring.

_____ 13. Atraumatic clamps are designed to hold while exerting the least possible crushing force.

_____ 14. The palm position of holding forceps gives the widest range of maneuverability.

_____ 15. When sewing, then tying, palming the forceps can save time.

_____ 16. To change from "hold" to "use" with the forceps, the palm should be turned up.

_____ 17. Forceps are a principal instrument for fine retraction during dissection.

_____ 18. When elevating a clamp for vessel ligation, the RN first assistant pulls gently on the vessel while showing the tip.

_____ 19. When holding soft viscera with a Babcock, the RN first assistant tightens down to the third ratchet.

_____ 20. When smooth-jawed forceps are used, more force or tissue compression is required to lift tissue against resistance without slipping.

Answers

1. F (Nursing practice, not medical practice, is what should be evaluated. Evaluation should be in relation to professional nursing practice standards as well as relevant statutes and guidelines.)
2. T
3. T
4. F (The tip technique of applying a curved hemostat clamps the open vessel while including the minimum surrounding tissue.)
5. F (Jaw clamping leaves the tip exposed beyond the tissue; this traps the ligature as it is placed around the vessel.)
6. F (Speed is the by-product of expert surgical technique rather than its primary goal; speed should not take the place of technique.)
7. T
8. F (To allow optimal rotation for placing the tie, hemostat handles should be held without fingers in the rings.)
9. T
10. F (Clamps are always removed gradually to prevent the tissue from escaping while the first half-hitch is tightened.)
11. T
12. T
13. T
14. F (The pencil grip, with the forceps' shanks against the index finger metacarpal-phalangeal joint, gives the widest range of maneuverability. The palm grip requires too much wrist flexion.)
15. T
16. F (With the palm up, gravity makes the grasp too far from the tips; turning the palm down allows gravity to assist the RN first assistant by moving the forceps from the palm. The index finger and thumb can then grasp the forceps in the desired place without extreme flexion.)
17. T
18. F (The clamp is elevated without pulling on the clamped structure.)
19. F (The ratchet should be tightened only enough to hold the tissue.)
20. T

REFERENCES

1. Association of Operating Room Nurses: Standards of Perioperative Professional Performance. AORN Standards and Recommended Practices, II:5-2. Denver, Association of Operating Room Nurses, 1992
2. American Nurses' Association: Standards of Clinical Nursing Practice, p 14. Kansas City: American Nurses' Association, 1991

13 Providing Hemostasis

Nancy B. Davis

Hemostasis occurs when blood stops flowing from an injured blood vessel. The achievement of hemostasis during surgical procedures is fundamental to surgical intervention as a form of treatment. Excessive or uncontrolled bleeding is life threatening. Controlling bleeding not only is important in relation to the patient's prognosis, but also is necessary for adequate visualization of the operative site. Prolonged bleeding also interferes with healing of the surgical wound.

The natural defense mechanism of blood clotting is not adequate to control bleeding during surgery (see Figure 13-1). The surgeon depends on this defense mechanism as an important factor, but also uses mechanical, thermal, or chemical hemostasis techniques.

Bleeding during or after surgical intervention is influenced by several factors: the type of surgical intervention, the patient's physical condition, coagulation mechanisms, and fibrinolytic activity. During surgery, the most frequent cause of bleeding is injury to blood vessels. The amount of bleeding depends on the amount of injury to blood vessels, the type of vessels injured, and the anatomic site of the injury to vessels. These factors, related to the vessel injury and the surgeon's technical skill, influence the achievement of hemostasis during surgery.

PATIENT ASSESSMENT

The RN first assistant implementing Standard I of the Association of Operating Room Nurses' (AORN) Standards of Perioperative Clinical Practice, related to collecting data about the patient's health status, may obtain information

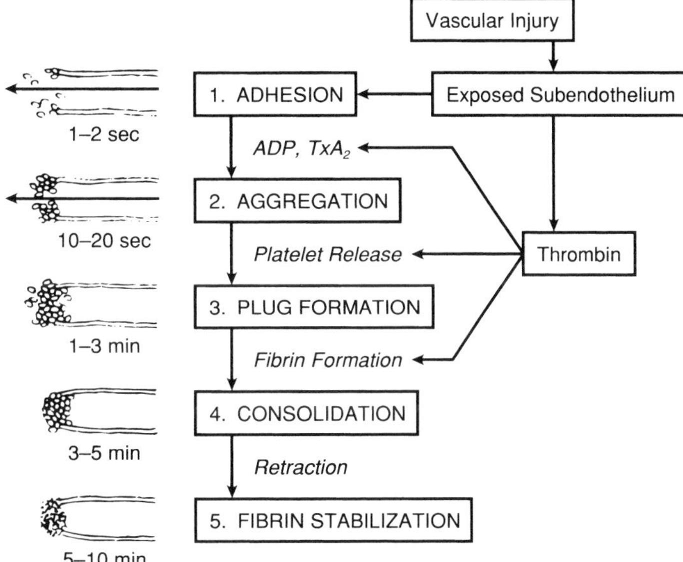

FIGURE 13-1
Formation of the primary and secondary (definitive) hemostatic plugs. *(Reprinted with permission from Harker LA: Hemostasis Manual, p 4 Seattle, University of Washington Press, 1970.)*

pointing to increased risk of intraoperative bleeding. All patients undergoing invasive surgical procedures face the risk of bleeding due to the traumatic nature of surgery.

Sepsis, deficiencies in blood clotting mechanisms, anticoagulant drugs, allergies, or diseases such as leukemia, thrombocytopenia, lymphoma, or multiple myeloma increase a patient's risk of bleeding. The history and physical examination provide information related to the patient's present condition, past history, and medication use. The patient should be queried about hemostatic responses to previous surgical interventions, as well as about easy bruising, epistaxis, gingival bleeding, and menorrhagia. Medication history should be reviewed for such drugs as anticoagulants, aspirin (and aspirin-containing drugs), or other nonsteroidal anti-inflammatory medications. Laboratory tests related to clotting factors must be reviewed for any abnormality; these may include tests of coagulation mechanisms (*i.e.*, activated coagulation time, partial thromboplastin time [PTT], prothrombin time [PT]), tests of platelet function (*i.e.*, platelet count, Ivy bleeding time, clot retraction time), and tests of fibrinolysis (*i.e.*, fibrinogen level). Any clotting defects must be communicated to the surgeon before surgery. Preparation of any needed clotting factors can then be done.

The operative procedure must be considered in relation to increasing the patient's risk of bleeding. The more extensive the operation, the greater the involvement with vascular structures. The need for blood transfusions, the use of cardiopulmonary bypass procedures, and the need to use heparin intraoperatively all increase this bleeding risk.

Preoperative assessment should also consider fluid balance. Fluid balance depends on normal volume and osmotic pressure in the intracellular, interstitial, and intravascular compartments; adequate fluid intake and output; normal renal function; a responsive endocrine system; and good nutritional status. The patient's general physiologic status should be assessed for establishment of outcome criteria. Specific data to be reviewed include the patient's normal intake and output and serum sodium, potassium, total protein, albumin, and glucose levels. The urinalysis should be reviewed to determine urine specific gravity. Body weight should be documented. The history should be investigated for evidence of preexisting illnesses involving the liver, pancreas, renal system, thyroid gland, adrenal gland, or respiratory system. The patient's use of diuretics or laxatives should also be noted.

Protein levels are important in relation to fluid volume; the liver manufactures albumin from amino acids, and albumin aids in the maintenance of colloidal osmotic pressure. Decreases in total protein cause fluids to shift from the vascular system to the tissues. It will be of concern to the RN first assistant if total plasma protein falls below 6g/dl and if albumin falls below 4g/dl. Careful preoperative assessment can identify treatable problems and assist in predicting the body's fluid preservation response to surgical stress.

The assessment phase concludes with the formulation of nursing diagnoses. One nursing diagnosis related to the possibility of bleeding during or after surgical intervention might be stated as "High Risk for Fluid Volume Deficit related to intraoperative or postoperative bleeding." AORN's Patient Outcome Standards of Perioperative Care can be used for postoperative evaluation of the patient's status in relation to the nursing diagnosis. Assessment of bleeding is ongoing during the intraoperative phase, and the RN first assistant must recognize abnormal or excessive bleeding during this phase. Also, the assistant must not inadvertently contribute to increased intraoperative bleeding through unnecessary tissue trauma or improper application of hemostatic techniques.

GENERAL CONSIDERATIONS IN HEMOSTASIS

Invasive operative procedures always injure tissue and interrupt the integrity of vascular structures to some extent. The RN first assistant must be knowledgeable about the normal blood supply to various tissues. Whenever possible, injury to blood vessels is avoided; the assistant must recognize vascular structures and be skilled in handling the structures without causing trauma. Some anatomic areas are more vascular than others; the scalp, face, and tongue are examples of highly vascular areas.

Excessive intraoperative blood loss is usually obvious. Arterial bleeding occurs more rapidly than venous bleeding because of the higher pressure in the arterial system. Arterial bleeding is bright red in the well-oxygenated patient, whereas venous blood is darker. Subtle blood loss can occur when there is a slow but continuous oozing of blood.

With sudden or rapid blood loss, the patient may develop signs of shock. Hypotension and tachycardia are significant findings. The hypotension can result in decreased urinary output. Vasoconstriction decreases tissue perfusion, and the patient's extremities may be cold, pale, or cyanotic.

Blood loss can be determined by weighing sponges that are soaked with blood (1 g = 1 cc) and by noting the amount of blood that has accumulated in the suction canister (minus any irrigating fluids or other body fluids). Blood lost on the drapes must also be estimated.

If hemorrhagic shock develops, it usually can be reversed by restoring the blood volume. Initially, this is done through rapid administration of intravenous fluids. Blood transfusions may be needed and are usually set up before surgery if the risk of bleeding is high. To decrease the administration of sodium, potassium, lactic acid, and other blood components, packed red blood cells combined with crystalloid or albumin are used to correct hypovolemia due to blood loss.

Excessive bleeding with the use of multiple blood transfusions or damage to the platelets through prolonged use of cardiopulmonary bypass can cause coagulation problems. Administration of platelets or plasma component therapy (fresh frozen plasma and cryoprecipitate) may be necessary.

To minimize intraoperative bleeding, the RN first assistant must know how hemostasis is achieved during surgery. Controlling bleeding and preventing hemorrhage are priorities, and the assistant facilitates this process by having the technical skills necessary to assist the surgeon in providing hemostasis.

MECHANICAL MEANS OF ACHIEVING HEMOSTASIS

An important goal for the RN first assistant is to prevent blood loss. A priority is anticipatory control of any vessels before they are ligated. The RN first assistant then uses many methods to quickly control any bleeding that does occur.

DIRECT PRESSURE

Direct pressure can be the simplest and the fastest method of controlling bleeding. During the skin incision, the RN first assistant should instinctively place his or her fingers or a moistened sponge against the ends of any transected and bleeding vessels. When this pressure is maintained for 15–20 seconds, small clots will usually form in the ends of small vessels. Digital pressure can be applied with a gauze sponge directly over the site of bleeding; however, care must be taken that the adherent surface of a gauze sponge does not dislodge fresh clots when the sponge is removed. The tip of an instrument, such as a suction tip, may also be used to initially cover and compress a bleeding point.

Indirect pressure might be applied to an area proximal to the bleeding area of the blood vessel, with the fingers or with a sponge on a sponge stick. Especially useful in a deep recess, the sponge stick should be held gently in position until lights and retractors are positioned for good visualization and suction clears away any free blood. Once a clamp is ready, the sponge stick is slowly rolled off the vessel to expose the end to be clamped. Packing can be used to exert pressure on bleeding surfaces, thereby achieving hemostasis.

In diffuse bleeding, pressure may be required for an extended time. When this is the case, a cool saline moist pack is pressed against the bleeding surface for 10–20 minutes while another aspect of the surgical procedure is undertaken.

When bleeding is extensive, it may be impossible to visualize the bleeding point by suctioning or sponging. In such a case, the bleeding can be slowed or stopped using pressure. With better visualization, the bleeding point can be identified and hemostasis achieved. The use of pressure to control bleeding has the advantage of being least traumatic to the vascular structures. The major disadvantage is that it is often only a temporary measure. When removing any sponge or pack, the RN first assistant should be ready to immediately control any renewed bleeding from larger vessels that have been controlled by pressure.

HEMOSTATS

Clamping instruments designed for temporary control of bleeding from small blood vessels, hemostats are available in various sizes, lengths, and shapes. The tips may be straight, angled, or curved, and jaws may be fine, pointed, or heavy, or blunt. Hemostats that are lighter in weight and construction are less damaging to tissue. Hemostats with fine and pointed jaws can be applied with more precision and less damage to the vessel or surrounding tissues. Hemostats with heavy, broad jaws can be used to clamp across larger amounts of tissue that may contain several small blood vessels (see Figure 13-2). The ser-

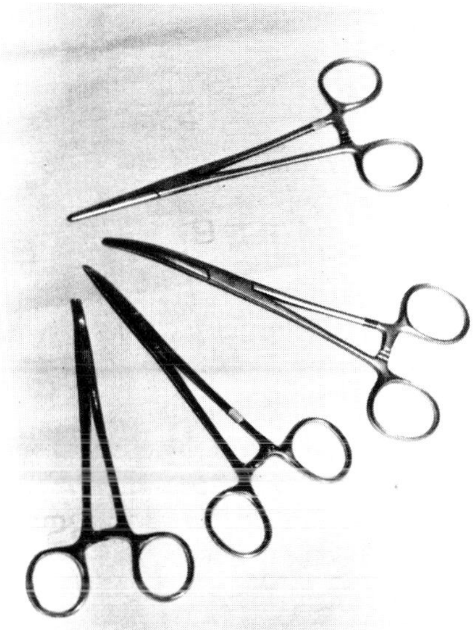

FIGURE 13-2
Examples of hemostats. (**Left to right, bottom to top**) Curved Crile hemostat; tonsil hemostat; curved-pean and straight-pean hemostats.

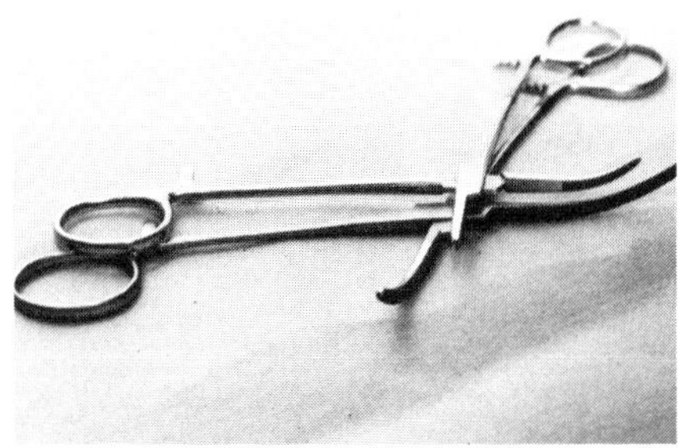

FIGURE 13-3
Kelly hemostat (partial serrations; **top**) and Crile hemostat (fully serrated; **bottom**)

rations in the jaws also vary. Serrations may cover only the lower portion of the jaws, or may cover the total jaw surface (see Figure 13-3). The extensiveness of serrations affects the security of the jaw's grip on the tissues when clamped. Hemostats should be clamped tightly enough to stop blood flow while maintaining the security of the clamp on the vessel, but without exerting excessive pressure, which can cause unnecessary tissue damage. The RN first assistant must be knowledgeable about the types of hemostatic clamps available and skilled in applying them to bleeding vessels.

To apply a hemostat, the open end of the bleeding vessel is grasped in the tip of the clamp. Only the minimal amount of the vessel is clamped. If the open end of the vessel cannot be held securely with the tip of the hemostat, it should be cross-clamped with the hemostat jaws (see Figure 13-4).

Whenever possible, blood vessels are clamped before being cut to decrease blood loss. Either the tips or the jaws may be used, depending on vessel size and location and on the content of surrounding tissues. The vessel is usually clamped with two hemostats, with space left between the clamps for cutting the vessel. The amount of vessel between the clamps must be sufficient to prevent the clamps from slipping off the vessel once it is severed. When placing a hemostat on a branch of a blood vessel, the assis-

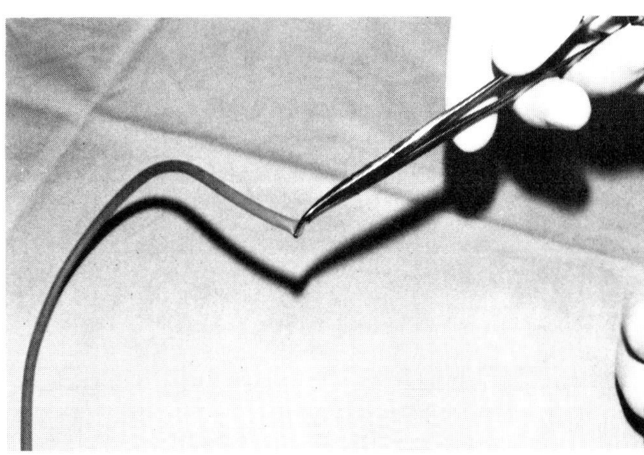

FIGURE 13-4
Method of clamping blood vessel (represented by rubber tubing) with hemostat.

tant should allow space on the branch between the clamp and the major vessel; this facilitates placing a ligature around the cut branch and prevents fracturing (or injuring) the major vessel (see Figure 13-5). If using curved hemostats, the tips of the two clamps should point toward each other. This facilitates cutting between the clamps and the subsequent placement of ligatures (see Figure 13-6).

Removing a hemostat during vessel ligation requires coordination between the person holding the clamp and the one tying the ligature. The hemostat handle is lifted so that the ligature can be placed behind the clamp (see Figure 13-7). This must be done carefully, so that the hemostat is not pulled off the vessel. The hemostat is then lowered or flattened to hold the ligature behind the clamp and elevate the point (tip) of the hemostat. The ligature is then brought around the tip of the hemostat, encircling the vessel to be ligated (see Figure 13-8). As the first throw of the ligature knot is being tightened, the hemostat is slowly and carefully opened, thereby releasing the end of the vessel. The hemostat should be removed in a direction that will not interfere with the placement of the ligature or obstruct the vision of the person doing the tying. The hemostat can be opened and removed with precise control by placing the third finger and thumb into the ring handles, although in many instances the hemostat can be removed with the use of leverage on the handle (see Figure 13-9). Although the release of the hemostat is not as precise, it is acceptable when ligature placement and tying are easy. The leverage method is quicker and easier once the skill is developed.

There are three basic techniques for clamping and ligating blood vessels deep within a wound. The method used, determined by the surgeon, is usually related to the accessibility, size, and fragility of the vessel or surrounding tissue structures. In one technique, the vessel is clamped with longer, fine hemostats and divided with a scissors or knife. The ligature is held at one end with a tissue forceps or a tonsil hemostat, and the free end of the ligature is passed around the handle of the clamp and held taut with the free hand. The

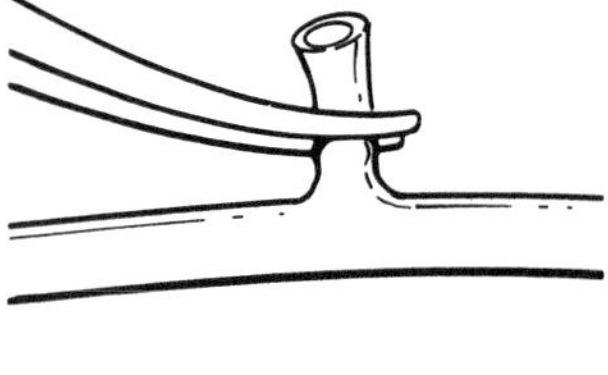

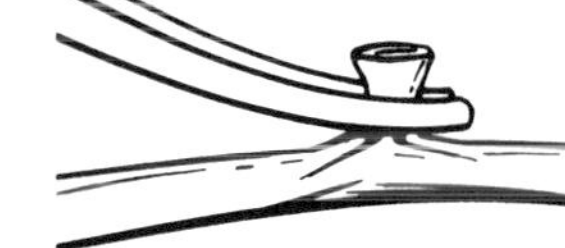

FIGURE 13-5
(**Top**) Proper application of clamp to branch of blood vessel allows room for ligating without injuring vessel. (**Bottom**) Improper placement of clamp on branch of blood vessel. Note injury to vessel.

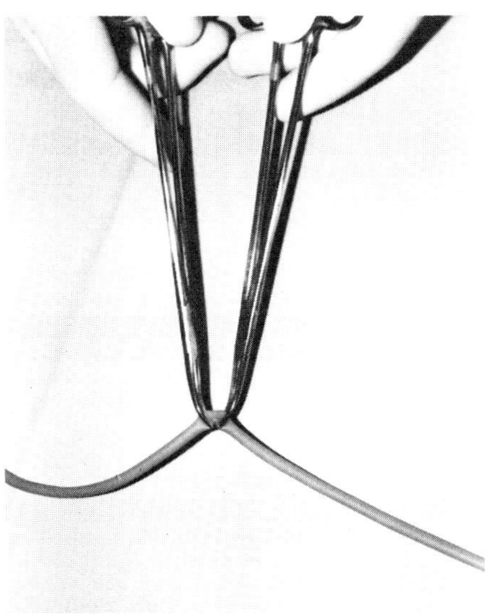

FIGURE 13-6
Method of clamping vessel (represented by rubber tubing) with hemostats curved toward each other.

clamped end of the ligature is then placed under the tip of the hemostat. The assistant, holding the hemostat, then tilts the hemostat tip downward and holds the ligature.

The hemostat's position must be changed very cautiously to prevent it from slipping off the end of the vessel. After the ligature is passed under the

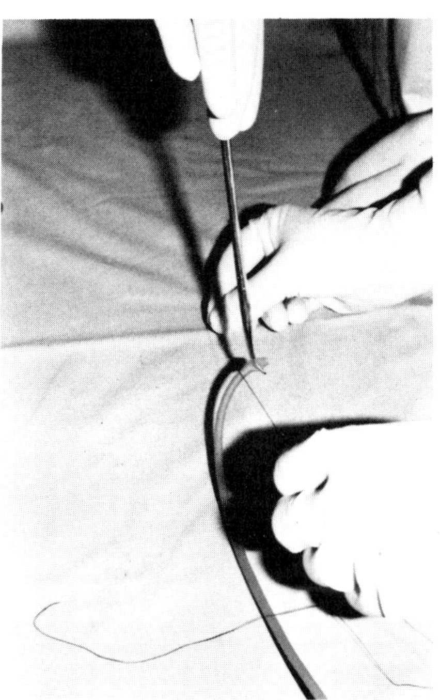

FIGURE 13-7
Lifting handle of hemostat for ease in placing ligature.

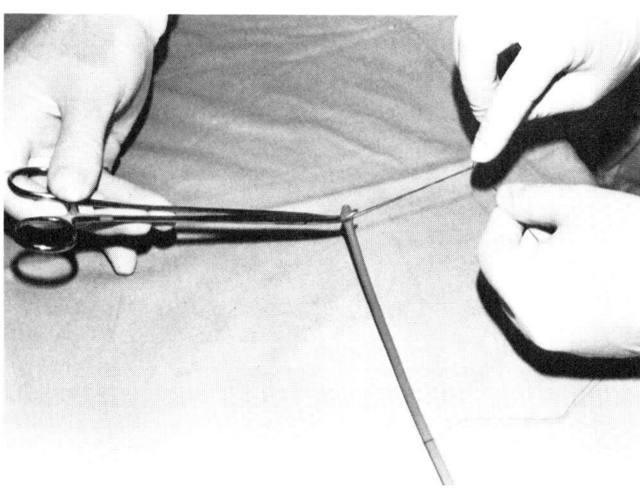

FIGURE 13-8
Flattening handle of hemostat and tying ligature.

tip of the hemostat holding the vessel, the ligature is pulled until enough length is available for ease in tying (see Figure 13-10). The ligature is released from the clamp or tissue forceps, and the first throw of the knot is slipped down behind or to the side of the hemostat clamped to the vessel as the hemostat is slowly removed by the assistant.

In another method, the blood vessel is clamped and cut in the same manner. Instead of using a free ligature, however, the surgeon uses a ligature on a

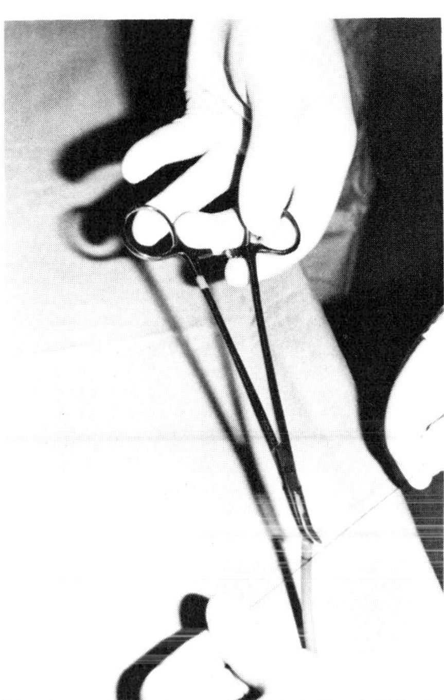

FIGURE 13-9
Releasing hemostat by leverage on handle.

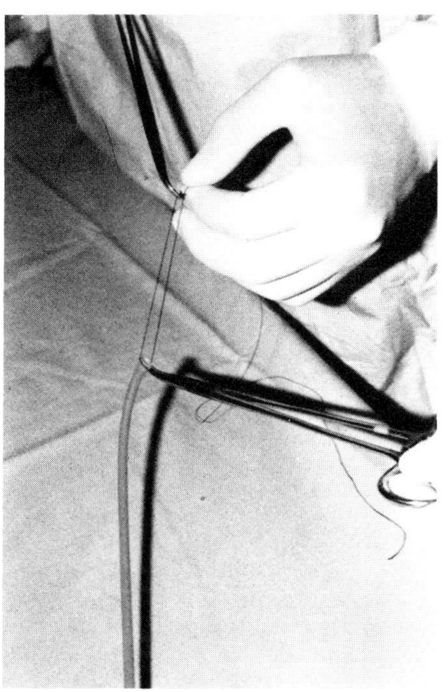

FIGURE 13-10
Using a hemostat to pass ligature around vessel (represented by rubber tubing).

needle (stick tie). The surgeon holds the hemostat clamped to the vessel as the suture needle is placed through the blood vessel behind the hemostat. The ligature is pulled through the vessel, leaving enough length on the free end for easy tying. The ligature is then tied behind and around the vessel as the assistant slowly removes the hemostat.

In the third technique, the ligatures are placed before the vessel is cut. The vessel is dissected free of surrounding tissue so that it can be visualized. An angled clamp of the appropriate length is used. The tip of the clamp is placed under the vessel and opened. The assistant then passes the ligature into the open tip of the angled clamp. It will be necessary for the assistant to hold the ligature with both hands; one hand to keep the ligature taut and the other hand to hold the end of the ligature that will be placed in the angled clamp. In deep wounds, a tonsil hemostat or tissue forceps can be used to hold the end of the ligature to be placed in the open clamp tip (see Figure 13-11). The angled clamp is closed so that the ligature is gripped securely between its jaws as the assistant releases the ligature. Care must be taken not to close surrounding tissue in the clamp jaws. The angled clamp is then withdrawn and the ligature passed under the vessel. Enough ligature is pulled under the vessel to allow it to be tied easily. The ligature is released from the angled clamp and tied securely around the vessel. The procedure is then repeated. Before the second ligature is tied, it is positioned such that space on the vessel is allowed between the two ligatures. The vessel is cut between the

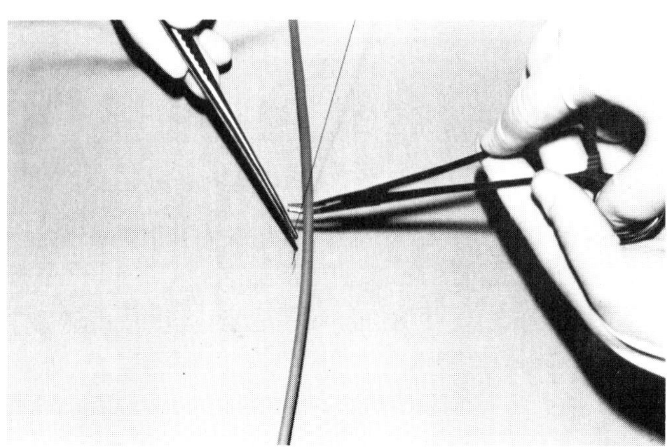

FIGURE 13-11
Using a forceps to pass a ligature into angled clamp.

two ligatures. The amount of vessel between the cut ends and the ligatures must be long enough so that the tie will not slip off. It is easier to cut the vessel if both ligatures are held taut, thereby pulling on the vessel. The ligatures are then cut (see Figure 13-12).

HEMOSTATIC CLIPS AND STAPLES

In deep, narrow areas, where tying may be difficult or the use of the electrosurgical unit inadvisable due to the potential for damage to adjacent structures, hemostatic clips may be used.

Clips. Clips for ligating vessels vary in size and are made from tantalum or stainless steel wire. Serrations across the inside keep the clip from slipping off the vessel after it is applied. Absorbable clips made of polydiaxanone are absorbed in approximately 210 days. Ligating clips are useful for ligating vessels that are difficult to clamp with a hemostat. They are easy and quick to

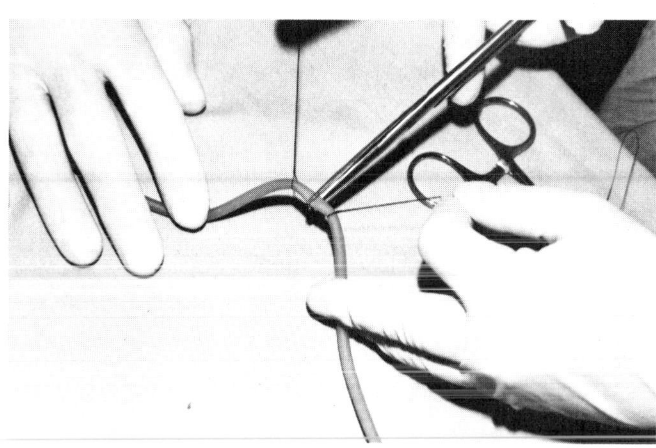

FIGURE 13-12
Cutting blood vessel between tied ligatures.

use and decrease the risk of foreign body reaction that may occur with sutures.

Although using ligating vessel clips is relatively easy, it must be done correctly. The correct clip size must be selected to ensure that the vessel is completely obliterated. Clip applicators are available in different lengths and are angled at the tip for ease in visualizing the vessel while the clip is being applied. Once the clip is in position around the vessel, the applicator handle is firmly squeezed and released. The applicator must be completely released before it is removed from around the clip, to avoid pulling on the clip. If the clip is accidentally pulled, it may come off the vessel or the vessel could be torn. The clip must be far enough back from the open end of the vessel to avoid slipping off the vessel later.

Scalp clips (*e.g.*, Adson, Raney) may be reusable or disposable. Designed to provide hemostasis of the scalp incision edges, these clips are applied with special applicators after the scalp incision has been made, left in place during the surgery, and removed when closing the incision.

Staples. Stapling devices provide hemostasis and closure of a transected organ such as the lung, bowel, or stomach. Staples are also available for vascular structures. Staples are available in various lengths and types and are selected according to the surgeon's preference. It is important to inspect the edges of stapled tissues to ensure adequate closure and hemostasis.

VASCULAR CLAMPS

Vascular clamps are designed to completely or partially occlude blood vessels with minimal injury to the vessel. The jaws have single or multiple rows of teeth, serrations, or cushioned inserts. Numerous variations in vascular clamp size, length, and configuration provide for adequate hemostasis in many different anatomic locations (see Figure 13-13). The RN first assistant can facilitate clamp placement by retracting surrounding tissues so that they do not interfere with the clamp's occlusion.

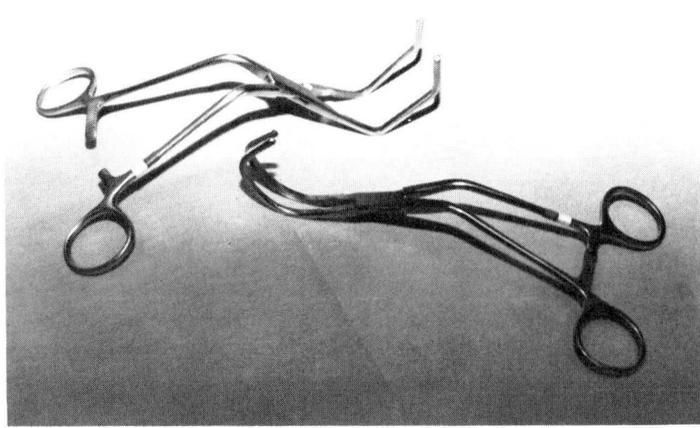

FIGURE 13-13
Examples of vascular clamps for aorta. Note different angles and curves of clamp jaws and handles.

Once the surgeon has placed the vascular clamp, the assistant usually holds it in position. This must be done in a manner that does not interfere with clamp position or cause vessel injury. By holding the clamp by the shaft rather than by the ring handles, the assistant is less likely to accidentally unlock the clamp ratchet. Excessive pulling or twisting of the clamp must be avoided, as the clamp may slip off the vessel or fracture the intimal wall of the vessel.

The vascular clamp provides a temporary means of hemostasis until the vessel opening is sutured. Before removing the clamp, it must be opened completely free from the vessel, to prevent accidental tearing of the vessel. Partial occluding clamps are usually removed by placing the fingers and thumb through the ring handles from behind the clamp (see Figure 13-14). This position is more comfortable for the assistant's hand, and it allows the clamp to be opened more easily and with less chance of it turning or twisting on the vessel. The clamp can also be released by unlocking it from above (see Figure 13-15).

SUTURES, KNOTS, AND KNOT TYING

Sutures provide hemostasis by permanently holding tissues or vessel walls together while they heal. Once the suture is placed and tied securely, the bleeding is stopped.

Sutures can be used as free ties to ligate vessels that have been clamped with a hemostat. Sutures are also used with needles to place single or multiple stitches. Stitches are indicated when there is a chance of the ligature slipping off the vessel or when the open area in the vessel is too large to ligate.

Regardless of how the suture is used to provide hemostasis, the RN first

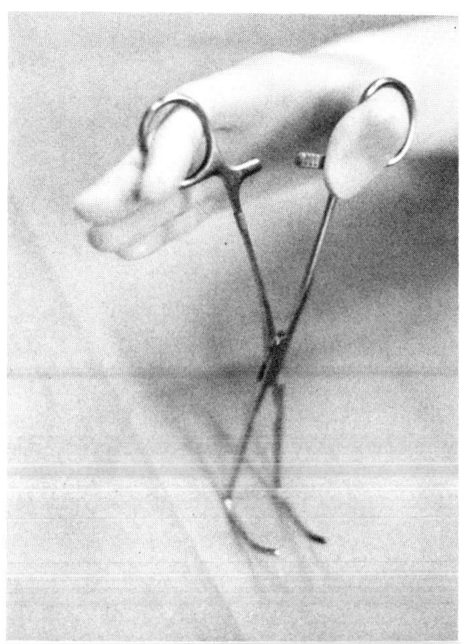

FIGURE 13-14
Removing a vascular clamp by opening from behind.

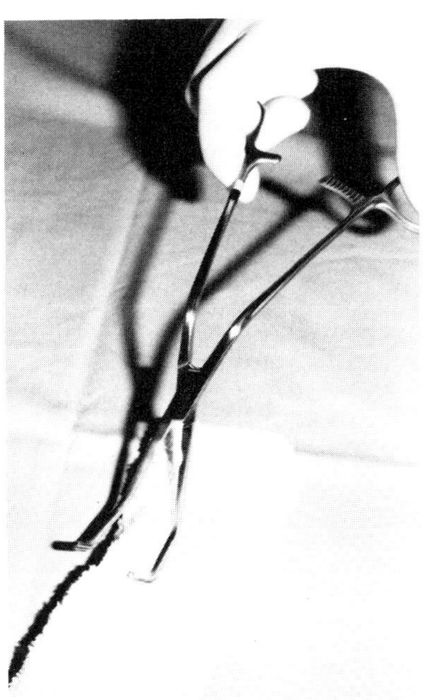

FIGURE 13-15
Removing a vascular clamp by opening from above.

assistant must be skilled in tying secure knots. To develop this skill, the assistant must become familiar with the various types of knots and must practice the techniques until dexterity is achieved.

Three basic types of knots are used in surgery: the square knot, the surgeon's knot, and the granny knot (see Figure 13-16). The *square knot* is used most frequently and is the most secure. The *surgeon's knot* is helpful when tying under a moderate amount of tension. By doubling the first throw, the suture will not slip while the second knot is being placed. The *granny knot*, or slip knot, is made by placing two identical throws of the suture. This knot can be slipped or cinched tighter and is especially useful in wounds with limited access. A square knot is tied upon the granny knot to keep it from slipping.

The three techniques for tying knots are two-handed, one-handed, and instrument ties.

(*text continues on page 274*)

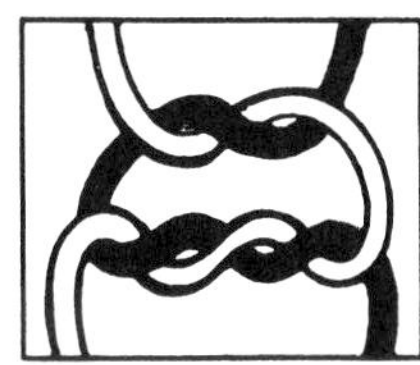 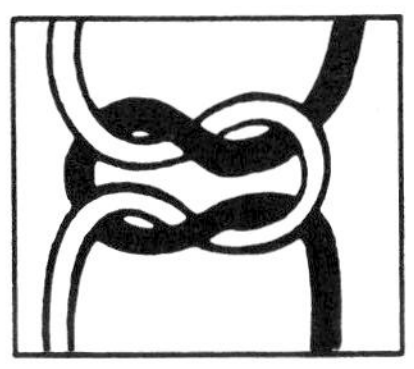

FIGURE 13-16
Types of surgical knots (**right**) Square knot, (**left**) surgeon's knot. *(From Ethicon Knot Tying Manual, 1983. Courtesy of ETHICON, Inc., a Johnson & Johnson Company, Somerville, NJ)*

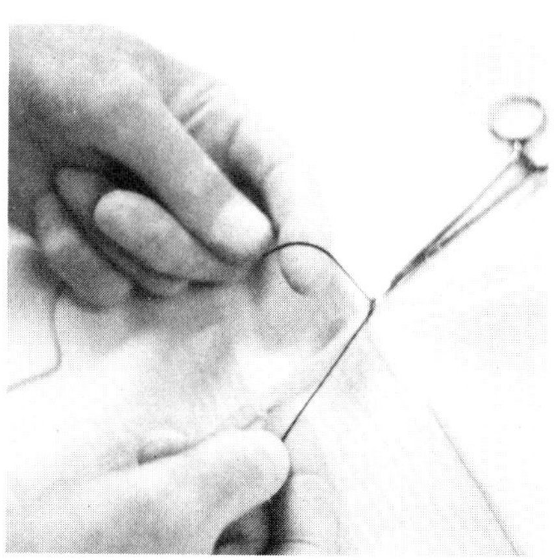

1. Grasp the short end of the suture with the right hand. Hold the long end of the suture in the left hand with the suture over the index finger.

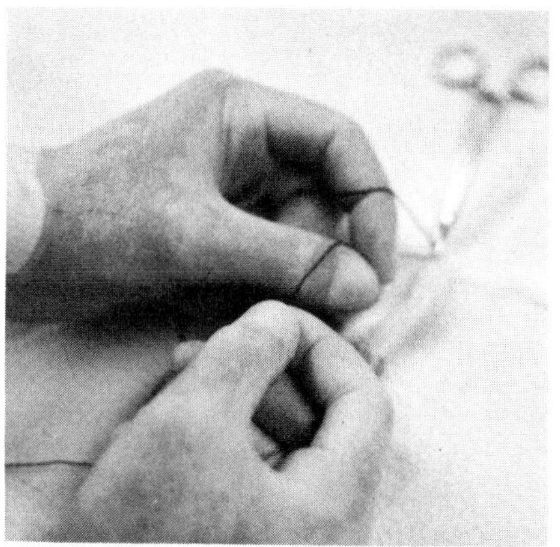

2. Bring the short end of the suture held in the right hand under the left index finger and over the left thumb.

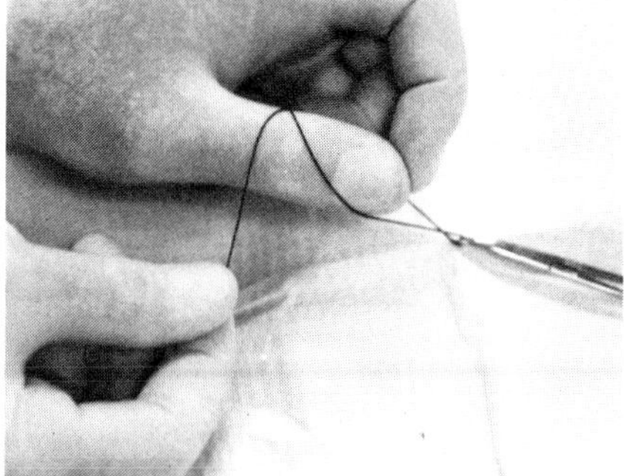

3. Slip the suture from the left index finger over the left thumb so that the thumb is through the loop.

FIGURE 13-17
TWO-HANDED TIE. Step-by-step instructions for completing the two-handed tie.

(continued

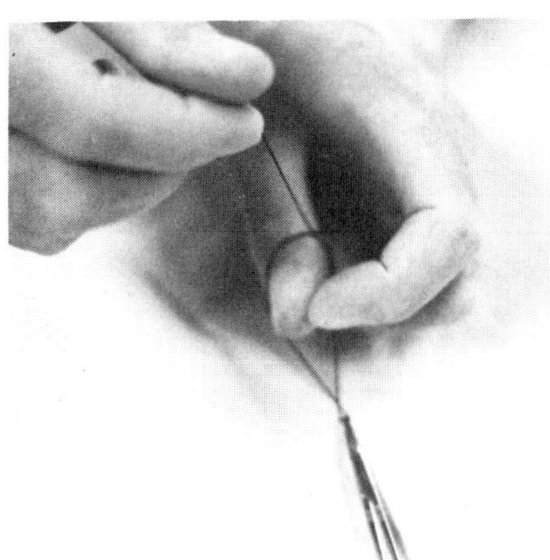

4. Bring the short end of the suture held in the right hand toward the left thumb and index finger.

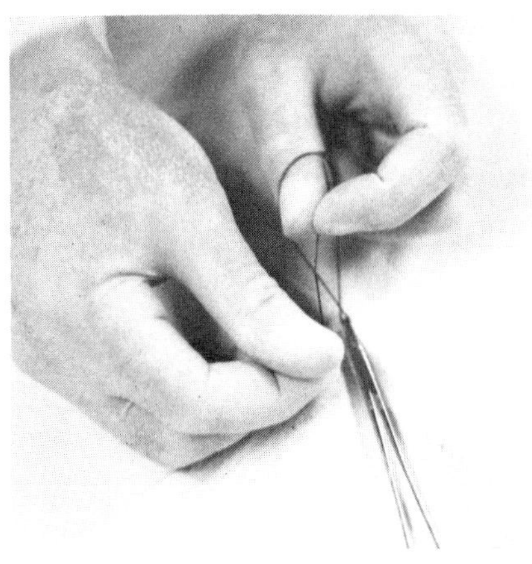

5. Grasp the suture in the right hand with the left thumb and the index finger.

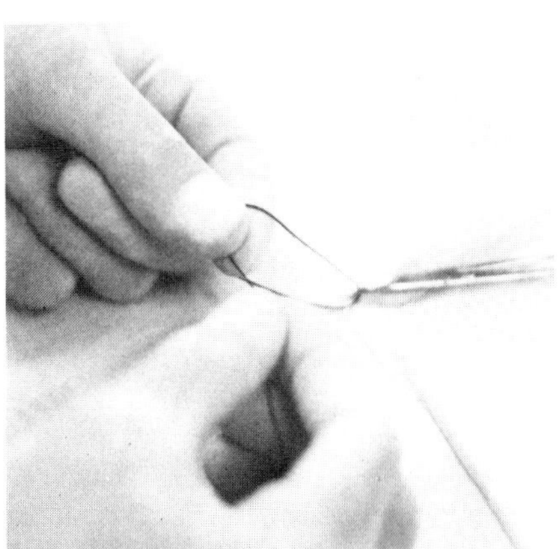

6. Rotate the wrist and push the short end of the suture through the loop while releasing the suture end from the right hand.

Figure 13-17 *(continued)*

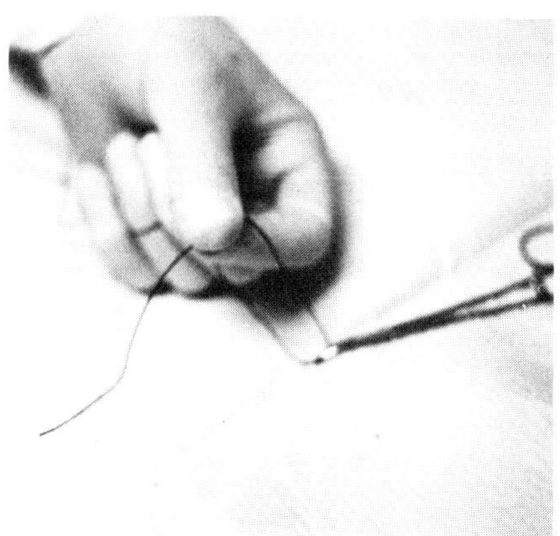

7. Short end of the suture passes through the loop and can be grasped by the right hand.

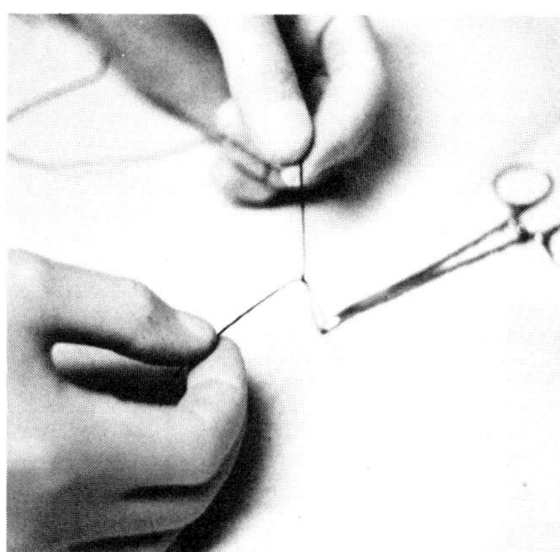

8. Secure the knot.

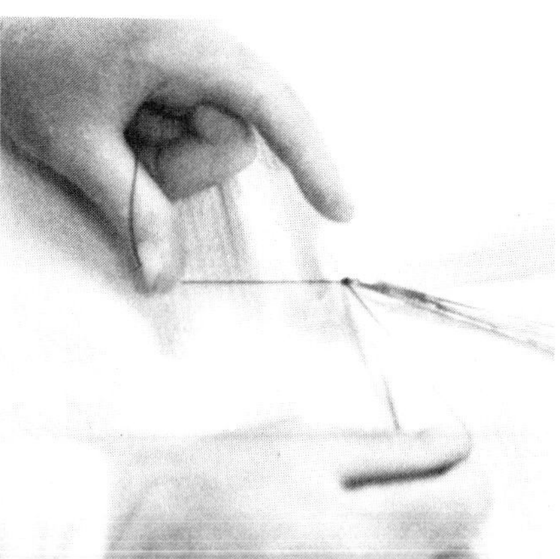

9. While holding the long end of the suture in the left hand, place the left thumb on the suture.

Figure 13-17 *(continued)*

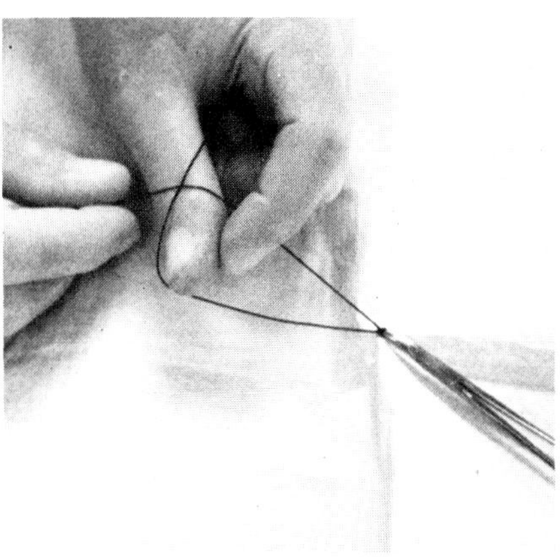

10. Bring the short end of the suture in the right hand over the thumb, and place the left index finger over the suture, touching the thumb.

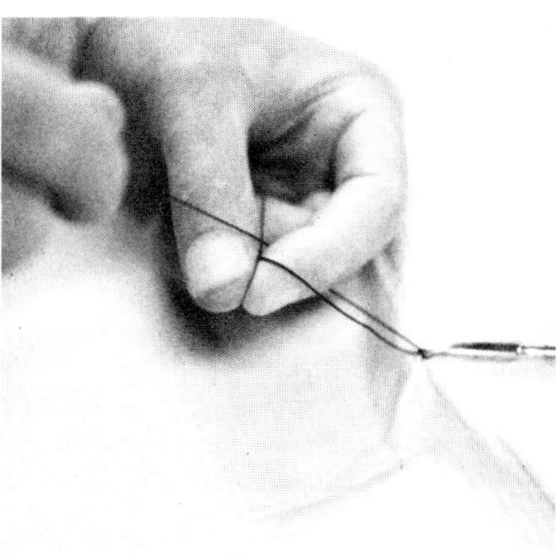

11. Rotate the left hand so that the suture slips off the thumb and the index finger is through the loop.

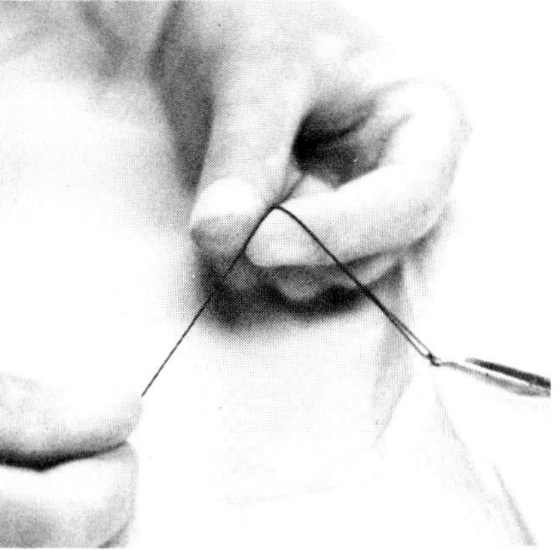

12. Place the short end of the suture that is held by the right hand between the thumb and index finger of the left hand.

Figure 13-17 *(continued)*

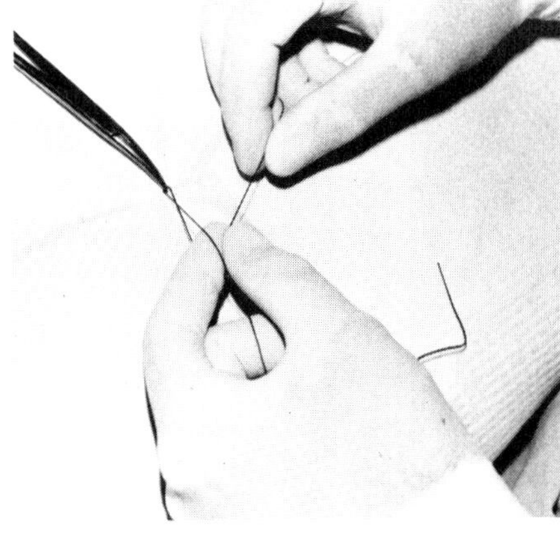

13. Hold the short suture with the thumb and finger while performing step 14.

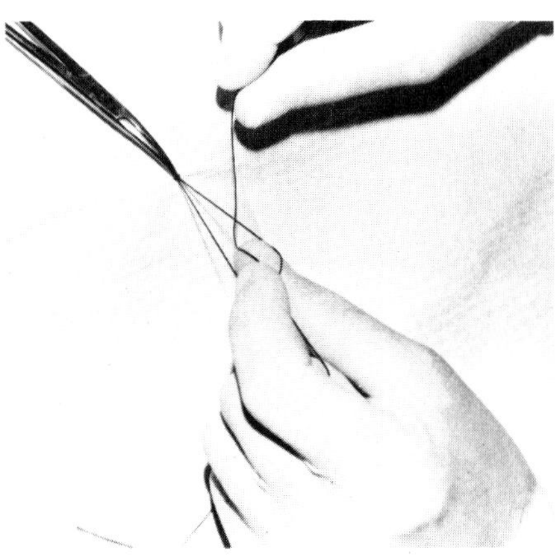

14. Rotate the left hand so that the thumb pushes the short suture through the loop.

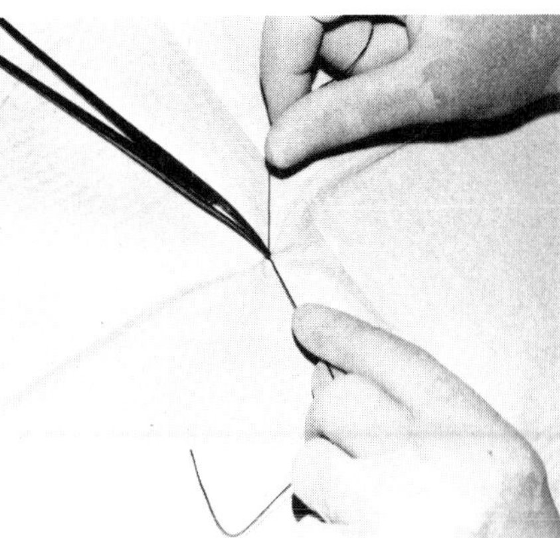

15. Regrasp the suture with the right hand after it passes through the loop, and secure the knot.

Figure 13-17 *(continued)*

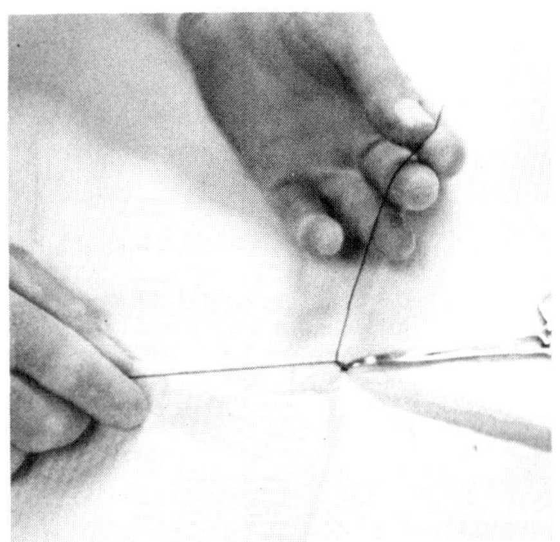

1. Grasp the short end of the suture with the thumb and index finger of the left hand.

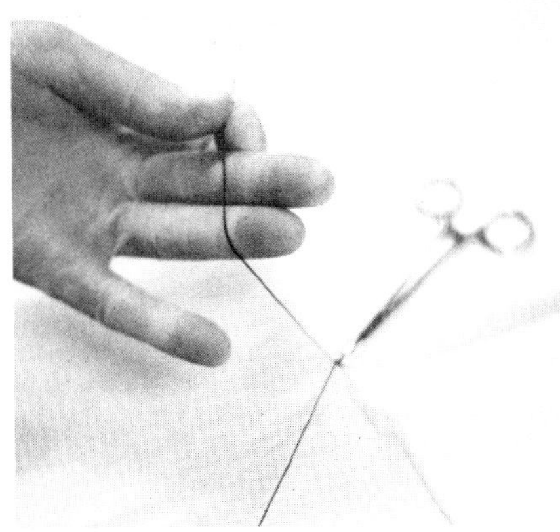

2. Rotate the left hand so that the suture rests across palmar surface of the long finger and the ring finger.

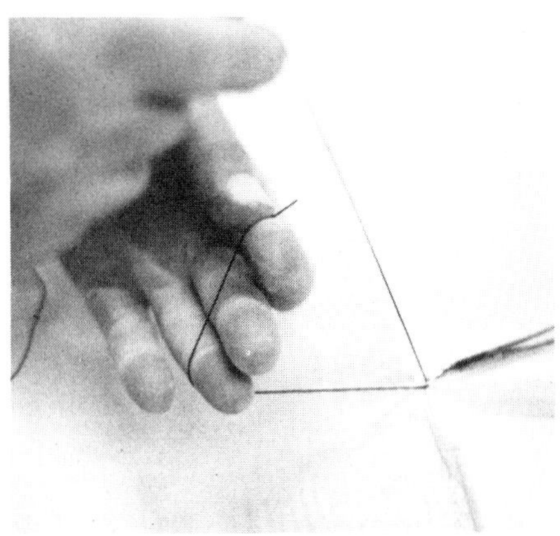

3. Bring the suture in the right hand over the left hand.

FIGURE 13-18
ONE-HANDED TIE. Step-by-step instructions for completing the one-handed tie.

(continued)

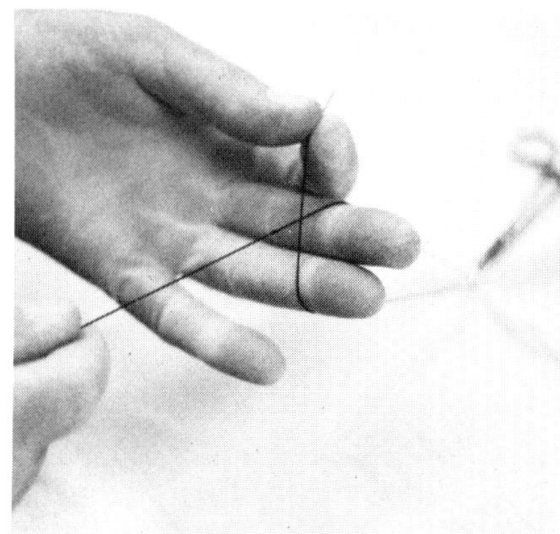

4. Place the suture in the right hand onto the long finger of the left hand, and across the suture being held in the left hand.

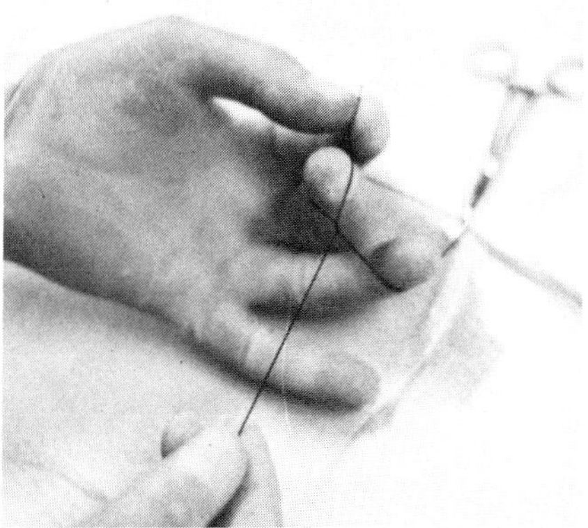

5. Flex the long finger of the left hand so that the tip goes under the short suture that is being held by the left thumb and index finger.

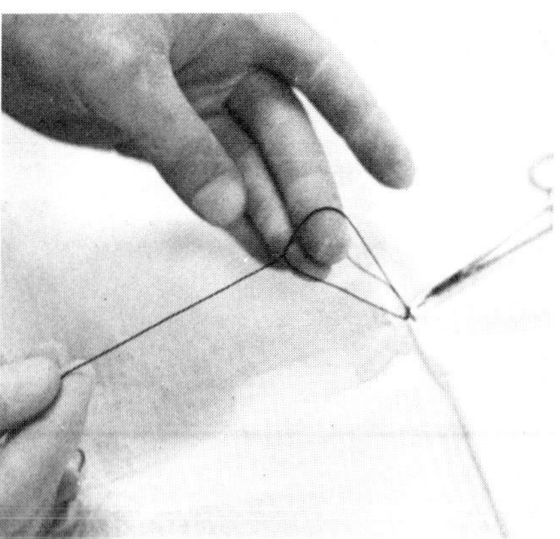

6. Release the short suture from the left thumb and index finger while extending the long finger and rotating the left hand. This flips the suture through the loop.

Figure 13-18 *(continued)*

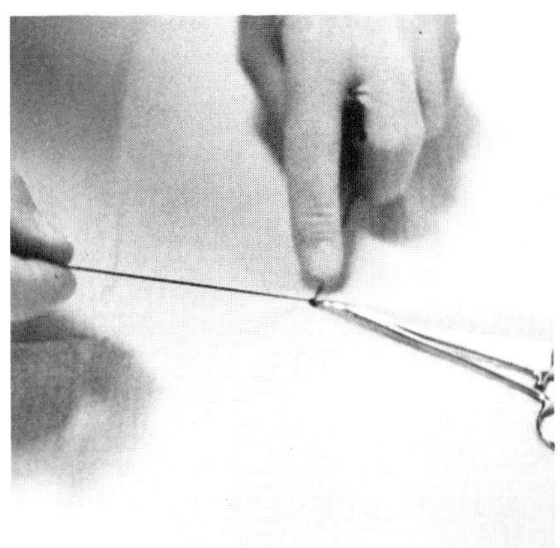

7. Secure the knot.

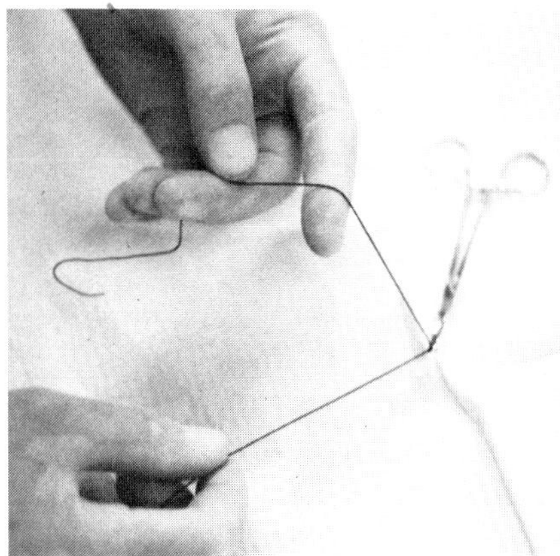

8. The short end of the suture is held in the left hand and over the extended index finger. The right hand holds the long part of the suture taut.

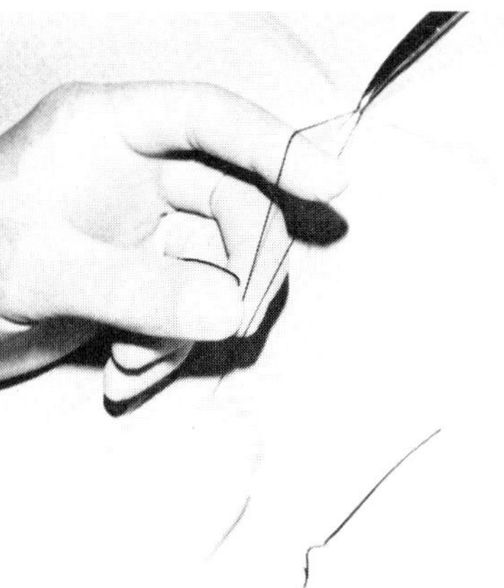

9. Bring the suture in the right hand under the extended left index finger.

Figure 13-18 *(continued)*

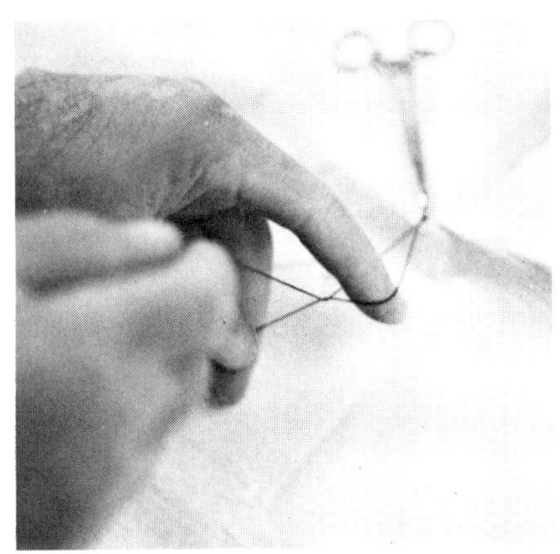

10. Lift the suture in the right hand while rotating the left hand so that the index finger passes through the loop.

11. Flex the left index finger under the suture held in the left hand.

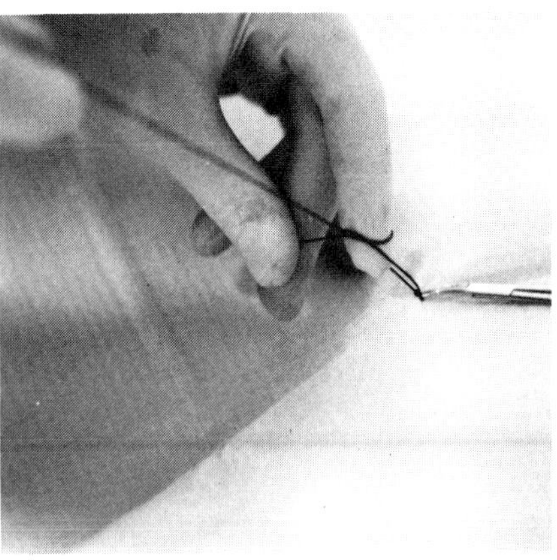

12. Extend the left index finger and release the suture from the left hand.

Figure 13-18 *(continued)*

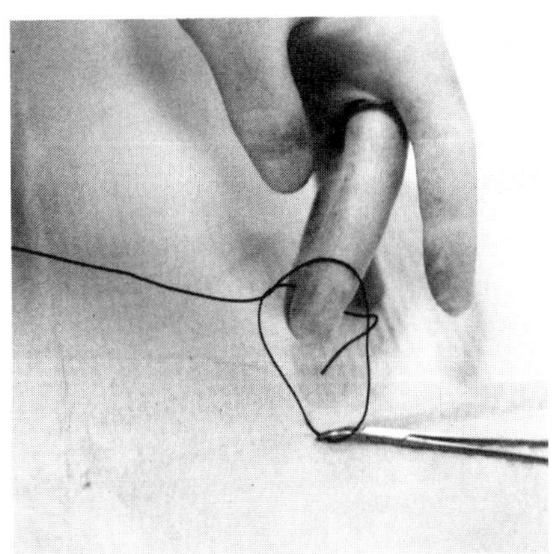

13. This flips the suture through the loop.

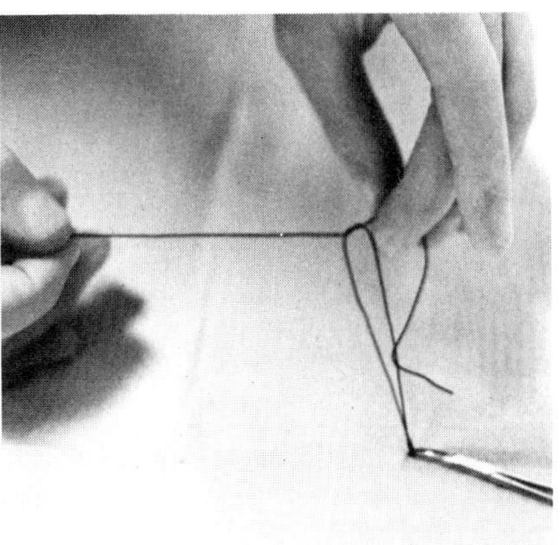

14. The suture is held in the left hand between the long-finger and third-finger tips after it passes through the loop.

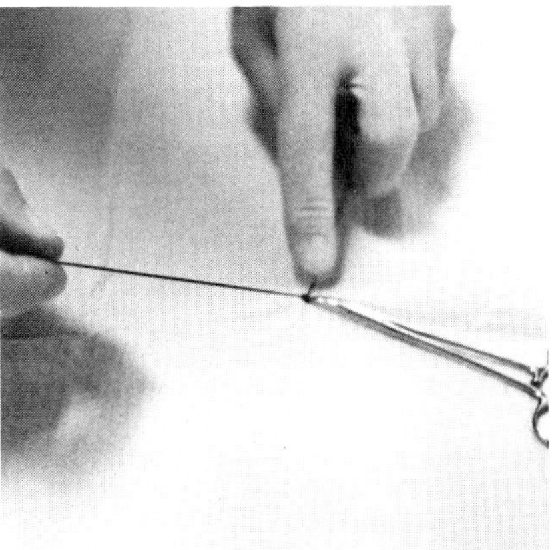

15. Secure the knot.

Figure 13-18 *(continued)*

The *two-handed technique* is usually the first one the assistant learns because it is easy to learn, provides control of the knot, and ties easily under tension (see Figure 13-17).

The *one-handed technique* is a little more difficult to learn, but it ties quickly (see Figure 13-18). An *instrument tie* is necessary when the free end of the suture is too short to tie by hand. It is also very useful for economizing on sutures (see Figure 13-19).

Regardless of the technique used, some basic principles guide knot tying. The free end of the suture must be of sufficient length to allow easy grasping; excessive length, however, is clumsy and interfering. The amount of tension exerted on the suture while the knot is being secured depends on the suture type and size. The knot should be tied tightly enough to hold securely without cutting through the tissue or breaking the suture. The knot is usually secured with three throws if the vessels are small or the tissues are not under tension. Four throws are advised for larger vessels or tissues under tension. Slippery or very smooth sutures (*e.g.*, nylon) require 5 to 10 throws for security. Fine, braided wire can be tied like suture, but heavier wire must be twisted for at least three complete turns. Suture material will weaken if strands are "sawed" against each other during tying. Care must also be taken to ensure that the suture is not partially cut with instruments.

BONEWAX

Made from refined beeswax, bonewax is used to control bleeding from bone marrow. It is gently pushed and rubbed into the edge of the bone where the marrow is exposed and bleeding. Foreign body reactions can occur from excessive bonewax application. Only just enough wax should be used to control the bleeding; excess wax must be removed.

TOURNIQUETS

Pneumatic Tourniquets. Used to control bleeding during extremity surgeries, a pneumatic tourniquet restricts both venous and arterial blood flow. It is inadvisable to use a tourniquet on patients who have vascular disease or problems with peripheral circulation.

A pneumatic tourniquet can cause neurologic or vascular injury if used incorrectly. Cuff selection is based on the size of the extremity. The cuff is placed around the largest circumference of the extremity, overlapping itself by 3–6 inches. It should not be placed around an elbow or knee, as injury can occur to the nerves and vascular structures. The skin under the cuff is padded with a stockinette. The padding should not have wrinkles, which could cause skin or nerve damage.

Venous blood is removed from the elevated extremity by wrapping it with a rubber bandage (*e.g.*, Esmark), starting at the toes or fingers. Once the venous blood is removed, the tourniquet cuff is inflated. The optimum pressure in the cuff depends on the patient's age, size, and blood pressure and is

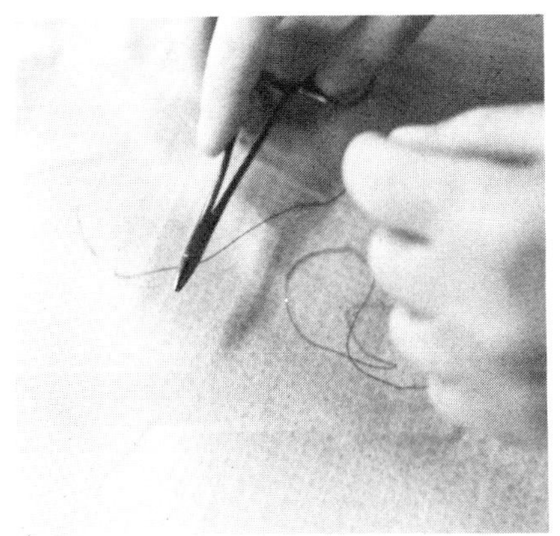

1. After the suture is placed through the tissue, pull the suture and leave a short end. Place the needleholder against the suture.

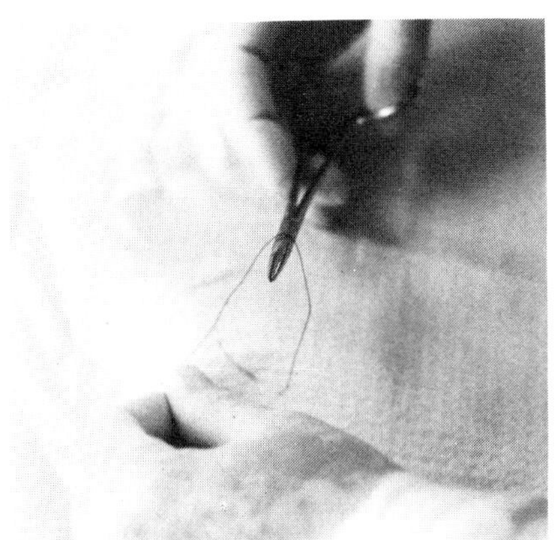

2. Wrap the suture around the needleholder (once or twice).

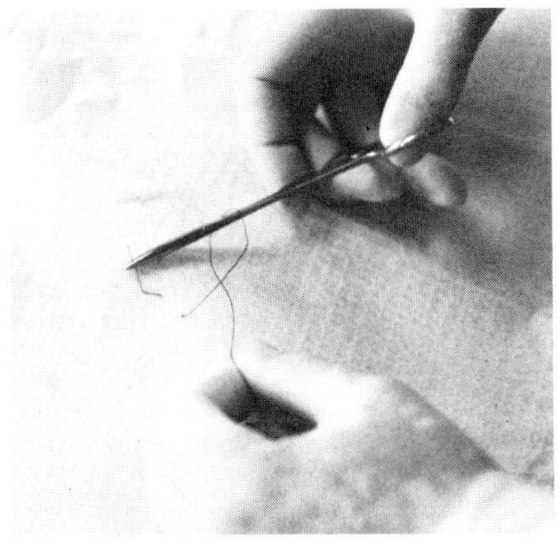

3. Grasp the short end of the suture with the needleholder and pull it through the suture wrapped around the needleholder.

FIGURE 13-19
INSTRUMENT TIE. Step-by-step instructions for completing the instrument tie.

(continued)

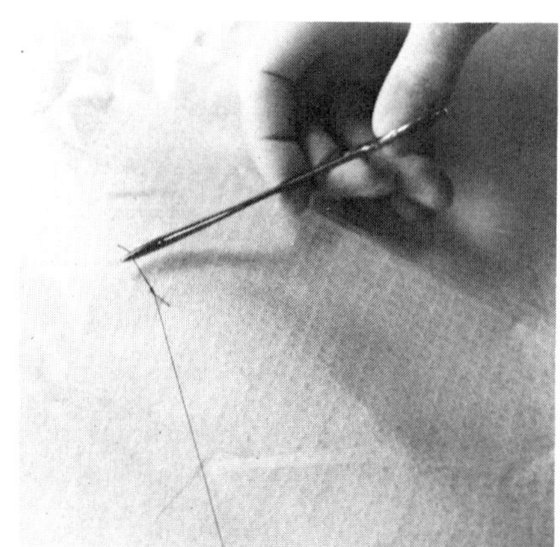

4. Secure the knot.

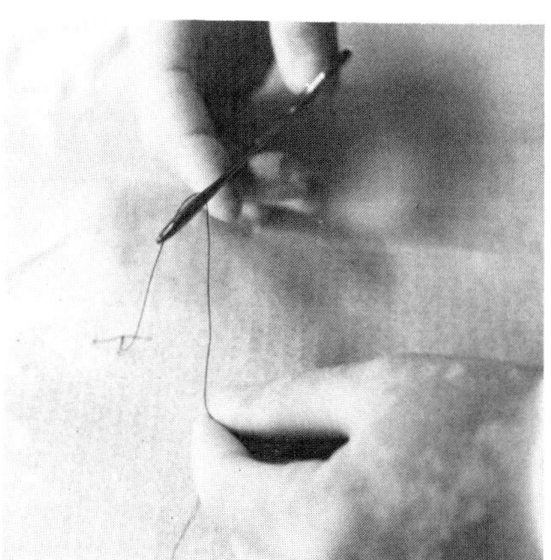

5. Wrap the suture over the needleholder in the direction opposite that of the initial wrap.

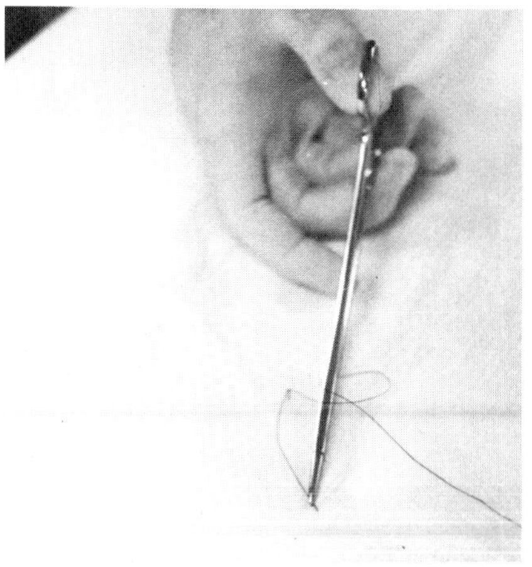

6. Again, grasp the short end of the suture with the needleholder and pull it through the suture wrapped around the needleholder. Secure the second half of the knot.

Figure 13-19 *(continued)*

determined by the physician. Usually, the pressure is 50–75 mm Hg above the patient's systolic blood pressure for the arm and 100–150 mm Hg above the systolic pressure for the leg. The inflated cuff should be left in place for only brief periods, a maximum of 1½ hours for the leg and 1 hour for the arm. If the surgery is not yet completed, the cuff can be deflated for 10 minutes and then reinflated. The periods of cuff inflation should be accurately documented, with the surgeon kept informed at 30-minute intervals.

Once the tourniquet is deflated, bleeding in the operative area will need to be controlled. Postoperative evaluation of the patient's extremity will be necessary to determine whether any injury occurred related to the use of the pneumatic tourniquet.

Vascular Tourniquets. Vascular tourniquets are used to control bleeding from vascular structures. The Rummel tourniquet is used to control the tightness of a purse-string suture in a blood vessel or heart chamber. Umbilical tapes are commonly placed around major arteries and veins to be used as tourniquets. The tourniquet effect may be accomplished by passing the umbilical tape around the vessel, tightening the tape until blood flow stops, and holding it secure with a hemostat. The umbilical tape can also be threaded through a piece of catheter tubing (using a stylet), then pulled tightly and held with a hemostat clamp above the tubing that holds both the tape and the tubing (see Figure 13-20). A vessel loop, pulled tightly around the vessel and secured with a hemostat, may be used instead of umbilical tape.

THERMAL MEANS OF ACHIEVING HEMOSTASIS

Wound hemostasis can be achieved quickly by applying electrical current to thrombose vessels. However, damage to adjacent tissue may be extensive if the correct technique is not used. Although the electrosurgical unit (ESU) is the most frequently used electrical unit for hemostasis, the argon beam coagulator may also be used for controlling hemorrhage from vascular structures. This unit uses argon gas, which flows through a handpiece, to clear fluid from the target site and then create a superficial eschar. The argon beam coagula-

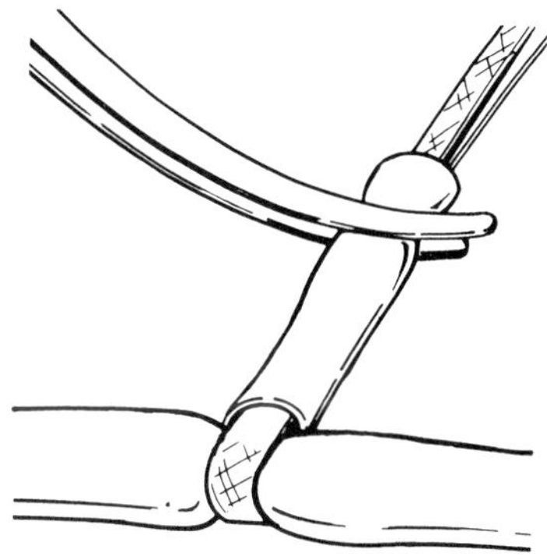

FIGURE 13-20
Umbilical tape is used to obstruct blood flow through the blood vessel. A rubber-tubing tourniquet is slid down the tape toward the blood vessel and held in place with a hemostat clamp.

tor may produce less necrotic tissue than is caused by high-current electrosurgery.

ELECTROSURGICAL UNITS

ESUs are used frequently during operative procedures. The electrical current creates heat that desiccates tissue and coagulates blood, occluding small blood vessels and providing hemostasis. Advantages of this type of hemostatic control are that it saves time, it can stop bleeding from vessels that are too small to clamp or ligate, and it helps control bleeding that is difficult to control by other methods, especially when accessibility is limited or the tissues are fragile.

Some problems may arise in using electrosurgery for hemostasis. Poor wound healing can occur with improperly performed electrosurgery. The depth of thermal injury to tissue is hard to control, and bleeding may recur from cauterized tissue. Accidental patient burns are common and can be avoided only when all members of the team understand and implement the necessary precautions. The ESU cannot be used in the presence of explosive anesthetic gases or to open a gas-filled bowel.

The ESU operator can choose among cutting, coagulating, or blended modes of electrical current. Cutting current is continuous and produces intense heat to vaporize tissue cells. The tissues separate because of the heat, and a shallow, devitalized, and desiccated area remains. Coagulating current is intermittent and produces less heat; tissues are charred rather than divided. Blended current combines the advantages of both cutting and coagulating currents.

The electrical current flows from the ESU through a wire to a tip held by a nonconductive handle. The handle, or active electrode, is called a "pencil" and may be disposable or reusable. Active electrodes should never be left lying unprotected on the surgical field; when not in use, the pencil should be placed in a clean, dry nonconductive holster. The electrode tip may be ball-shaped, flat, and narrow; have a needlepoint; or be a wire loop. After the current enters the tissues, it is returned to the patient through a dispersive wire. This wire may be attached to a plate or dispersive pad (grounding pad) that has been properly placed on the patient's skin. Because improper dispersion of electric current is a major cause of burns during electrosurgery, all operating room personnel must know the principles of proper pad positioning, characteristics of the particular pad used in the institution, skin assessment factors, and the warning system used in the particular unit. Various ESUs are available, each with its own particular warning system and user instructions. The importance of reading instructions and familiarity with the equipment and electrosurgical accessories cannot be overemphasized. Prevention of patient injury depends primarily on a knowledgeable perioperative team.

Two basic units are used with electrosurgery: monopolar and bipolar. The bipolar unit is the safer of the two and does not require a patient plate. In bipolar units, the current flows from one side of an accessory forceps, passes through the tissue, and enters the other side of the forceps. The risk of burns is decreased with these units, because the current's path is confined to the tip of the forceps and lower power settings are used. Bipolar instruments should be inspected regularly for defective insulation and other damage. Caution must be exercised in thinking that only bipolar units use forceps accessories; there are also monopolar forceps. Monopolar forceps must be used with a patient dispersive pad (grounding pad). The RN first assistant must be able to distinguish between monopolar and bipolar forceps. If monopolar forceps are used without a patient plate, the potential is created for an alternate current path burn. Familiarity with equipment and with the AORN's recommendations for electrosurgery application is essential for the safe use of any ESU.

The operator uses electrosurgery for tissue layers beneath the epidermis. The "pencil" is held comfortably like a pencil. The on/off switch, when located on the pencil, can be controlled easily with the index finger. A foot-controlled on/off switch may be used as an alternative to the hand-actuated pencil. To prevent accidental burns, the current should be on only when cutting or coagulating. Only the very end of the electrode tip should be used to ensure precision and minimal tissue damage. The sides of the tip will burn any tissue they contact; careful observation and precise control are necessary. The current can be conducted through metal, so care must be taken to avoid touching instruments that could burn another area. For larger vessels, a hemostat may be placed on the vessel. When the clamp is touched with the activated tip, current is conducted down the metal instrument, coagulating the vessel (See Table 13-1).

The active electrode is more effective if the tip is kept clean and charred tissue is removed periodically. The area to be cut or coagulated must be kept dry, as the electrical energy is ineffective if dispersed through fluid or blood. By blotting with a sponge immediately before using the active electrode, the operator can identify bleeding points. The active electrode should be used only on the ends of bleeding vessels to avoid unnecessary tissue damage. The ESU should be activated only long enough to stop the bleeding. If prolonged activation is necessary, the power setting may be too low, the patient circuit (ground) may be inadequate, or the vessel may be too large for this mode of hemostasis. Power settings should never be increased without first assessing pad placement and unit connections.

TABLE 13-1

Key Points in Using Electrosurgery for Hemostasis

1. Power settings should be set at the lowest level commensurate with rapid, localized vessel thrombosis.
2. A minimal amount of tissue should be lifted with the vessel.
3. Tissue around the vessel should be dry before activating current.
4. Coagulation power should be activated immediately before lightly touching the active electrode to an instrument.
5. The electrical circuit should be immediately broken on seeing the first darkening of tissue as coagulation begins about the vessel.

Extreme care must be taken when using electrosurgery around vital organs or tissues that should not be injured. In these cases, lower power settings and adequate retraction help prevent accidental injury.

When using the cutting mode, the operator applies only just enough pressure to allow the tissues to fall away from the tip as they are cut. Excessive pressure will not allow the cutting action, and coagulation of vessels will be inadequate.

It is not uncommon for RN first assistants or surgeons to report receiving a shock during ESU use. This may be especially true when the current is applied to an instrument during electrosurgical coagulation. Holes in gloves may be present as a manufacturing defect or occur during the surgical procedure. When the RN first assistant is engaged in a long surgical procedure, consideration should be given to regloving before using electrosurgical equipment. If heat is felt in the hand holding the instrument to which the current is being applied, current flow should be discontinued.

HYPOTHERMIA

Hypothermia causes vasoconstriction and decreases bleeding. However, generalized hypothermia is not effective unless the temperature is lowered to 35° C, and shivering and ventricular fibrillation may occur at this temperature, making hypothermia a poor choice as a method for hemostasis. Localized cooling has been effective for controlling esophageal or gastric bleeding, but this is not usually done intraoperatively. Cryogenic surgical procedures affect bleeding by causing necrosis of the vascular structures at extreme cold temperatures (-20° C).

CHEMICAL METHODS OF ACHIEVING HEMOSTASIS

Chemical methods useful in achieving hemostasis include blood pressure regulation with medication or anesthetic agents, the use of topical agents, and appropriate treatment of coagulation defects.

BLOOD PRESSURE REGULATION

Regulating blood pressure can be very effective in controlling bleeding. This is considered a chemical method of providing hemostasis, because medications or anesthetic agents are used.

Hypertension. Hypertension is controlled medically whenever possible. Intraoperative and postoperative bleeding can increase when blood pressure is elevated. Blood pressure is monitored frequently, and hypertension is treated with appropriate medications. Pain can cause hypertension and is controlled as much as possible postoperatively. Intraoperatively, pain occurs when the anesthesia is inadequate. A rise in blood pressure may be one of the first signs that the patient is experiencing pain.

Hypotension. Hypotension during the intraoperative period may be induced to decrease bleeding. The hypotensive state is closely monitored and controlled by the anesthesiologist. Medications and anesthetic agents are used intraoperatively to induce hypotension for procedures that are highly vascular (*e.g.*, hip surgery) or when surgery involves vascular structures (*e.g.*, cerebral aneurysms). Complications from hypotension can arise when the perfusion of vital organs is inadequate.

TOPICAL AGENTS

Thrombin. Thrombin is used topically to promote hemostasis by directly clotting the fibrinogen in the blood. It is useful in controlling bleeding or oozing from small blood vessels or capillaries.

Thrombin most commonly comes in solution but may come as a dry powder, to which isotonic saline or sterile distilled water is added to make a solution. The speed with which the thrombin acts to coagulate blood depends on solution concentration. Solutions should be prepared immediately before use.

When using absorbable gelatin sponges soaked in thrombin, it is important to squeeze the sponge gently to remove any trapped air so that the sponge is completely saturated with thrombin and more effective in promoting hemostasis.

Thrombin must never be injected into the bloodstream or allowed to gain access through opened, large blood vessels. Extensive intravascular clotting and possible death may ensue.

Excess blood should be removed by sponging or suctioning the operative area before applying thrombin. Once the area has been treated, it should not be sponged, as the clots will be removed.

Gelatin Sponges. Absorbable gelatin sponges (trade name Gelfoam) are prepared from a purified gelatin solution that has been whipped into a foam, dried, and then sterilized. Gelatin sponges can be applied to the bleeding surface either dry or moist. The sponge can be moistened by dipping it in normal saline solution that may have thrombin or epinephrine added to it. The sponge absorbs many times its own weight in blood, which then clots within the sponge. The blood is drawn into the sponge by capillary action, but it can be suctioned into the sponge if the sponge is protected with a gauze sponge or cotton pledget.

The gelatin sponge liquefies in 2–5 days following application to bleeding mucosal areas; it is absorbed completely in 4–6 weeks. A gelatin sponge should not be used in the presence of an infection that could localize in the sponge. When used in cavities or closed tissue spaces, care must be taken not to overpack; swelling of the sponge could cause pressure, injuring surrounding tissues, nerves, and vascular structures. The sponge is often cut into the desired size and, if used moist, immersed in the solution, squeezed to remove air, and stored in the solution until used.

Microfibrillar Collagen. A hemostatic agent derived from bovine dermis, microfibrillar collagen (trade name Avitene) can help provide hemostasis when other methods are ineffective or impractical. Collagen promotes hemostasis by causing platelets to aggregate and activate by releasing substances that initiate the coagulation mechanisms. Collagen is available in a loose fibrous form and in a compacted, "nonwoven" web form. Collagen adheres to wet surfaces and therefore is applied with dry, smooth forceps to the bleeding site. The bleeding site is compressed with a dry sponge, the collagen is applied, and then pressure is applied with a sponge placed over the collagen. Pressure should be continued for 1–10 minutes, depending on the severity of the bleeding. If bleeding continues through the collagen, the application can be repeated. Any excess collagen should be removed by gently teasing it away, because excess collagenous material could later cause complications such as bowel adhesions or mechanical pressure on ureters.

Absorbable Collagen Sponges. Absorbable collagen sponges (trade name Collastat) are made from collagen derived from bovine flexor tendon. The sponge can be cut to size and applied directly to the bleeding area. It will not disperse like the microfibrillar collagen and is easier to handle and place. It, too, is handled with dry smooth tissue forceps. After placement on tissue, the sponge controls bleeding in 2–4 minutes by causing platelet aggregation and clot formation.

Oxidized Cellulose. Oxidized cellulose (trade names Oxycel and Surgicel) is available impregnated in treated gauze or cotton. Applied directly to a bleeding surface, it promotes clotting of capillaries and small vessels that cannot be controlled by other means. The gauze can be cut into strips or to the size desired and placed on the bleeding site dry, with a dry sponge to hold it in place. The oxidized cellulose is absorbed in 2–7 days. It must not be packed tightly because it swells; also, it must never be left in the patient if used near the spinal cord, optic nerve, or any area where swelling can seriously damage surrounding tissues or nerves. Oxidized cellulose is not used as permanent packing in bone fractures, because it interferes with bone regeneration. It should never be used with thrombin, because it interferes with thrombin action.

Fibrin Glue. When hemostasis cannot be obtained with the usual measures, fibrin glue might be used. This substance is useful for controlling generalized oozing of blood, but it will not control vigorous bleeding. The glue is prepared with 25–50 cc of cryoprecipitate in one container and two ampules of thrombin (10,000 u/ampule) mixed with 500 mg of calcium chloride in a separate container. Each solution is drawn into a separate syringe with a #18 gauge hypodermic needle attached. The two solutions are then sprayed simultaneously on the bleeding site.

Albumin. Albumin is frequently used to coat vascular prosthetic grafts to prevent bleeding through the porous graft surface. This not only contributes to hemostasis, but also makes the luminal surface of the graft smoother, decreasing postoperative thrombosis formation inside the graft. The graft is prepared by soaking it in albumin, wiping off any excess, and then steam sterilizing for 3 minutes at 270° F.

Epinephrine. Epinephrine is used frequently with local anesthetic agents because it causes vasoconstriction, prolonging the effect of the local anesthetic and decreasing bleeding. Topically, gelatin sponges may be soaked in epinephrine and applied to a bleeding surface. Epinephrine should never be used for finger or toe surgery; sloughing may occur. It should not be used in patients with peripheral vascular disease for the same reason. Because epinephrine can cause increased blood pressure, tachycardia, and vasoconstriction, it is not usually recommended for patients with cardiac conditions.

CONCLUSION

Perioperative nurses have long recognized the many potential risks facing patients during the intraoperative period. The RN first assistant, acting in the expanded perioperative nurse role, continues to monitor and ensure patient safety. The potential for patient injury exists even when nursing interventions are directed at the achievement of a positive outcome, such as assisting with hemostasis and using hemostatic adjuncts. A review of the critical elements of providing hemostasis elucidates the following potential nursing diagnoses and consequent safety considerations:

1. Fluid Volume Deficit (intraoperative) related to inadequate control of bleeding
2. High Risk for Injury related to the use of electrical equipment (the ESU)
3. Altered Tissue Perfusion related to surgical interruption of blood vessels, the use of hypothermia, the tourniquet, controlled hypotension, and vasoconstrictive drugs
4. High Risk for Infection related to the use of vasoconstrictive drugs, electrosurgery, and tissue-reactive suture materials
5. Fluid Volume Deficit (postoperative) related to inadequate volume replacement or slippage of knot or suture.

The RN first assistant, through the application of knowledge and skill, directs efforts toward providing patients with injury-free postoperative outcomes. When wounds are dry and hemostasis is achieved, attention has been paid to meticulous detail and the correct decisions have been made. Using a sound knowledge base, the RN first assistant has implemented techniques that prevent potential patient injury and wound complications.

REVIEW QUESTIONS

1. The RN first assistant initially seeks to prevent blood loss by
   a. appropriate use of the ESU and argon beam coagulator
   b. anticipatory control of blood vessels
   c. learning how to use the square knot
   d. using digital compression before other methods
2. The body's natural defense of blood clotting will produce adhesion, aggregation and initial plug formation within
   a. 1–2 seconds
   b. 1–3 minutes
   c. 5–10 minutes
   d. 1–2 hours
3. During assessment, the RN first assistant notes that the patient is undergoing cancer chemotherapy. This places the patient at risk for
   a. deficiency in factor X concentration
   b. hemolytic transfusion reaction
   c. thrombocytopenia
   d. disseminated intravascular coagulation
4. Which of the following would be the most appropriate question to ask a patient regarding any bleeding problems?
   a. "Can you tell me your normal clotting time?"
   b. "Have you had any problems with bleeding following dental extraction?"
   c. "Have you ever had a problem with a blood transfusion?"
   d. "Do you have problems with GI bleeding or hematuria?"
5. Prothrombin time measures
   a. the coagulant activity of the "extrinsic" system, including fibrinogen, prothrombin, and factors V, VII, and X
   b. the presence of immune globulin on the surface of erythrocytes or in the plasma
   c. disorders of platelet function
   d. deficiencies of all plasma coagulation factors except VII and XIII
6. Albumin aids in the maintenance of colloid osmotic pressure. An albumin level below ________g/dl is of concern in assessing risk for fluid imbalance.
   a. 3
   b. 4
   c. 5
   d. 6
7. Initial attempts at reversing hemorrhagic shock will be made by transfusing
   a. plasma
   b. red blood cells
   c. crystalloid albumin
   d. intravenous fluids
8. An example of the application of indirect pressure is applying it
   a. with a sponge on a stick
   b. between two fingers (bidigitally)
   c. to an area proximal of the bleeding vessel
   d. with the tip of an instrument, such as the suction tip

9. If a moist pack is used in an area of diffuse bleeding, it should be moistened with _______ saline.
   a. cool
   b. warm
10. When curved hemostats are used to clamp a vessel before transection, the hemostat tips should point _______ each other to facilitate cutting between the clamps.
   a. toward
   b. away from
11. When the RN first assistant must deal with multiple clamps as tying is about to proceed, he/she should
   a. take two or three in the hand at a time to speed the process
   b. suggest using the ESU rather than tying
   c. pick them up for tying in the order that they were placed
   d. take the most accessible one first and proceed in a logical order
12. Once the ligature is slid down the heel of a clamp, the clamp is lowered to a horizontal position and the tips are _______ without pulling.
   a. directed downward
   b. elevated
13. In general, during knot tying, the strand that is actively passed through the loop is held in which hand?
   a. dominant
   b. nondominant
14. Despite the type of knot to be used, a basic principle of knot tying is that
   a. the free end of a suture strand should be short
   b. the free end of a suture strand should be long
   c. suture strands should not be sawed against each other
   d. knots are secured with three throws
15. Keeping the suture strands loose and equal, forming a round loop as the knot is snugged down, prevents formation of an unwanted half hitch and
   a. the need to turn the body to properly orient the hands
   b. the need to alternate throws
   c. sawing and fraying of the suture
   d. tying away from the body
16. To prevent pulling up on the structure being tied (and to prevent reversing the throw into a half hitch), the RN first assistant should learn to complete the throw by putting the _______ finger of the hand holding the suture strand closest to the body down on the strand.
   a. middle
   b. long
   c. ring
   d. index
17. The first step of every throw is the formation of a loop over a finger or instrument; keeping the finger _______ the structure being tied prevents twisting of the loop and crossing.
   a. parallel to
   b. perpendicular to

c. away from
d. pointing towards

18. A pneumatic tourniquet applied to a patient's arm is usually inflated to ______ mm Hg above the patient's systolic blood pressure.
    a. 25–50
    b. 50–75
    c. 75–100
    d. 100–150

19. When using an ESU, the RN first assistant should deactivate the current immediately on noting ______ of tissue about the vessel.
    a. reddening
    b. charring
    c. darkening
    d. erythema

20. Vascular prosthetic grafts may be coated with ______ to prevent bleeding through porous graft surfaces.
    a. albumin
    b. thrombin
    c. fibrin glue
    d. oxidized cellulose

Answers

1. b
2. b
3. c
4. b
5. a
6. b
7. d
8. c
9. a
10. a
11. c
12. b
13. a
14. c
15. c
16. d
17. a
18. b
19. c
20. a

Bibliography

American College of Surgeons: Care of the Surgical Patient: Vol I, Critical Care. New York, Scientific American Medicine, 1989

Anderson R, Romfh R: Surgical Tools. New York, Appleton-Century-Crofts, 1980

Association of Operating Room Nurses: Recommended Practices for Electrosurgery. Denver, Association of Operating Room Nurses, 1992

Association of Operating Room Nurses: Standards and Recommended Practices for Perioperative Nursing. Denver, Association of Operating Room Nurses, 1992

Cardiovascular, Thoracic, and General Surgical Pilling Instruments. Fort Washington, PA, Narco Scientific, 1980

Doty D: Cardiac Surgery. Chicago, Year Book Medical Publishers, 1985

ETHICON Knot Tying Manual. Somerville, NJ, ETHICON, Inc, 1983

Groah L: Operating Room Nursing, Perioperative Practice. Norwalk, CT, Appleton & Lange, 1990

Kneedler J, Dodge G: Perioperative Patient Care. Boston, Blackwell Scientific Publications, 1987

McShane R, Perry A: Skin lacerations: Suturing and caring for the wound. In Clinical Nurse Practitioner, Vol 2, No 2, pp 8–10. Providence, RI, Pfizer, 1984

Meeker M, Rothrock JC: Alexander's Care of the Patient in Surgery. St Louis, Mosby–Year Book, 1991

Physicians' Desk Reference, 45th ed. Oradell, NJ, Medical Economics, 1991

Swartz S, Shires GT, Spencer F, Storer E: Principles of Surgery, 4th ed. San Francisco, McGraw-Hill, 1984

Symonds P: Skin sutures and principles of suture removal. In Point of View, Vol 2, No 1, pp 6–9. Somerville, NJ, ETHICON, Inc, 1983

Vaiden R, Fox V, Rothrock J: Core Curriculum for the RN First Assistant. Denver, Association of Operating Room Nurses, 1990

Van Way C, Buer C: Surgical Skills in Patient Care. St Louis, CV Mosby, 1978

Wound Closure Manual. Somerville, NJ, ETHICON, Inc, 1985

14 The RN First Assistant and Collaborative Practice

Patricia C. Seifert

Although not widely discussed in the literature, the concept of collaborative practice in the operating room is not a novel one to perioperative practitioners. As early as 1894, an operating team consisting of surgeons, nurses, and assistants was recommended and introduced at the Johns Hopkins Hospital in Baltimore.[1] Since then, the team approach has remained a vital working relationship in all operating rooms. It is still considered one of the best examples of cooperative efforts displayed by nurses and physicians.

BACKGROUND

It should not be inferred that the interactions among physicians and nurses have always been uniformly or consistently collaborative. Historically, the nurse–physician relationship has been characterized as a unilateral one, with most of the authority and decision making assumed by the physician. Nurses were not actively involved in planning patient care, nor were they privy to physicians' decision making rationales. They were expected not to question orders and not to communicate to patients the reasons for those orders.

Exceptions did occur. At the end of the 19th century in Rochester, Minnesota, the Mayo brothers were among the first to provide an opportunity to expand the role of nurses in the operating room and to include them in patient care by training them to provide anesthesia to their patients.[2] More commonly, however, the operating room nurse's duties at that time centered on maintaining instruments, supplies, and equipment; managing the sterilizing room; preparing dressings; and passing instruments.[3] But even in the confines of the operating room, the team concept did foster shared responsibilities and a growing mutual respect.

By World War I, operating room nursing had evolved into a distinct specialty with formal education programs and specialized training. The nurse's focus shifted from largely technical concerns to more patient-centered activities. Responsibility for maintaining an aseptic environment, supervising nonnursing personnel, and preparing the surgical patient were added. First assisting was occasionally performed, and became increasingly more common as World War I progressed. The shortage of qualified medical first assistants influenced the decision to train nurses for this role.

First assisting was further promoted during World War II, when the demand for assistants became so great that even nonnursing technicians were trained to assist. After the war, the shortage of nurses forced hospitals to hire technicians trained in the armed forces. This increased use of technicians for scrubbing and first assisting, along with the concurrent reduction in the requirement for operating room rotations in student nursing programs, had the effect of producing a somewhat technical and isolated image of the operating room nurse. It also had the unfortunate effect of limiting communication between nurses inside and outside the operating room. Of special significance for nurses outside the operating room was that deletion of an operating room rotation denied them contact with patients in surgery. It also reduced the interaction with nurses who had the special knowledge and skills necessary for aseptic technique. That knowledge is still crucial to many nursing functions in all practice areas. In addition, first assisting by registered nurses, with its potential for increasing firsthand the nurse's knowledge of anatomy, physiology, and the impact of surgical interventions, was largely delegated to technicians.

The formation of the Association of Operating Room Nurses (AORN) in 1954 signaled operating room nurses' concern for defining and promoting a high level of professional practice during surgery. AORN's formulation of the perioperative role in 1978, and its revision in 1985 describing perioperative nursing practice, addressed the nurse's responsibility for providing care in the preoperative, intraoperative, and postoperative phases of the patient's surgical experience. According to AORN, the perioperative nurse "works in collaboration with other health care professionals to determine and meet patient needs and has primary responsibility and accountability for nursing care of patients having surgical intervention."[4] By 1992, AORN recognized that with changing practice patterns and care delivery settings, the focus of care could no longer be easily delimited by geographic boundaries (*i.e.*, perioperative care was being delivered in settings other than traditional "operating rooms") or time boundaries (*i.e.*, the traditional preoperative, intraoperative, and postoperative phases of care had become blurred).[5] As care delivery routines and practices change, the need for collaboration between and among health care professionals intensifies.

The scope of perioperative nursing includes a variety of roles, including the practice of first assisting. This represents an expanded role.[6] Thus, RN first assistants are first and foremost perioperative nurses and are responsible not only for assisting the surgeon intraoperatively, but also for preoperative patient assessment and postoperative patient evaluation.

It is crucial that the RN first assistant fulfill the perioperative role, because first assisting *in and of itself* is not nursing[7], but rather a medically supervised supportive service. This distinction has serious ramifications for the development of collaborative relationships. Joint or collaborative practice can be achieved only among persons or groups with accountability, responsibility, and authority for their own profession and practice. As H. Robert Cathcart, Chairman of the National Commission on Nursing, noted in 1981, "collaborative practice demands a complementary relationship between nurses and physicians, not an unequal supervisor–subordinate type of relationship."[8]

As a perioperative nurse, the RN first assistant operates within the framework of nursing even though during the act of assisting he/she is supervised by the surgeon. This is similar to any interdependent nursing function that necessitates a physician order, such as giving medications or prescribed treatments. If a first assistant's practice did not also incorporate those independent nursing functions that the RN first assistant is legally licensed to perform (*e.g.*, assessment, evaluation), there would be no basis for a collaborative working relationship. Nurses and physicians each offer areas of expertise, making them interdependent for providing a total plan of care. Neither medicine nor nursing alone can totally meet a patient's needs. Quoting Dr. Marc Hansen, Ingeborg Mauksch addressed this attitudinal change by physicians who have come to the realization that nurses' contributions provide a "missing component in effective care and fill a gap in the care of and caring for patients and their families."[9] This change was influenced by a number of social and cultural factors.

CHANGES IN NURSING PRACTICE

The impact of two world wars, the women's movement, technological advances, and the growth of specialization have profoundly affected nursing practice and practice relationships in the operating room and throughout the health care field. In addition, federal reimbursement policy changes (*e.g.*, prospective payment and diagnosis-related groups [DRGs], as well as physician payment reform and resource-based relative value scales) necessitating the delivery of cost-efficient as well as quality care have been influential in altering traditional nursing roles. Nurses and other professionals have had to become more specialized to keep abreast of rapid technologic advances. New responsibilities have prompted the need for increased knowledge and new skills. As a result, the nurse's role has expanded and changed, producing greater expertise within a particular area of practice.

Although these developments have provided exciting opportunities for first assistants and other specialists, they have also fostered professional fragmentation, not only between nurses and physicians, but also among nurses themselves. Moreover, many nurses continue to function in a traditional role that offers little stimulation or opportunity to develop professionally; these nurses may experience varying levels of dissatisfaction and "burnout." Those nurses attempting to make a concerted effort to deal with these problems have had to contend with concerns about differing educational preparation, authority, power, role ambiguity, incongruent expectations, money, and status.

DEVELOPMENT OF COLLABORATIVE PRACTICE

In an effort to address some of these problems and to improve nurse–physician relationships, the American Nurses' Association (ANA) and the American Medical Association (AMA) established the National Joint Practice Commission (NJPC) in 1972 with funding from the W.K. Kellogg Foundation. The creation of this national commission, consisting of equal numbers of nurses and physicians, had been recommended in *An Abstract for Action,* a 1970 report by the National Commission for the Study of Nursing and Nursing Education. Known as the Lysaught Report (after the commission's director, Dr. Jerome P. Lysaught), the findings proposed, among other recommendations, institutional joint practice committees representing medicine and nursing. They also proposed the recognition and reward of increased competence in nursing practice.

The NJPC focused on the need for more collaboration and used the terms "joint practice" and "collaborative practice" interchangeably. Joint practice was defined as "nurses and physicians collaborating together as colleagues to provide patient care."[10] Reference to a collegial relationship represented a departure from the traditional notion that nurses had little to contribute to decision making in patient care management.

To be accepted as colleagues, nurses must achieve clinical credibility and have it recognized by physicians, administrators, peers, and patients. In the past, reward systems in nursing encouraged competent nurses to move away from direct patient contact and into administration or education. The more recent emphasis on clinical performance has led to the development of performance standards and clinical ladders, which have fostered and rewarded clinical competence. Another benefit has been that nurses have increased their self-esteem and become more confident in their contribution to patient management. In addition, there has been the need and a willingness by nurses to accept a greater share of responsibility and accountability for nursing actions. The growing realization by nurses and physicians that each profession makes a unique contribution to the welfare of patients has been a major step toward achieving collaborative working relationships.

Such a relationship is nurtured in a climate of open communication, trust, and mutual respect. These characteristics cannot be mandated, but they can be fostered and encouraged under the right circumstances. Many individual examples of cooperative efforts exist, whether formally labeled "collaborative practice" or not, and they are usually distinguished by the presence of people working to create an environment conducive to such conduct.

ELEMENTS OF COLLABORATIVE PRACTICE

Communication, trust, and mutual respect were highlighted in the NJPC's 1981 *Guideline for Establishing Joint or Collaborative Practice in Hospitals.* In addition, five elements for the formal implementation of a collaborative practice model were recommended:

1. primary nursing
2. a joint practice committee of equal numbers of doctors and nurses who practice on the unit
3. unit doctors and nurses jointly evaluating their patient care
4. integrated patient records
5. encouragement of nurses' individual clinical decision making.[11]

These elements were established (or already in place) on nursing units in four pilot hospitals selected to implement the NJPC guidelines. Papers published by those involved in the pilot study describe success in implementing the commission guidelines within their practice settings.[12] Although none of the selected units included the operating room, collaborative practice as outlined is feasible and practical.

PRIMARY NURSING

Definition

As defined by the NJPC, primary nursing is the performance of clinical nursing functions by RNs with minimal or no delegation of nursing tasks to others. Nurses who are individually responsible for patients' comprehensive nursing care are able to enter into a collegial relationship with physicians who provide the patient's medical care.[13]

Zander noted that primary nursing can succeed in all clinical settings, including the operating room.[14] Since the inception of the surgical team, perioperative nurses have accepted responsibility for providing primary nursing care to patients. The reaction to the threat of technicians being allowed to circulate has demonstrated the perioperative nurse's concern for maintaining primary responsibility for the surgical patient.

Complementarity

Primary nursing does not imply that all patient care activity and responsibility is subsumed under the role of nursing. Rather, the primary nurse and the physician complement one another. This complementary relationship is particularly evident between the surgeon and the first assistant. For example, a patient's preoperative assessment data are used by the RN first assistant for proper positioning to prevent or minimize muscle or nerve injury. Patient and family support and education are strengthened by the first assistant's specialized knowledge of the procedure and its impact on patient outcomes. Information sharing by the first assistant and other nurses facilitates improved discharge planning and home care by providing information pertinent to activities of daily living, learning needs, and psychosocial concerns.

Intraoperatively, the RN first assistant engages in a cooperative effort with the surgeon to achieve a successful surgical intervention. Although responsible for supervising the first assistant's performance, the surgeon is nevertheless dependent on the first assistant for help with the operation. The first assistant must assume responsibility for self-performance. It is during this period that the surgeon and the first assistant are most closely associated and need most to rely on one another. Some of the factors necessary to accomplish this include:

- ☐ possessing the requisite knowledge and experience related to anatomy, physiology, microbiology, pharmacology, and behavioral sciences
- ☐ knowing the procedure and the rationale for it
- ☐ acquiring the manual skill and dexterity to perform the required maneuvers
- ☐ being familiar with the individual surgeon's preferences
- ☐ anticipating the needs of the surgeon and the patient
- ☐ communicating information relevant to the procedure
- ☐ concentrating on the operative field throughout the procedure
- ☐ protecting the patient from injury
- ☐ maintaining flexibility and adaptability when emergencies or unanticipated events occur
- ☐ possessing creativity in solving problems or dealing with difficulties during the procedure
- ☐ knowing one's limits as required by experience, conscience, professional responsibility, and legal and jurisdictional constraints.

The RN first assistant's contributions extend beyond the immediate sterile field. One of the major benefits to be derived from assisting is the knowledge gained from directly observing and participating in the surgery itself. Sharing this knowledge with nonassisting nurses enhances these nurses' levels of practice. Not only is "routine" patient care improved, but a greater appreciation of the possible dangers and complications inherent in the procedure enables clinicians to work collaboratively to anticipate and plan for these potential occurrences. Standardized care plans are certainly useful, but each patient is unique and requires individualized attention and planning based on his actual and potential needs. Moreover, knowledgeably communicating with the surgeon from his frame of reference encourages active participation by staff and also improves staff morale and self-esteem.

Postoperative evaluation provides an opportunity for the RN first assistant to investigate areas for improvement and to confirm the adequacy of aseptic technique, preoperative teaching, and prevention of thermal, chemical, or mechanical injury.

The primary nurse not only is responsible for the completion of tasks but also is accountable for the planned outcomes of care[15]; for example, the patient's demonstrated ability to perform deep breathing and coughing exercises or to describe and be able to act on potentially harmful side effects of a prescribed anticoagulation regimen. To clarify this last example, when a patient requires a mitral valve replacement, the first assistant in cardiac surgery should know that of the two main types of valvular prostheses (biological and mechanical), the latter requires constant anticoagulation postoperatively. Anticoagulation therapy requires that the patient have routine follow-up blood tests to ensure and maintain adequate coumadin levels. Suppose that the RN first assistant learned from the preoperative assessment that where the patient lived made it difficult to arrange for frequent follow-up blood tests. This aspect of the patient's lifestyle would be important in the surgeon's determination of which type of prosthesis to insert. If either a biological or mechanical valve were indicated, the surgeon would be more likely to implant the former, given the constraints on follow-up care imposed by the patient's residential location. This information would be part of the nurse's psychosocial assessment. Sharing this assessment data with the surgeon can favorably alter the patient's outcome. If only a mechanical valve was indicated, then the RN first assistant would be able to plan with the patient for home health care providers or visiting nurses to meet the need for follow-up blood tests.

Primary nursing requires a broad knowledge base that incorporates both "nursing" and "medical" knowledge. The boundaries between the two areas are arbitrary; it is how the information is used that differentiates practice. Although some knowledge is more pertinent to one profession than to the other, an increasing amount of shared knowledge fosters interdependency and collaboration. It is not surprising that research has shown collaborative efforts to be more effective in situations where nurses are familiar with medical policies and protocols[16] and in situations where nurses are better educated.[17]

JOINT PRACTICE COMMITTEES

According to the NJPC, "a joint practice committee equally representing practicing nurses and physicians, and supported by the administration, will continuously monitor nurse–physician relationships and recommend appropriate actions supporting joint practice."[18]

Nurse–physician committees consisting of perioperative nurses and surgeons have flourished on the national level for years. The AORN and the ACS hold conferences that provide an opportunity to discuss and find solutions to operating room problems.[19] Joint boards of medicine and nursing on the state level have addressed practice questions and in some instances have jointly recommended guidelines for the role of the first assistant.[20] Locally, hospital-wide and unit-based committees have been formed to foster communication, shared problem-solving, and exploration of the scope of nursing practice.

In the operating room, committees consisting of nurses, surgeons, and anesthesiologists have been successful in encouraging joint practice. In addition to specific patient care questions, agenda items specific to the operating room have included cost containment, scheduling of cases, recommended practices, medical student orientation, aseptic technique, assignment of specialty personnel, and problem solving at the level of occurrence. The Joint Commission for Accreditation of Health Care Organizations (JCAHO) has stated the expectation that "there are policies and procedures, approved by the hospital administration and the medical staff, designed to assure effective collaboration among departments/services providing and those supporting surgical and anesthesia services."[21]

By providing a forum for physicians and nurses to clarify their roles, a joint practice committee enables the participants to communicate, to discuss questions of competence and accountability, and to foster trust and mutual respect. Nursing must be represented, because it is ultimately in the practice setting itself that true collaborative practice can succeed.

RN first assistants can provide pertinent insights into practice problems encountered in the operating room. Their familiarity with the surgeons' perceived needs and requirements specific to operative procedures can be invaluable in bridging the knowledge gap and promoting understanding between the professions. Interactive roles of nurses and physicians on joint practice committees underscore the value of discussion, negotiation, and compromise.

Even with the best intentions, joint practice committees cannot succeed without administrative support. The workplace culture should support an environment conducive to positive physician–nurse relationships, provide efficient and sufficient ancillary services, and include nursing in decision making committees that affect the delivery of services. In addition, committee discussions pertaining to practice issues that focus on licensure laws and hospital policies may require professional advice from risk managers and attorneys. For example, the questions of what a nurse does, and more specifically what an RN first assistant does, may not be easily defined. It is essential that committees addressing the role of the first assistant familiarize themselves with state nurse practice acts and institutional policies.

Committee sessions need not always be harmonious. Complex subjects require careful exploration, frank appraisal, and sometimes reappraisal of roles and duties. This can lead to arguments. As long as disagreements focus on issues rather than on personalities, conflicts can form the basis for better understanding and teamwork. The important point is that communication be ongoing. Committee members approaching difficult issues in an open-minded manner foster trust and respect. Moreover, they are as likely to gain as they are to give.

JOINT EVALUATION OF PATIENT CARE

The NJPC has stated that "nurses and physicians together will review the patient care which they have collaborated in providing. This review will supplement separate medical and nursing audits."[22]

The purpose of the joint review is to examine the nursing and medical care given to patients and to ascertain whether documentation reflects the care described. This creates a learning opportunity for physicians to discuss pathophysiology and the treatment provided; it also offers nurses the occasion to describe nursing interventions based on patient responses to the disease and the medical therapy instituted. Yeston noted that "a physician-nursing partnership is the key to a successful quality assurance program."[23] He described collaborative research that focused on such patient practices as admission and discharge from a critical care unit, decubitus ulcers, incidental blood loss due to arterial lines, the occurrence and prevention of self-extubation, indwelling catheter infection rates, and prolonged ventilator times. The salient point of such collaboration in research is the ability to function together to change practice and effect positive patient outcomes. Group success, rather than individual reward, is the focus of a well-functioning team.

As part of the evaluation process, the joint review enables RN first assistants to assess the results of their own work within the overall team effort. Attention might be focused on the patient's skin healing, the development of postoperative infections, nerve injury secondary to improper manipulation of extremities, or other complications. Problems jointly discussed provide an avenue for mutually supportive actions.

Successful procedures without morbid complications would be useful as learning experiences as well. Learning each other's rationale for treatment is in itself a beneficial aspect of the review. The value of joint reviews as teaching sessions is appreciated not only by practicing clinicians, but also by medical and nursing students. In addition, students are exposed to role models after whom they can pattern their own professional behavior.

Joint patient care conferences, morbidity and mortality conferences, trauma reprises, and specialty meetings are all useful forums for fostering increased understanding among professionals and promoting integrated patient care.

Informal meetings between the primary nurse and the physician also facilitate comprehensive care. Postoperative discussions focusing on surgery just performed are useful for future planning. The insights gained from each operation contribute to the first assistant's store of knowledge and experience.

INTEGRATED PATIENT RECORDS

According to the NJPC, "a patient record system integrating the observations, judgments, and actions of both nurses and physicians will reflect collaborative practice and contribute to it, and will provide a formal means of doctor–nurse communication in the care of patients."[24]

Initially, this element of the joint practice guidelines aroused the greatest concern in physicians and nurses on pilot units. The former feared increased legal liability risk; the latter expressed anxiety about the quality of their charting. Once nurses developed the necessary skill in writing notes and physicians came to appreciate the information documented, integrated progress notes and flow sheets fostered coordination of patient care.[25] One obvious benefit is the reduction of duplicate information; another is a better mutual understanding of the care and concerns of nurses and physicians. This leads to improved continuity of care and has the potential for reducing errors.

Complete integration of the patient record may not be feasible or advisable. Surgeons may not wish to read through the numerous items charted on operative nursing notes; perioperative nurses may not need to know that a 3-0 suture ligature was used. However, documentation of a patient's preoperative mental status or ability to participate in activities of daily living is of importance to the surgeon and could justifiably be noted in the progress notes or assessment forms. Surgeons also want to be aware of intraoperative activities such as correct sponge, needle, and instrument counts; and they ought to know what actions are taken for the preparation and protection of patients during surgery. The RN first assistant should be aware of the admitting diagnosis and indication for surgery, as well as pertinent laboratory data and the results of the history and physical. Knowing that the patient has been taking aspirin, for example, allows the RN first assistant to anticipate the possible need for platelets.

The RN first assistant anticipates the possibility of prolonged bleeding. A low hematocrit indicates the possible need for blood replacement. The patient with a history of arthritis will have special positioning needs. By documenting individualized nursing care, the RN first assistant educates others and accepts responsibility for her actions. The surgeon's operative reports provide the same learning opportunities and reflect his responsibility.

Postoperative evaluations should be documented as well. The RN first assistant will want to assess and note the effects of her interventions, the adequacy of preoperative preparation and teaching, and the need for additional support and education.

In hospitals where integrated nurse–physician records are not yet a reality, integrated records are certainly appropriate for nurses themselves. Where charting commonly includes "Patient to OR via stretcher," only to be immediately followed by "Patient returned from OR via stretcher," continuity of care would be facilitated by the inclusion of a perioperative note. This would benefit both unit nurses and perioperative nurses by increasing awareness of their individual roles. Collaboration must begin in nursing practice before it can be fully achieved between nurses and physicians.

This was emphasized by Jordan, who noted that nurse–physician collaboration will be more effective if we first have "close identification and collaboration with other nurses"; it was further emphasized by JCAHO's expectation that "nursing staff members collaborate, as appropriate, with physicians and other clinical disciplines in making decisions regarding each patient's need for nursing care."[26] Given the increasing complexity and specialization that exist in health care provision, the need for cooperation, mutual understanding, and unity is greater now than ever before.

ENCOURAGEMENT OF NURSES' INDIVIDUAL CLINICAL DECISION MAKING

To exercise their professional skills to the fullest, nurses must be encouraged to make individual clinical nursing decisions using both medical and nursing consultations. These decisions will lie within the "scope of nursing practice" defined within the hospital. Individual decision making is essential for the collegial practice of nurses and physicians.[27]

Probably no other element of the NJPC guidelines tests the level of trust and respect as greatly as does the encouragement of nurses' individual clinical decision making. Physicians must trust and respect their nursing colleagues, but so too must supervisors, administrators, patients, and peers. These attitudes are derived from the recognition of clinical competence, and this fact is the basis for any form of collaborative practice. Because the focus of all our efforts is ultimately the patient, nurses and patients cannot afford to accept anything less than the highest level of practice.

For the RN first assistant, clinical competence incorporates experience, an educational/intellectual component, and demonstrated manual skill and dexterity. Not all perioperative nurses have such skill, nor will they choose, for whatever reason, to assist during surgery. While first assisting is considered to be an acceptable expanded role, it is not necessarily *integral* to perioperative practice. Rather, it is an option, and a nurse's choice not to assist must be respected. Surely no surgeon nor supervisor can expect the highest level of performance from a nurse who is forced to engage in this activity.

For those nurses who desire to assist competently, the importance of highly developed technical surgical skills cannot be overstressed. Many areas of clinical nursing require technical skills, whether they be critical care units or perioperative care units. The RN first assistant's clinical competence demands such skill in conjunction with knowledge. There is little merit to the unfortunate notion that the performance of technical skills is somehow demeaning to the image of professional nursing. The high public esteem for surgeons is due in no small part to surgeons' technical skill, and physicians are no less admired because they work with their hands as well as their minds.

A surgeon's competence is judged mainly on his ability to produce a successful operative repair. This entails mental as well as manual ability in both preparation and execution. The RN first assistant accepts the same dual demands. The reward is the satisfaction of participating in what can be an esthetically pleasing creation as well as a meticulously scientific therapy. Appreciating our work from different aspects yields greater satisfaction and pride. This in turn inspires continued efforts for improvement.

Competence depends also on a secure knowledge base. Although nursing is still in the process of developing and defining a unique scientific body of knowledge, this limitation does not prevent the display of clinical competence. Conscientious practitioners are aware of their limitations and the need for greater understanding. Knowing what you don't know, and practicing accordingly, is a sign of wisdom, maturity, and professional responsibility. Asking questions or requesting assistance should not be rebuked; it should be encouraged and respected for the courage it entails. The RN first assistant with a secure self-concept accepts such risk-taking as necessary for the coordination of joint practice.

Questions about practices, procedures, and patient outcomes can be translated into researchable hypotheses. If supported by empirical data, these hypotheses add to the body of nursing knowledge. The operating room is a fertile field for investigating clinical problems ranging from asepsis to job-related stress. Collaborating with experienced researchers can provide a proper framework and methodology. Joint physician–nurse research projects can also foster collaborative practice.

Professionals who realize their limitations and seek to fill knowledge gaps better understand the learning needs of others. Taking the opportunity to share expertise with students and visitors often turns into a beneficial experience for the teacher as well. The selection and synthesis of information required to teach tests the educator's grasp of the subject. The RN first assistant can provide learning experiences and foster collegiality in interactions with students by offering formal and informal educational sessions.

Learning to relate to and interact with other health care professionals is one positive outcome. Practical benefits are evident from the perspective of better cost containment, fewer surgical wound infections, and improved time management.[28]

According to the NJPC guidelines, defining the boundaries of nurses' clinical performance is accomplished by the "scope-of-practice" statements outlined jointly by hospital practice committees. The scope is determined by hospital and professional nursing standards and by state nurse and medical practice acts.[29] Even within the constraints of scope-of-practice statements, the nurse is afforded considerable independence. With this comes the same burden of responsibility borne by physicians. Independent practice decisions must be accompanied by responsibility and accountability for the results of those decisions. Obviously the primary nurse cannot fulfill all patient needs, nor solve all patient problems. Physicians accept this fact and have referral systems and consultation mechanisms for problem-solving. Nurses also need to develop such systems to tap the rich diversity of resources available to them. For example, medical nurses caring for occasional preoperative patients might call on perioperative and surgical nurses for insights and information relating to their patient's problems, concerns, and knowledge deficits.

The RN first assistant's wealth of knowledge about anatomy, surgical technique, and indications for a particular procedure is more than just intellectually interesting to critical care or trauma nurses facing emergency thoracotomies. The RN first assistant's background in aseptic technique is helpful for nurses instituting universal precautions or investigating the increase in urinary tract or wound infections.

RN first assistants have much to gain by consulting pediatric or psychiatric clinicians about reducing preoperative fear or anxiety in children or adults. Surgical intensive care nurses can provide a greater appreciation for a well-delivered postoperative report by explaining the rationale for including baseline pulmonary or ventricular function studies or preoperative mental status assessments.

The need for consultation may not always exist, but when it does it should be available. This not only encourages better patient care, it also creates a feeling of mutual respect for the knowledge and skills that nurses have to offer one another. This in turn fosters self-esteem and pride in one's accomplishments and promotes professional growth. Turning to a colleague, nurse or physician, for professional advice reflects strength and a desire to use all the resources available to provide the best care possible.

Experts in other areas should be consulted for their expertise as well. It is appropriate to call on not only surgeons, anesthesiologists, and other physicians, but also on physician assistants, or social workers, or microbiologists, or epidemiologists, or physiotherapists. Health care delivery has become highly complex and specialized. Fragmentation can at least be lessened by fostering communication and accepting the need for interdependence. The RN first assistant, by virtue of a close and constant interaction with the patient, is well positioned to view the patient as a whole and to integrate and coordinate available resources.

Decision making in nursing is achieved through the nursing process and the formulation of nursing diagnoses. These diagnoses represent the identification of patient needs or problems and provide direction for both independent and interdependent nursing interventions. The classification of some patient needs as "collaborative problems" defines situations in which the RN first assistant uses both physician-prescribed and RN first assistant-prescribed interventions.[30] During the operative period itself, nursing and medical diagnoses focus mainly on patients' physiological needs. Clinical decision making entails the setting of priorities. The acuteness of the anesthetized patient's status during surgery necessitates first meeting basic physical demands. In these types of collaborative care situations, the RN first assistant focuses on monitoring for onset or noting changes in status of physiologic complications and responding to these with both physician-initiated and RN first assistant-initiated interventions. A patient under local anesthesia has additional needs for emotional and spiritual support; families and loved ones also require support. Physical, emotional, and spiritual needs all must be met, but the essence of decision making is ranking these needs in order of priority in a given situation. Assessment, outcome identification, planning, evaluation, and reassessment must be ongoing and continuous.

Emergency situations illustrate well the ability to plan, anticipate, and set priorities appropriately. The RN first assistant's insights and abilities are especially helpful, because they increase awareness not only of the order of surgical requirements, but also of the individual surgeon's preferences.

During emergencies, the smoothest, quickest, and most efficient intervention is commonly the one known and practiced by the participants. Unessential movements are minimized.

Although acute patient demands may rearrange nursing routines, they need not obviate the necessity for those procedures. Emergencies require maximal efficiency, flexibility, and integration of roles and functions. In the operating room, this is accomplished by each team member anticipating and performing interventions deemed necessary by the circumstances. As a key facilitator, the RN first assistant can contribute special knowledge and understanding to non-first assisting nurses. Consequently, confidence in the ability to anticipate needs is greatly improved and overall performance enhanced.

Fagin and Lamberton could have been describing the operating room when they wrote that the "crucial element of professional collaboration . . . is the development of a strong relationship built on sharing of knowledge, confidence, and, most important, trust."[31]

CONSIDERATIONS AND IMPLICATIONS OF COLLABORATIVE PRACTICE

The previous discussion of the NJPC guidelines offers suggestions for their implementation in the perioperative setting by physicians, perioperative nurses, and specifically RN first assistants. The knowledge and experience gained from observing and participating in the surgery itself offer additional advantages as well.

Managers and administrators are more apt to encourage and reward this expanded role when cost savings and better productivity can be achieved. Job satisfaction conserves costs because it reduces staff turnover and the subsequent expense of orienting new personnel. Greater efficiency in the delivery of care and increased flexibility in job performance are facilitated by the presence of RNs who can scrub, circulate, and assist. The benefit of this is especially evident during emergencies.

The expertise of the RN first assistant can also have an impact on the judicious use of supplies and better inventory control. Familiarity with surgeons' preferences reduces confusion and uncertainty about which items to make available for a procedure, and this in turn reduces waste. Better time management is another consequence of knowing preferred positioning and prepping.

Capital equipment expenditures can be controlled more efficiently if staff and supervisors are aware of innovations in surgical technique. These are often accompanied by the requirement for expensive special instruments, supplies, and equipment. Selecting and purchasing the appropriate items and providing inservice staff training on their use helps ensure proper use of equipment and minimizes the possibility of damage.

First assisting offers advantages in both material management and personnel management. Although the advantages provide sufficient justification for developing and extending the role, some potential and actual problems must be considered. One is the danger of inadequate education and supervision. Ensuring the competent performance of assisting functions requires careful selection of candidates with suitable personal and professional qualities, as well as adherence to the guidelines outlined in AORN's Official Statement on RN First Assistants (see Appendix I) and AORN's Core Curriculum for the RN First Assistant.[32]

Interpersonal relations can be jeopardized when there is inequitable distribution of assigned procedures to assistants or inadequate compensation for the increased responsibilities associated with the role. Scrubbing and circulating duties must continue to be integrated into performance duties, and supervisors must be alert to prevent resentment against first assistants in the midst of staffing shortages. Ideally, adequate staff should be available to supply all needs. Effective leadership can also prevent negative interactions between nurses and residents or physician assistants.

CONCLUSION

The experience of first assisting during surgery is unlike any other in nursing. It involves a unique form of collaborative practice between the RN first assistant and the surgeon based on trust in one another's abilities, respect for each other's capabilities, and mutual concern for the patient undergoing surgery. The essence of such a patient care partnership is that the people in it perceive one another as equally important peers who mutually contribute to the same desired outcome–excellence in perioperative patient care. The rewards of instituting joint practice in the NJPC's pilot units are attainable in the operating room. The NJPC noted that, first and foremost, patients received better nursing care and were more satisfied with their care. Communication between doctors and nurses improved, mutual respect and trust increased, and job satisfaction was greater for both nurses and physicians. Additional studies have begun to focus on the correlation of these improvements in the quality of relationships between physicians and nurses and patient outcomes.[33]

These results can be encouraged by the establishment of joint practice committees, but committees in and of themselves are neither necessary nor sufficient for true teamwork. Working together in a collaborative framework brings forth a joint intellectual effort, a sharing in planning, making decisions, solving problems, setting goals, and assuming responsibility, as well as cooperation, coordination, and communication. Teamwork can be achieved only when physicians and nurses each decide that working together in the interest of consistent, quality patient/family care will bring them to their fullest professional potential.

REVIEW QUESTIONS

1. List four reasons why RN first assistants are cost-effective.
   1. ______________________________
   2. ______________________________
   3. ______________________________
   4. ______________________________

2. The RN first assistant role should be integrated into the perioperative nursing role because
   a. perioperative nursing provides the collegial foundation for collaborative practice
   b. it is necessary for the performance of the perioperative nursing role
   c. it provides a rationale for reimbursement
   d. the surgeon will not have to assume responsibility for the RN first assistant
3. Benefits of the RN first assistant role include (1) achieving new dimensions of clinical competence, (2) having greater responsibility and accountability, (3) allowing participation in collaborative practice, and (4) maintaining positive nurse–physician relationships.

   Which of these statements are true?
   a. 1, 2, and 4
   b. 1, 2, and 3
   c. 1 and 3
   d. 1, 2, 3, and 4
4. Factors necessary for successfully fulfilling the RN first assistant role include (1) knowing the reason for the operation, (2) being familiar with a surgeon's preference, (3) anticipating the patient's needs, (4) communicating relevant information to the postoperative care unit, and (5) possessing manual skills.

   Which of these statements are true?
   a. 1, 3, and 5
   b. 1, 2, 3, and 4
   c. 2, 4, and 5
   d. 1, 2, 3, 4, and 5
5. One of the independent nursing functions that an RN first assistant performs is
   a. determining the necessity for surgery
   b. performing patient assessment
   c. positioning the patient for optimal exposure
   d. suturing and dressing the surgical incision site
6. One of the initiating factors for the development of the National Joint Practice Commission (NJPC) and its subsequent work was to improve
   a. role ambiguity for professional nurses
   b. incongruent expectations between nursing education and service
   c. nurse–physician relationships
   d. the positional status of hospital-employed nurses
7. The NJPC definition of collaborative practice is
   a. to work together in a mutual undertaking
   b. to work together, side-by-side, in a cooperative effort
   c. a process whereby a nurse works with a physician to deliver health care services within the scope of the practitioner's professional expertise
   d. nurses and physicians collaborating together as colleagues to provide patient care
8. The interpersonal milieu for collaboration must be founded on
   a. self-esteem and professional confidence
   b. truth, active listening, and sincerity
   c. open communication, trust, and mutual respect
   d. negotiation, compromise, and working within one's sphere of influence

9. An essential element in establishing nurse–physician collegiality is
   a. clinical credibility
   b. advanced educational preparation
   c. advanced, specialty certification
   d. joint attendance at professional meetings (like the AORN/ACS meeting)
10. The NJPC recommended that five elements be present for the formal implementation of joint practice models. Which of the following was *not* part of their recommendations?
   a. joint practice committees
   b. team nursing
   c. joint care reviews
   d. integrated patient records
11. The RN first assistant who is appointed to a joint practice committee should expect that the committee will focus on
   a. clinical outcomes
   b. critical pathways
   c. practice guidelines
   d. nurse–physician relationships
12. In preparing for a JCAHO accreditation team visit, the RN first assistant should know that JCAHO expects to see
   a. confirmation that the state Board of Nursing has determined that first assisting is within the scope of nursing practice
   b. medical bylaws that define the institutional role of the RN first assistant
   c. policies and procedures ensuring effective collaboration among departments providing surgical services
   d. peer review by RN first assistants and surgeons
13. When involved in committee discussions, the RN first assistant should be careful to avoid
   a. having to compromise
   b. discussing personalities
   c. negotiating on patient care issues
   d. conflict and disagreements
14. In joint care reviews, one way of examining care provided is to review
   a. documentation on the patient care record
   b. survivor rates
   c. nurse job satisfaction
   d. success of PPOs
15. If collaborative practice aims to truly promote joint efforts and communication about patients, then
   a. clinical ladders should include advancement opportunities for RN first assistants
   b. nurses should use the medical model, not nursing diagnoses
   c. RN first assistants should learn to do histories and physical exams
   d. RN first assistants and surgeons should write on the same progress notes

16. For the RN first assistant, clinical competence incorporates (1) experience, (2) an intellectual component, (3) the ability to assist in any surgical procedure, (4) demonstrated manual skills, and (5) cross-training in postanesthesia care.

Which of these statements are true?

a. 1, 2, and 5
b. 1, 3, and 4
c. 1, 2, and 4
d. 1, 2, and 3

17. In the preoperative admitting area, the RN first assistant is reviewing the history of a 20-year-old female who is the mother of an 8-month-old child. While discussing postsurgery discharge plans and whether the patient will be able to manage decreased activity for the next 24 hours, the patient expresses her frustration over her baby's crying behaviors, revealing her fears of harming the baby. The most appropriate action of the RN first assistant would be to

a. instill confidence in the patient that she is experiencing normal frustrations with a teething infant
b. determine whether the mother, as a child, was physically abused by her parents
c. provide empathy, support, and therapeutic touch
d. request a consult with the psychiatric nurse clinical specialist

Indicate whether each of the following statements is true (T) or false (F).

18. _______The RN first assistant has an obligation to share knowledge derived from assisting with perioperative nursing colleagues.
19. _______If quality improvement is really the goal of joint care reviews, then the committee should focus on correcting problems; quality improvement efforts don't need to focus on what already is working well.
20. _______Probably no other element of the NJPC guidelines tests the level of trust and respect as much as the encouragement of nurses' individual clinical decision making.

Answers

1. Some of the reasons include: decreased staff turnover from increased nurse satisfaction; improved OR efficiency from using a flexible RN staff (RNs can scrub, circulate, first assist); more effective and efficient use of costly supplies; improved time management; less potential for damage to instruments and supplies.
2. a
3. b
4. d
5. b
6. c
7. d
8. c
9. a
10. b
11. d

12. c
13. b
14. a
15. d
16. c
17. d
18. T
19. F
20. T

REFERENCES

1. Kneedler JA, Dodge GH: Perioperative Patient Care: The Nursing Perspective, p 20. Boston, Blackwell Scientific Publications, 1987
2. Clapesattle H: The Doctors Mayo, p 429. Garden City, NJ, Garden City Publishing, 1941
3. Groah LK: Operating Room Nursing: Perioperative Practice, pp 5–8. Norwalk, CT, Appleton & Lange, 1990
4. A model for perioperative nursing practice. AORN J 41:188–194, 1985
5. Members discuss important issues. AORN J 55:1401, 1406–1408, 1992
6. Task force defines first assisting. AORN J 39:404–405, 1984
7. Davis NB: Charting a course for the first assistant. AORN J 32:1032–1038, 1980
8. A share of decision-making and equal education. Surgical Rounds, 69–71, 1982; Nursing Commission issues preliminary report. Hospitals 55(18):20, 1981
9. Mauksch I: Nurse-physician collaboration: A changing relationship. J Nurs Admin, 6(6):37, 1981
10. National Joint Practice Commission: Guidelines for Establishing Joint or Collaborative Practice in Hospitals, p 2. Chicago, National Joint Practice Commission, 1981
11. National Joint Practice Commission, p 7
12. Vaughn RA: Collaborative practice. Nurs Manage 13(3):33–35, 1982; Devereux PM: Nurse/physician collaboration; Nursing practice considerations. J Nurs Admin, 11(9):37–39, 1981; Notkin MS: Collaboration and communication. Nurs Admin Q 8:1–7, 1983; Steel JE: Putting joint practice into practice. Am J Nurs, 81:964–967, 1981; See also Baggs JG, Schmitt MH: Collaboration between nurses and physicians. Image, 20:145–148, 1988
13. National Joint Practice Commission, p 11
14. Zander K: Second generation primary nursing: A new agenda. J Nurs Admin 15(3):18–24, 1985
15. Zander, p 19
16. Alt-White AC, Charns M, Strayer R: Personal, organizational, and managerial factors related to nurse–physician collaboration. Nurs Admin Q 8:8–18, 1983
17. Weiss SJ, Davis HP: Validity and reliability of the collaborative practice scales. Nurs Res 34:299–305, 1985; Thiele J: Guidelines for Collaborative Research. App Nurs Res 2:150–153, 1989
18. National Joint Practice Commission, p 11
19. Palmer P: Perioperative nurses, surgeons, anesthesiologists discuss challenges of today's OR environment. AORN J, 50:424, 1989
20. Joint Practice Committee of the Virginia Nurses' Association and the Medical Society of Virginia: Recommended Revisions of Guidelines for Registered Nurses as First Assistants in Surgery. Virginia, 1978
21. Joint Commission on Accreditation of Health Care Organizations: Accreditation Manual for Hospitals, p 170. Chicago, Joint Commission on Accreditation of Health Care Organizations, 1992

22. National Joint Practice Commission, p 12
23. Denholm B, Lehr P: Physician–nurse cooperative efforts. AORN J 55:262, 1992
24. National Joint Practice Commission, pp 11–12
25. Ibid, p 18
26. Jordan C: Keynote address emphasizes universal caring. AORN J 42:774–781, 1985; Accreditation Manual for Hospitals, p. 79. Chicago, Joint Commission on Accreditation of Health Care Organizations, 1992
27. National Joint Practice Commission, p 11
28. Boegli EH: Teaching some ORs new tricks: Surgical asepsis. Surgical Rounds, September 17:78–81, 1984; Webster D: Medical students' views of the role of the nurse. Nurs Research September/October 34:313–317, 1985
29. National Joint Practice Commission, p 17; Gregory B, Lewis J, Ward S: Quality Improvement in Perioperative Nursing, pp 2-2–2-3. Denver, AORN, 1992
30. Carpenito LJ: Nursing Diagnosis: Application to Clinical Practice. Philadelphia, JB Lippincott, 1992
31. Fagin CM, Lamberton MM: Nurse–physician collaboration: Evaluation of nursing school–medical school joint practice. In Aiken LH (ed): Health Policy and Nursing Practice. New York, McGraw-Hill, 1981
32. Vaiden R, Fox V, Rothrock J: Core Curriculum for the RN First Assistant. Denver, Association of Operating Room Nurses, 1990
33. Knaus WA, Draper EA, Wagner DP, Zimmerman JE: An evaluation of outcome from intensive care in major medical centers. Ann Int Med 104:410–481, 1986; Kerfoot K: Nurse/physician collaboration: A cost/quality issue for the nurse manager. Nurs Econ, 7:335–338, 1989

15 Clinical Applications

Denise Jackson, RN, BSN, RNFA, CNOR
Christine Espersen, RN, CNOR, RNFA
Jacqueline Daly, RN, MSN, RNFA, CNOR

THE RN FIRST ASSISTANT IN ENDOSCOPIC SURGERY*

Endoscopic abdominal surgery, often called operative laparoscopy, is fast becoming a routine method of treating patients with gynecological as well as general surgical disease. A skilled assistant is essential for smooth completion of laparoscopic procedures. An in-depth knowledge of the procedures, instrumentation, and technical equipment provides the RN first assistant with the necessary skills to first assist effectively. This section of Chapter 15 provides an overview of gynecological and general laparoscopic surgery as it relates to the RN first assistant's role.

Laparoscopy had its beginnings as far back as the 1800s, with the development of cystoscopy. The viewing of abdominal contents using pneumoperitoneum was first reported by Dr. Jacobaeus in Sweden. Carbon dioxide was first used to insufflate the abdomen in 1924.[1] Over the next few decades, great strides were made in the development of laparoscopic equipment and diagnostic techniques. Until the 1970s and early 1980s, however, laparoscopy was limited to diagnostic examination of the abdomen or female sterilization procedures.

Dr. Kurt Semm from West Germany played a significant role in the development of operative laparoscopy, designing and developing the first generation of most operative laparoscopy equipment used today. Accredited to Dr.

* *This section was prepared by Denise Jackson, RN First Assistant, Shannon Medical Center, San Angelo, Texas.*

Semm is the endocoagulator or thermal coagulator; endosuture, endoligature, endoloops, and endoloop passers; early techniques for intracorporeal and extracorporeal knot tying; and design of such instruments as the claw, spoon, biopsy, and grasping forceps, the Aquapurator for irrigation and aspiration, and an insufflator that monitors intraabdominal pressures and gas flow. He also designed hook and microscissors and the first morcillator, which made possible the removal of large specimens through trocars. To facilitate teaching and learning operative laparoscopic techniques, he went on to develop the pelvic trainer, which allows for simulated practice inside the abdomen with endoscopic instruments.[2]

Laparoscopic surgery had its beginnings in gynecological surgery. Procedures frequently performed pelviscopically include adhesiolysis, ovariolysis, salpingolysis, fimbrioplasty, salpingostomy, myomectomy, salpingectomy for ectopic pregnancy, oophorectomy, coagulation or laser ablation of endometriotic implants, and cystectomy. More recent advances include laparoscopically assisted vaginal hysterectomy and the laparoscopic Marshall–Marchetti–Krantz procedure for bladder suspension. In general surgery, the most commonly performed procedure is laparoscopic cholecystectomy, with intraoperative cholangiography. Laparoscopic appendectomy has become an accepted method of removing both the normal as well as the acute appendix; clinical research has supported this approach in most cases of appendicitis.[3] Laparoscopic procedures such as hernia repair, lymphadenectomy, bowel resection, and thoracoscopy are not done as frequently as cholecystectomies; however, more surgeons and RN first assistants are acquiring the necessary skills to master these more advanced procedures.

For perioperative patients, laparoscopic surgery has some significant advantages over open laparotomy. Patients experience less postoperative discomfort and incisional pain, a shortened hospital stay, and earlier return to normal activity. Potential postoperative complications from abdominal incisions, such as dehiscence, are decreased, as are possible indirect cardiovascular and respiratory complications resulting from delayed early ambulation. The cosmetic result is also a benefit.

PATIENT PREPARATION

Preoperative patient preparation varies with the disease being treated. A complete history and physical examination, along with normally required diagnostic studies and preoperative evaluation of the blood and urine, remain part of the patient workup. If the procedure is gynecologic, a serum pregnancy test is often done to ensure that an unsuspected uterine pregnancy is not disturbed. Sometimes coagulation studies are ordered as well. If the procedure is being done to evaluate and treat a pelvic mass, a sonogram is also done. For laparoscopic surgery of the biliary tract, liver function studies and a gallbladder sonogram are commonly prescribed. For laparoscopic-guided colectomy, a preoperative abdominal x-ray, followed by placement of metallic clips proximal and distal to the lesion via a colonoscope, may be done the day before or the day of surgery.[4] Chest x-ray and electrocardiography may be required for the patient undergoing laparoscopic surgery, depending on age and physical status.

Significant information such as previous abdominal surgery, presence of abdominal or pelvic mass, or hepatosplenomegaly are important to note on the history and physical examination. Previous abdominal surgery will alert the surgeon that adhesions may be present and may alter the surgical technique; possible alterations in technique are discussed later in this chapter. The RN first assistant should carefully note any contraindications to laparoscopic surgery, such as severe intestinal distention, severe cardiopulmonary disease, shock, cardiac or respiratory failure, third trimester of pregnancy, abdominal carcinoma, massive obesity, or generalized peritonitis.[5]

Preoperative counseling by the RN first assistant can provide the patient with the opportunity to clarify information and ask questions. The patient should know what to expect during the surgical experience. The RN first assistant should explain the purpose of showering with an antimicrobial soap the evening or morning before surgery, pointing out the need for special attention to the umbilical area, an incisional site often overlooked while bathing. The patient also should be prepared for preoperative intravenous line insertion, preoperative enema (to empty the bowel and decrease the risk of injury), and the possibility of waking up with an indwelling urinary catheter after surgery. In general surgery laparoscopy, the stomach is often decompressed with a nasogastric tube intraoperatively; the patient also should be prepared for this. The possibility of referred shoulder pain also should be discussed. Carbon dioxide and water on the peritoneal surfaces combine to make carbonic acid. When this occurs in the right hemidiaphragm, the peritoneum becomes irritated. The shoulder pain occurs because the phrenic nerve innervates both this portion of the diaphragm and the shoulder.

The RN first assistant also should tell the patient that although postoperative pain is significantly decreased with laparoscopic surgery, some is to be expected. The assistant also may explain where the incisions will be made and how many small incisions to expect. For most laparoscopic procedures, the patient can anticipate going home the day of surgery, or within 24 hours if no complications occur. When the patient can tolerate a regular diet and bowel and bladder function have resumed, he usually is ready for discharge.

INTRAOPERATIVE CONSIDERATIONS

Patient positioning varies with the operative procedure to be done. (See Chapter 7, Anesthesia and Patient Positioning, for a thorough discussion of patient positioning requirements.) Before positioning the patient for surgery, sequential compression stockings are often applied. For gynecologic surgery, the patient is put in a low lithotomy position, and her arms are padded, protected, and secured on padded armboards. If the surgeon insists on tucking the patient's arms at her sides, extreme caution should be taken to protect her hands and fingers when changing the position of the footpiece of the operating room bed. The addition of Trendelenberg position helps displace the bowel out of the pelvis. The anesthesiologist determines the maximum degree of Trendelenberg that the patient can tolerate. The RN first assistant stands across from the surgeon. The television monitor is positioned between the patient's legs and is viewed by both the surgeon and the RN first assistant.

For laparoscopic cholecystectomy, the patient will be supine on the operating bed, in reverse Trendelenberg with the right side elevated. This permits optimal visualization by causing the bowel to fall away from the gallbladder. The patient's arms can be abducted at less than 90 degrees on armboards, or the right arm may be padded, protected, and tucked at the patient's side. The RN first assistant will stand on the patient's right side. Television monitors are placed so that the surgeon and RN first assistant each view a separate screen across the operating room bed.

General endotracheal anesthesia is preferred for laparoscopic procedures, because maximum relaxation is necessary to minimize insufflation pressures in the abdomen. In some cases, however, local anesthesia with systemic analgesia or spinal or epidural anesthesia may be administered.[6]

There are two basic techniques for laparoscopy: the Hasson or open laparoscopy technique and the percutaneous method. In the Hasson technique, a small infraumbilical incision is made to allow visualization of the peritoneum before trocar insertion. After the trocar is inserted and secured, insufflation is done directly through it. Trocars used for this technique are designed so that pneumoperitoneum is not lost around the incision. The stay sutures, placed one on each side, can be used to close the peritoneum and fascia at the end of the procedure. This technique is often used on extremely obese patients and on patients with suspected adhesions along the anterior abdominal wall from previous surgery.

The second and most commonly used technique is the percutaneous method. After making a small skin incision, the surgeon blindly inserts the veress needle through the abdominal wall into the peritoneum and insufflates the abdominal cavity before inserting the larger trocar. Towel clips may or may not be used to put the umbilical skin on traction. Common sites of veress needle insertion are umbilical, infraumbilical, and periumbilical and in the cul de sac. The veress needle can be reusable or disposable; which type used is usually a matter of surgeon preference. The needle should be checked for sharpness, for patency, and for its spring action before each use. After the veress needle is inserted, its position is checked before the carbon dioxide is turned on. Then, 10–20 ml of normal saline is injected into the veress needle. If the needle is in the peritoneum, the saline should drop quickly as it is pulled into the peritoneal cavity by negative pressure.

In a patient with suspected dense abdominal wall adhesions, the surgeon may choose to insert the veress needle into the upper right abdominal quadrant. After insufflation, a 5 mm trocar is inserted, followed by a 5 mm laparoscope. The umbilical area is visually inspected for adhesions before 10/11 mm trocar insertion. This technique decreases the chance of puncturing omentum or bowel adhered to the abdominal wall.

Another technique to test for adhesions on the abdominal wall is to insert the veress needle in the routine fashion and establish pneumoperitoneum. If the veress needle is in the bowel, abdominal pressures will be unusually high and insufflation is stopped immediately. Once proper pneumoperitoneum is obtained, a 20 gauge needle attached to a 20 ml syringe half filled with normal saline is inserted lateral to the midline. This area should be free of adhesions, because a previous abdominal incision would have been in the midline. It will establish where adhesions begin if they are present, and will reveal the abdominal wall thickness. Then the needle is inserted in various locations along the lower midline. If bubbles are aspirated, then the needle is in the peritoneal cavity and that location should be free of adhesions. If blood is aspirated, or if there is no return, then the needle is probably in the omentum. If a brownish liquid is aspirated, then the bowel likely has been punctured. A puncture wound of this size does not require repair, whereas a puncture made by a 10/11 mm trocar would require a laparotomy to suture the bowel puncture. An alternate location for 10/11 mm trocar insertion must be chosen if aspiration yields brownish liquid.

Initial insufflation should not exceed 1 L/min until the surgeon determines that pneumoperitoneum is being achieved. The flow rate is then increased to a higher rate of 4–6 L/min. Before insufflation, the intraabdominal pressure monitor is set for a 12–16 mm Hg upper limit. Pressures above this limit could increase the risk of air embolism, diaphragmatic damage, and hemodynamic instability. Excessive intraabdominal pressure decreases diaphragmatic excursion and venous return. This causes decreased ventilation, which results in decreased cardiac output due to decreased cardiac filling. The CO_2 insufflator should automatically regulate gas flow and monitor intraabdominal pressure. Although frequent monitoring of flow rate and intraabdominal pressure is usually the responsibility of the scrub nurse, the RN first assistant should have a working knowledge of normal parameters. If the pressure alarm should sound, the RN first assistant should first check the insufflation tubing for kinks and verify that the trocar has an open valve. Other common causes of increased intraabdominal pressure are inadequate patient relaxation, abdominal compression as secondary trocars are inserted, and extraperitoneal placement of the veress needle.

If the irrigator–aspirator is driven by CO_2, the irrigator can push CO_2 into the peritoneal cavity if the irrigating solution bottle becomes empty during use.

Once adequate pneumoperitoneum is established, a larger trocar (at least 10 mm in diameter) is inserted in the same site as the veress needle. Then the scope with attached camera is inserted, and placement of secondary trocars is accomplished under direct visualization. The RN first assistant inserts these secondary trocars through small skin incisions.

Correct trocar placement is essential to facilitate manipulation during the procedure. The trocar tip should be visualized as it passes into the peritoneum. If visualization is lost for any reason, downward pressure on the trocar should be immediately stopped until visualization is regained. For gynecological procedures, the secondary trocars are usually placed in the right and left lower abdominal quadrants. Trocar size depends on the type of procedure to be done. For laparoscopic cholecystectomy, 5 mm trocars are inserted—one placed in the midclavicular line two finger widths beneath the right costal margin, and the second placed in the anterior axillary line, three finger widths below the right costal margin. The 11 mm trocar is inserted by the surgeon one-third of the distance between the xiphoid and umbilicus, just to the right of the midline.

The RN first assistant should be familiar with the equipment needed to provide visualization. The fiberoptic light cord provides the necessary light to view the abdominal cavity. It attaches to the laparoscope and to a light source. Certain precautions should be taken with the light cord. Careful handling will help prevent breakage of the fibers that transmit the light. Black spots on the end of the cord indicate broken fibers. To avoid loss of light and color distortion, cable connections should be checked for cleanliness before each patient procedure. When in use, many light cords become very hot on the ends and can burn disposable drapes quickly. It is best to wait until the light cord is attached to the scope before it is turned on. The laparoscope can also burn internal organs if prolonged contact occurs. Light cords and sources that remain cool throughout use are now available.

Different cameras are available for viewing endoscopic procedures. A one-chip end-viewing camera with 450 horizontal lines per inch of resolution provides good visualization; the newer three-chip camera with 700 horizontal lines per inch of resolution provides an even sharper image. The camera and the television monitor should have equal resolution to ensure the best image possible. The RN first assistant should verify that the camera has been "white balanced" before use. This procedure, necessary each time the camera is turned off and then on again, is done by focusing on a pure white object and pushing a button either on the camera source or on the camera itself to set it to an absolute white.

When the laparoscope enters the peritoneal cavity, the rapid temperature and humidity change can fog the laparoscope's lens. Rinsing the scope in warm water before inserting it into the abdomen helps reduce fogging. A special telescope warmer manufactured for this purpose also may be used. Sterile antifog solutions can be applied to the lens before scope insertion and after cleaning during the procedure. Applying Phisohex to the lens also may help reduce fogging.[7]

The RN first assistant should be familiar with the type of irrigating–aspirating device used in the institution. There are several types available, and smooth operation of the device is essential to provide good visualization and prevent injury to surrounding organs.

Use of an electrosurgery unit or a laser is common during laparoscopic surgery. The RN first assistant must know the special precautions needed when using these devices. For instance, in endoscopic electrosurgery, injury to adjacent organs from the spark-gap effect can be avoided by ensuring that the tip of the probe is touching the tissue before applying the power. Some electrosurgery probes use a foot pedal to activate the current; others are controlled at the hand piece. If reusable metal trocars are used, care must be taken not to touch the tip of the probe to the trocar; contact could cause injury via conduction.

When using a free-beam laser, careful control of the fiber's focal point must be maintained. The RN first assistant must make sure that retracted adjacent organs do not fall into the path of the beam during laser operation. When operating the camera, the assistant must provide visualization of the beam at all times. The contact-tip laser must come into direct contact with the target tissue. It is not as effective at coagulation as it is for dissection, and changing to a free-beam laser may be necessary if bleeding is encountered.[8] As with any laser, appropriate safety measures must be maintained.

Hemostasis and tissue approximation can be accomplished through many endoscopic techniques. Endoligatures are pretied loops of suture that can be passed around pedicles to ligate vessels or can be used to close holes in cystic structures to prevent leakage into the abdominal cavity. After the loop is positioned over the structure to be ligated, the RN first assistant goes through the loop with graspers and pulls the structure through the loop, enabling the surgeon to tighten the knot down around the pedicle. The assistant then releases the structure, replaces the graspers with the hook scissors, and cuts the suture, leaving about a 1/4-inch tail. (This is using a three- or four-trocar technique.) Two or three loops are passed, depending on what is being ligated.

In advanced laparoscopic procedures, the RN first assistant should learn to do intracorporeal and extracorporeal suturing and knot tying.

Intracorporeal or intra-abdominal suturing can be done with a straight, curved, or ski needle, and all knots are tied with instruments inside the abdominal cavity. Extracorporeal knots are tied outside the abdomen, and the knot is slid down the trocar with the assistance of a knot pusher and secured intraabdominally. Access to a pelvic trainer for practicing is essential to master this type of suturing and knot tying.

Instrumentation needed for endoscopic suturing includes a suture introducer, 5 mm needle driver, 3 mm needle holder, hook scissors, and tissue graspers. Many types of sutures, endoligatures, pretied suture knots, and needles are available.[9] The surgeon's preferences will determine what instruments and equipment the RN first assistant needs to become most familiar with.

Many endoscopic instruments, some disposable and some reusable, are available. Basic instruments include traumatic and atraumatic tissue graspers of varying diameters, the most common being 5 mm, 10 mm, and 11 mm; dissecting forceps, which have finer jaws and also come in various forms; and four types of scissors: hook scissors, microscissors, mayo scissors, and straight or paper cutting scissors. Electrosurgery probes are available in various forms. Some of these probes have the ability to irrigate and aspirate as well as cauterize and cut. Suction tips vary as well.

When handling endoscopic instruments, the RN first assistant needs to make adjustments for using elongated instruments and to compensate for altered depth perception and tactile sensation in video-controlled laparoscopic surgery, where everything is seen in two dimensions instead of three. Hands-on practice is the only way the assistant can learn to manipulate the instruments skillfully. A good rule to follow is never grasp, cut, or coagulate what cannot be seen extremely well. Movements should be slow and determined; quick, jabbing movements only increase the risk of injury. While practicing, the RN first assistant should have the camera operator follow the instrument in and out of the trocar.

During a procedure, the camera will probably be focused on the surgeon's instruments. The RN first assistant holding graspers not in camera view should keep them in position until he/she can reposition them under direct visualization. If the assistant loses the orientation of an instrument in the abdomen, he/she may regain it by looking at the abdomen from the outside to determine where the instrument should go, then heading the instrument in that direction while the camera operator follows. The assistant should never hesitate to ask the operator to show him/her where the instrument is in the abdomen. It is far better to take the time to be sure of instrument location than to move blindly, possibly inflicting damage.

The RN first assistant should be familiar with potential complications of laparoscopic surgery. These include thermal or puncture injury to the bowel, urinary tract injury, common bile duct or common hepatic duct injury, retained common duct stones, gas embolism, injury to blood vessels, subhepatic abscess, bile peritonitis, and pneumomediastinum. There is always a possibility of the need for laparotomy. The perioperative nursing team should have an open setup readily available whenever laparoscopic surgery is being done.

CONCLUSION

Five years ago, laparoscopic cholecystectomy and laparoscopically assisted hysterectomy were being performed by only a handful of surgeons. Today, these procedures are becoming routine for many operating room teams around the country. As technological advances continue to improve the instrumentation and surgical techniques, it appears that more and more procedures that required laparotomy will be done through trocars with the use of a laparoscope and video camera. As new approaches to general surgical operations are developed, RN first assistants should participate in studies to improve the evaluation, management, and health outcomes for surgical patients. Implications for access to these procedures, quality of care, and health care costs need to be studied. Minimally invasive surgery is the trend of the future, and mastering the knowledge and skills necessary to assist at these procedures will ensure that the RN first assistant moves into the future with endoscopic surgery.

*THE RN FIRST ASSISTANT IN CARDIAC SURGERY**

Cardiac surgery has become a common therapeutic modality. The adult cardiac surgery patient population has increased in terms of both the chronological (age in years) and the physiological age (presence of risk-factors) of patients considered appropriate candidates for surgical intervention.[10] This in and of itself presents challenges for the RN first assistant involved in preoperative, intraoperative, and postoperative care of the patient undergoing cardiac surgery. The RN first assistant in a cardiac service has the opportunity—and indeed, the responsibility—to contribute to the quality of patient care and the achievement of optimal patient outcomes. Collaboration with nursing colleagues, physicians, and other members of the surgical team in the operating room and within the health care facility can effect the smooth running of a cardiac service, with consequent improvements in patient care. In some major cardiac surgery centers, the RN first assistant's job responsibilities are designed with such collaboration in mind. They may encompass multiple aspects of perioperative patient care, as well as staff education and development within the cardiovascular surgery department. In addition to first assisting during surgery, the RN first assistant may act as clinical consultant, educator, and researcher.[11]

Due to economic and scheduling factors, most patients undergoing elective cardiac surgery have already been evaluated for their cardiac disease, as well as any concurrent medical or surgical conditions, before admission for cardiac surgery. The RN first assistant should not assume, however, that such a patient is completely prepared, either physically or psychosocially, for surgery. Careful attention should be given to medical records from previous admissions and also to any physical or emotional changes that the patient might have experienced in the interim.

PREOPERATIVE PATIENT PREPARATION

Preoperative assessment and preparation of the cardiac surgery patient is extremely important. Common routine diagnostic studies include chest x-ray, electrocardiography (ECG), stress test, angiography, carotid Doppler study, gated equilibrium heart scan (MUGA), pulmonary function tests, and room air arterial blood gas analysis. Among other diagnostic studies performed on a selected basis are echocardiography, venous Doppler studies, venography, electrophysiologic studies, and any other patient-specific studies deemed necessary (*e.g.*, gastroscopy examination for the patient with a past history of gastric ulcer disease).

In addition to these diagnostic studies, routine laboratory data are also vitally important. Traditional preoperative laboratory studies include complete

* *This section was prepared by Christine C. Espersen, RN First Assistant, Cardiac Surgery, Buffalo General Hospital, Buffalo, New York.*

blood count (CBC), electrolytes, coagulation studies, blood urea nitrogen (BUN), creatinine, and urinalysis. (See Appendix II for information on these and other laboratory studies.) Other important laboratory studies for the patient undergoing cardiac surgery might include medication levels (*e.g.*, digoxin), cardiac enzymes, blood chemistries, and lipid levels.[12] Unfortunately, these laboratory data are sometimes given less priority than the results of cardiac diagnostic studies. For the cardiac surgery patient whose routine laboratory data is not within normal limits, overlooking these data can have disastrous consequences. Thus, the RN first assistant must carefully review all laboratory data.

Review Of History And Physical Examination

The admission history and physical examination are very important elements in the preoperative assessment of cardiac surgery candidates. Identifying previous surgical procedures is essential. For example, consider vein stripping and ligation, commonly performed 10–20 years ago. Although the act of stripping does not necessarily destroy incompetent perforators or remove varicosities of the branches[13], today it is recognized that preservation of the long saphenous vein for coronary artery or peripheral vascular conduits is advisable.[14] But because vein stripping was once so common, many of today's cardiac surgery patients underwent the procedure. In such a patient, consideration may need to be given to using the lesser saphenous vein, bilateral internal mammary arteries, or the gastroepiploic artery[15], or possibly using a homograft saphenous vein. Other important history information includes medication use (including cardiac medications, anticoagulant/antiplatelet agents, antiarrhythmics, and birth control pills), allergies, smoking history, height and weight, activity intolerance, and any concurrent medical problems.

During the physical examination, particular attention should be paid to the respiratory and cardiovascular systems. The patient's general appearance, breathing pattern, respiratory rate, skin color, nail bed and nail configuration, chest wall configuration, and tracheal position should be inspected. Chest percussion should note areas of resonance, hyperresonance, tympany, dullness, or flatness. Chest auscultation should be performed to detect normal breath sounds (vesicular, over most of the lung fields; bronchovesicular, over the main bronchus and upper right posterior lung; and bronchial, over the trachea) and abnormal breath sounds (decreased breath sounds, crackles, wheezes, rales). The presence of murmurs, rubs, or gallops should also be documented. Patients undergoing cardiopulmonary bypass are subjected to hemodynamic changes that are not generally seen in other major operative procedures. For these patients, careful respiratory and cardiac assessment are therefore essential.

Patient Education

A large research base supports the importance and effectiveness of psychological and educational interventions on a patient's postsurgical outcomes.[16]

Even in today's post-DRG environment, with decreased lengths of stay, research on psychoeducational intervention continues to document such positive patient benefits as use of fewer sedatives, antiemetics, or hypnotics, as well as earlier hospital discharge.[17] Modern medicine and the sophisticated technology that allows complex surgical intervention does not completely "cure" a patient's illness. These major advances may allow a longer life and enhance the quality of that life; however, they are not fully adequate in dealing with the psychosocial issues that underlie the disease process. The RN first assistant is well positioned and educated to assist patients and their families in meeting these psychosocial needs.

Research on the timing of preoperative education of cardiac surgery patients indicates that patient knowledge, postoperative mood states, and improved physiologic recovery result when such education is initiated 5–14 days before surgery.[18] If it is not possible for the RN first assistant to participate this early in the preoperative phase, a collaborative patient education program could be designed. Educational interventions might be begun by nursing staff in the angiology laboratory. Postangiography, patient education should continue after the patient is referred for surgery. This requires collaboration between the surgeon and the RN first assistant. As the RN first assistant becomes involved in patient and family education, a positive relationship can be established and lines of communication opened.

Although much media attention has been given to cardiac surgery, the patient still may have misconceptions about the actual surgery and the recovery period. Before patient teaching can begin, it must be determined what the patient knows and how much the patient wants to know. Information included in preoperative teaching has often been determined by health care professionals and assumed to be important for all patients. Although there is certain general information that all patients should have access to, the patient and the RN first assistant may not have the same perceptions of what is stressful. Identifying the perioperative events and conditions that the patient considers stressful and anxiety-producing allows the RN first assistant to determine which are amenable to nursing intervention and to design a plan of care accordingly.

Cardiac surgery and recovery from it may elicit mental distress, such as anxiety and fear about outcomes; the physical and physiological demands of the diagnostic workup may magnify psychological stress. Preliminary research on the rank order of perceived stressors by coronary artery bypass surgery patients indicates that, in severity of stress, having the surgery is followed by such concerns as resuming lifestyle, pain and discomfort, dying due to illness or surgery, absence from home/business, progress in recovery, activity level, and the interval before the surgery.[19] Elucidation of individual stress-generating events can guide psychoeducational preparation.

Patient education should involve the family and significant others, as appropriate, and work from a baseline of their understanding. Explanations regarding the procedure itself, location of the incision, and anticipated length of recovery need to be reinforced. Usually, when a patient understands the reason for a request, he will comply with it. Perioperative events may be described in the order of their occurrence. The importance of showering using antimicrobial soap should be explained. The scheduled start time of the operation should be reviewed, along with the possibility of postponement and cancellation. The routine for transporting the patient to the operating room should then be explained. Presurgery procedures, such as the insertion of monitoring lines in a holding area or in the operating room, possibly under local anesthesia, need to be reviewed. Relaxation techniques, such as guided imagery and deep breathing, can be reinforced at this time. The patient needs to know that perioperative staff will be in constant attendance, reexplaining and supporting him during this period.

Postoperative care regimens should be reviewed and explained preoperatively. The patient should understand that he will "wake up" in a special care unit, and special monitoring equipment should be described in terms that the patient can understand. Explaining methods for communicating while intubated is very important, as is reassuring the patient that the tube in his throat will be removed as soon as he is awake enough to breathe on his own. Simple but factual information regarding intravenous or blood replacement therapy, oxygen therapy, monitors, and drainage tubes and devices will help prepare both the patient and family for what they will see and hear. The patient and family also should be reassured that the nurses in the special care units are very attuned to taking care of postoperative heart patients and able to discern their needs. A qualitative study of coronary artery bypass patients' experiences showed that many patients had fears of mistakes by health care providers.[20] Preoperative preparation can alleviate such fears by increasing patients' confidence in nursing expertise.

Postextubation, the patient should be taught that this is the time when he can really "help himself" by performing deep breathing and coughing, incentive spirometry, foot and leg exercises, and frequent positional changes. These maneuvers should be demonstrated and time allowed for the patient to practice them. Because anxiety regarding postoperative pain is common, and some degree of pain or discomfort is inevitable after cardiac surgery, the patient should be reassured that medication is available for any discomfort related to the surgery and should be taken if needed. If patient-controlled analgesia (PCA) is available, this should also be explained. (Studies of PCA following cardiac surgery indicates, however, that it may not be most effective in the early postoperative period.[21]) The stay in the special care unit is usually 1–2 days. The urinary catheter, invasive monitoring lines, and chest tubes are usually removed before transfer from the special care unit to a postsurgical unit.

After moving to the postsurgical cardiac unit, the patient should be instructed to gradually increase activities as tolerated. Depending on the institution, the patient may be enrolled in a cardiac rehabilitation program that could extend postdischarge. Such programs assist cardiac patients to regain physical abilities and resume functional and productive lives. High-risk cardiac surgery patients, including patients who develop ventricular arrhythmias or marked ischemia with exercise, appear to benefit the most from cardiac rehabilitation services.[22]

Home care requirements and needs should be reviewed. With decreased lengths of stay, many patients may not be able to master self-care requisites during hospitalization. A study of anticipatory guidance for home recovery revealed that patients who received special instruction, counseling, and follow-up telephone calls to discuss problems reported better ratings at 3 months postsurgery.[23] Telephone teaching programs for at-home follow-up can reinforce previous teaching, clarify information, and provide additional information to enhance home health maintenance posthospitalization.[24] An important point for the cardiac surgery patient to understand is that although he might have days when he does not feel quite as good as he did the day before, in general he should experience an upward trend during recovery. Postoperative recovery is a dynamic time during which changes in physical activity and emotions may provoke some patient anxiety. The RN first assistant can develop a follow-up program with the patient to provide information and interpretation of both physiologic and psychologic reactions to enhance performance of recovery behaviors.[25]

INTRAOPERATIVE PATIENT CARE

The overall quality of patient care has increased dramatically due to the development of invasive monitoring techniques and the increased knowledge and skill of those professionals involved in their use. Routine invasive monitoring lines include the arterial pressure line (peripheral or central), central venous pressure (CVP) line, and pulmonary artery catheter. The pulmonary artery catheter may be omitted if the patient is hemodynamically stable and has good (> 50%) left ventricular function and if the benefits of catheter insertion do not outweigh the risks. During placement of these lines, the ECG should be monitored closely for any dysrhythmias. In addition to the ECG, other monitoring devices include a urinary catheter (with temperature probe attached) and a blood pressure cuff. Transesophageal echocardiography (TEE) is increasingly used to evaluate functional repair of the mitral valve; it allows evaluation of regurgitation and stenosis at the time of repair. Residual mitral regurgitation, as assessed by transesophageal color flow mapping in the operating room, correlates highly with the ultimate mitral regurgitation by cineangiography.[26] TEE is also useful for assessing function of the tricuspid and aortic valves and for measuring the aortic root size and valve annulus to aid in determining the size of the prosthesis required. Perioperative TEE is a primary tool for assessing the chambers for air after valve replacement.[27]

The supine position is the position of choice for most cardiac procedures. However, the left lateral position might be used for a redo coronary artery bypass graft (CABG), depending on the vessels to be grafted and the patency of existing grafts.[28] Also, the right lateral position could be used for a redo mitral valve repair or replacement. The rationale for these deviations is primarily the presence of fewer adhesions as well as the preservation of existing grafts.

During routine patient positioning (see Chapter 7, Anesthesia and Patient Positioning, for a full discussion of patient positioning), special attention is given to the hand. If a radial line is used care must be taken to position the hand so that the arterial pressure trace is not dampened. The elbows must be in a forward position to prevent stretching of the nerve trunks and padded to protect the ulnar nerve and the radial artery as it crosses the inner aspect of the humerus. In addition, the occiput must be protected from dependent pressure. The patient's head may be positioned on a piece of foam and turned from side to side every half hour to prevent alopecia or necrosis, which might arise from a low perfusion state and a certain degree of hypothermia. Care also must be taken when positioning the legs to ensure that the heels are well padded and that the "frog leg" position is not so acute as to cause peroneal nerve injury, resulting in footdrop.

First Assisting Skills

An analogy can be made between first assisting and a beautiful dance. Each member of the operative team performs in a manner that enhances the performance of the others. To do this, all members must have perfected their skills. The RN first assistant must know the operative procedure as well as the special preferences of the individual surgeon. Procedures that are inherently difficult become easier when the individuals involved are familiar with each others' routines.

The importance of exposure during cardiac surgery can not be overemphasized. Good visibility and illumination of the field are essential. The proper method of exposure needs to be selected at the right time. As with any type of surgery, instrumentation and techniques used for exposure during cardiac surgery vary depending on the procedure. Adjustable fixed instrumentation for sternal retraction has evolved from the Burford rib retractor, normally used for thoracotomy approaches, to the Kuyper or Pilling retractor. The sternotomy incision should not be too widely retracted with these retractors, especially in elderly patients or in female patients with osteoporosis; either the sternum or the ribs and costal margins could be fractured. Unnecessarily wide retraction may lead to bleeding in the costovertebral articulation and consequent intercostal nerve injury. The retractor blades also need to be placed carefully; cephalad placement may fracture the first rib. Retractors for dissecting the internal mammary artery (IMA) have progressed from hand-held army–navy and rake retractors to such self-retaining devices as the Favalaro, Rultract, and Pilling. Proper exposure for mitral valve surgery, previously gained by using two green retractors (or hand-held atrial retractors) to retract the left atrium, can now be achieved using modified Carpentier-type sternal/atrial retractors. Although these fixed retractors are a real benefit, especially during mitral valve repair, the RN first assistant needs to use clinical judgment in helping to determine when a self-retaining retractor might be better replaced by hand-held retractors, such as atrial retractors.

Providing exposure during CABG surgery is another critical RN first assistant nursing behavior. During this procedure, the RN first assistant assumes very important tasks. The assistant retracts the heart with his/her hand; using gentle pressure with fingers on either side of the coronary artery, an experienced assistant is able to expose the wall of the incised coronary artery for the surgeon. Utmost care must be taken when doing this so as not to lacerate the epicardium or injure the myocardium. The hand of the assistant should be positioned as flat as possible. Maintaining a clear and dry field requires thoughtful and deliberate suctioning. The suction should be placed as far as possible from the artery to avoid damage to the vessel and provide the surgeon with an unobstructed view. The use of medical air, passed through a sterile filter and tubing, can also be useful in providing exposure in certain cases.[29] Hemostasis is achieved in cardiac surgery using the same techniques described for all surgeries. (See Chapter 13, Providing Hemostasis, for a thorough discussion of achieving hemostasis during surgery.) The cardiac surgery patient, however, is heparinized and hemodiluted. If an incision is closed (*e.g.*, vein harvest site in the leg) before cardiopulmonary bypass, even though the heparin has been given, then the amount of drainage from that site is less at the conclusion of the procedure. The fact that the wound is closed and not open to air decreases the risk of wound infection.

Gentleness is the key word when discussing tissue handling. During any procedure, all of the operating surgeon's skill cannot make up for rough handling of tissues by an assistant. This is particularly true when harvesting a saphenous vein. The RN first assistant must be constantly aware of the ramifications of his/her actions. Vein branches left long and untied are much easier to deal with than are those torn by rough dissection. Branches tied too far away from the vein are easier dealt with than are those tied too close to the vein, compromising the vein lumen.

The RN first assistant needs skill in suturing and assistive behaviors during suturing to ensure smooth teamwork and prevent problems. For example, if the first assistant follows the suture too closely, the second assistant and scrub nurse will not be able to see the operative field. All members of the team need to be able to see to anticipate the next step in the procedure. The first assistant must follow the suture in a manner that gives due respect to the needs of other team members. The same principle applies to suctioning, suturing, retracting (with or without the use of instruments), and dissection. Practice, practice, and more practice is essential to attain the skills necessary for quality first assisting. The RN first assistant must be diligent about maintaining proper technique in the operating room and must constantly assess his or her efforts as part of quality improvement efforts and professional performance standards for nursing.

CONCLUSION

The future promises many exciting changes for cardiac surgery and for RN first assistants involved in the care of cardic surgery patients. Trends include increasing performance of valve repair rather than valve replacement[30], increasing use of cardiac assist devices, more heart and heart and lung transplantation, and increasing involvement of nurses with issues affecting them and their practice. RN first assistants need to share their experiences, not only with their colleagues in the operating room but also with colleagues throughout the institution in which they practice. There is much research that needs to be done and many studies that need replication. Physiological and psychological factors often affect the cardiac surgery patient's anxiety about surgery and perceived self-confidence about his ability for postoperative recovery. The RN first assistant can be a critical intervener during the preoperative, intraoperative, and postoperative recovery process, providing the help and assistance the patient requires from a nurse caregiver.

THE RN FIRST ASSISTANT IN ORTHOPEDICS*

The skeletal system provides the anatomic and physiologic framework for the human body. Continuous use, misuse, trauma, or disease can negatively affect this framework. The specialty of orthopedics deals with a wide cross-section of patient populations. The term "orthopedics" is derived from two Greek words that, when translated, yield "straight child." Early orthopedists were concerned with correcting deformities in children. However, diseases previously responsible for large numbers of orthopedic surgeries have become uncommon in the 1990s. Instead, changes in demographics and in health care delivery systems have broadened the scope of orthopedics; age, gender, lifestyles, and economic status are all factors that may affect treatment and prognosis. In this era of cost-containment, endoscopic and outpatient surgical procedures are thriving, with the rapid development of arthroscopic approaches to surgery minimizing the need for "open" procedures. Such trends have increased the RN first assistant's need to understand the patient, the wide variety and scope of problems amenable to surgical intervention, and the complicated surgical devices and procedures that are common in the modern orthopedic surgical suite.

The RN first assistant faces the challenge of balancing technical advances with personalized, humanistic care. In the specialty of orthopedics, the RN first assistant must maintain skills in the tried-and-true techniques (*e.g.*, inter-

---

** This section was prepared by Jacqueline Daly, Assistant Director, Perioperative Education, Nursing Operating Room Services, Cedars-Sinai Medical Center, Los Angeles, California.*

nal and external fixation, total joint replacement), while also acquiring knowledge and assisting expertise with new interventions and advancements (*e.g.*, arthroscopy, laser surgery, advanced manufacturing techniques for implants). The RN first assistant must participate in the evaluation of patient outcomes and assist patients in meeting home care recovery requirements, contributing to data bases that measure effectiveness and provide cost-benefit analyses of the delivery of required patient care services.

PREOPERATIVE PATIENT MANAGEMENT

Preoperative management of the orthopedic patient requires the RN first assistant to first consider the type of procedure planned for the patient and then identify any special needs or patient care requirements. Orthopedic procedures may include arthroplasty (construction of a new movable joint), arthrodesis (joint fusion), osteotomy (cutting of the bone or creation of a surgical fracture), synovectomy (removal of the inflamed lining of a joint), bone grafting (for stabilization and encouragement of bone regeneration), tendon grafting or transplantation, arthroscopy (exploration of a joint with a lens and light, for both diagnosis and treatment), or multiple treatments for the trauma patient. The planned procedure may guide the RN first assistant's review of the history and physical, or the RN first assistant may initiate the history and physical to assist in determining the planned treatment.

Review Of History And Physical Examination

The RN first assistant uses the preoperative evaluation findings to determine the appropriate plan of care. Whether the RN first assistant actually performs the history and physical examination or just uses the information obtained by another nurse, an evaluation of all body systems is necessary.

The history should begin with a review of subjective data and the patient's description of specific complaints (*e.g.*, pain, edema, weakness in affected part, activity and movement limitations, gait disturbance). Pertinent background information should include any concurrent diseases or conditions, past illnesses and surgical procedures, family and social history, current medication use, allergies, and so forth. For the orthopedic patient, a complete social and family history is important to help the RN first assistant develop an appropriate discharge plan. During the assessment, the RN first assistant needs to ascertain to what degree, if any, the patient's condition has disrupted activities of daily living. This information will aid in determining the patient's motivation to participate in the discharge plan, which specifies necessary postoperative activities.

The RN first assistant will then focus on the nature of the existing condition, injury, fracture, or disability. A description of the onset, the progression of symptoms, and any limitations on mobility must be included. The physical examination includes a thorough inspection of the functions of all body systems, with a particular focus on the affected extremity or joint. An inspection of posture, gait, body movements, and the degree of mobility/immobility (both active and passive range of motion [ROM]) is performed. The skin of the affected body part is assessed for color, temperature, and sensation, with the degree of edema, nature of bruises, rashes, or lesions documented, if present. Pain or tenderness is also assessed and documented, including extent, nature, onset, and any exacerbating or relieving factors.

With his/her advanced physical examination skills, the RN first assistant brings considerable knowledge to patient assessment. For example, for a suspected injury as simple as a meniscal tear, the RN first assistant will understand common mechanisms of injury, the incidence of tears (*i.e.*, the medial meniscus is torn much more commonly than the lateral meniscus, and is frequently associated with anterior cruciate ligament tears), and the classification of tears according to shape (longitudinal, transverse, flap, horizontal, complex), location (peripheral versus central), and extent (complete versus incomplete). Evaluating the patient's history will help the RN first assistant determine whether the tear is traumatic (following a twisting injury) or degenerative (often following a minor twist or squat) and confirm symptoms such as pain, swelling, sensation of "giving way," and mechanical symptoms (*e.g.*, locking, catching, clicking). On physical examination, the RN first assistant will assess for joint line tenderness, effusion (using ballottement to determine the presence of excess fluid or an effusion in the knee), quadriceps atrophy, and certain signs such as McMurray's sign (manipulation of the tibia with the leg flexed produces a pronounced click and sometimes actual locking of the joint if the meniscus has been injured) or Apley's sign (clicks, locking, and pain in the knee on prone examination, with the knee flexed 90 degrees and rotated externally and internally).[31,32,33]

Patient Education

The RN first assistant is well prepared to augment preoperative patient teaching. In the immediate postoperative period, the importance of coughing and deep breathing and safe movement must be stressed. Coughing and deep breathing techniques, ROM exercises to unaffected extremities, and postoperative restrictions and limitations should be discussed and taught to the patient and family/significant others. For a patient undergoing total hip arthroplasty, additional teaching requirements would include gluteal and abdominal contractions, quadriceps setting, dorsiflexion and plantar foot flexion, hip spiking, isometric exercises, use of assistive devices such as a trapeze, and continuous passive motion, as well as the importance of leg abduction or adduction postoperatively.[34] The correct use, and rationale for use, of antiembolism stockings and sequential compression devices should be included on the preoperative teaching checklist. Pain management strategies, including the use of patient-controlled analgesia (PCA) and continuous epidural analgesia, should be reviewed as appropriate. Preoperative physical therapy instruction on safe and effective methods of postoperative movement is important in preparation for discharge planning. The patient's anxiety and fear of pain and functional ability postoperatively may confound postoperative participation in rehabilitation. Specific teaching plans can assist the patient in structuring a self-care program.[35]

Diagnostic Studies

One common diagnostic study for orthopedic patients is the x-ray. Minimally, the orthopedic patient will have x-rays taken of the affected extremity or joint. If the patient is scheduled to receive a general anesthetic, the facility may require a chest x-ray if he is over age 60 or in ASA (American Society of Anesthesiologists) category III, IV, or V, which includes most patients undergoing total joint replacement/revision. Magnetic resonance imaging (MRI) has become a valuable orthopedic diagnostic tool, especially for knee and shoulder complaints. MRI facilitates the examination of both osseous and soft tissue structures, which was not possible on older imaging methods such as plain x-ray and computed tomography (CT) scanning.

Preoperative laboratory work also is required. The specific tests may vary but should include as a minimum a CBC, urinalysis, electrolytes (sodium, potassium, carbon dioxide, and chloride), and, for total joint procedures, blood type and cross match. Renal function is assessed by obtaining a BUN and serum creatinine. For the orthopedic patient undergoing extensive surgery, such as a total joint revision, coagulation studies (bleeding time and platelet count, prothrombin time [PT] and partial thromboplastin time [PTT]) are usually obtained. Most institutions require an ECG for patients over age 45 or with a history of cardiac problems.

The diagnosis of prosthesis infection is occasionally obvious (as when an abscess presents around the prosthesis), but is more often accompanied by nonspecific signs and symptoms. Pain is a principal sign of infected total hip prostheses. Sinus tracts that communicate with the prosthesis may be present in either late or chronic infection. Contrast arthrography can demonstrate loosening of the prosthesis and the presence of abscesses and sinus tracts; plain x-rays are helpful in detecting osteomyelitis associated with an infected joint prosthesis. CT scan and conventional ultrasonography are of limited usefulness due to the artifacts generated on the scan by the implant components. Combined technetium and gallium scanning may help distinguish joint prosthesis infection from aseptic loosening. An erythrocyte sedimentation rate (ESR) will be requested. Normally, the ESR returns to normal preoperative levels within 3–6 months following arthroplasty; if infection occurs, it remains elevated. C-reactive protein levels are likely to also be elevated with prosthetic infection.[36] This is a very weak determinant of infection, however, and there is no accurate noninvasive test to detect infection. The best method of detecting infection and identifying the organism is biopsy, either by open capsular biopsy or by aspiration of the joint fluid.[37] Because infection of a total joint prosthesis nearly always necessitates removal of the prosthesis, preventing infection is a primary nursing consideration.

Preoperative Measures To Prevent Infection

The patient should bathe or shower with an antimicrobial soap containing hexachlorophene or an iodophor, beginning 1 to 2 days preoperatively. A patient undergoing a major orthopedic procedure will receive prophylactic antibiotic therapy preoperatively. An initial dose of a cephalosporin is administered at least 1 to 2 hours before surgery, to ensure adequate tissue levels are present at the start of the operation. If a tourniquet is used, its inflation should be delayed for at least 5 minutes following IV administration of an antibiotic, to allow achievement of adequate tissue levels. Antibiotic prophylaxis may be continued every 6 hours for a 48-hour treatment window. It is important for the RN first assistant to note any patient allergies before the administration of any perioperative medication.

INTRAOPERATIVE PATIENT CARE

The choice of anesthesia is determined not only by the nature of the procedure, (*e.g.*, the length, extent, position of the patient, and location of the incision), but also by the age, physical condition, and history of the patient. Pediatric, trauma, arthritic, and elderly orthopedic patients each present special anesthesia requirements. For procedures involving an extremity and the use of a tourniquet, the choice between a regional anesthetic technique (specific nerve blockades, IV regional anesthesia, plexus anesthesia, spinal or epidural blockade) and a general anesthetic is usually determined by the usual interplay of patient and surgical parameters listed previously. For orthopedic procedures involving soft tissue, a local infiltration may be selected. For orthopedic procedures involving the bone, a regional or general anesthetic is desirable. During administration of a local anesthetic agent, awareness of the signs and symptoms of an overdose or allergic reaction and monitoring for their onset must be closely carried out. The use of epinephrine should be avoided in digital blocks or other areas where circulatory compromise to the tissues is a concern.

Probably no other specialty uses as many varied surgical positions as orthopedics. Positions for orthopedic surgery are usually variations on supine, lateral, and prone. For procedures involving the extremities, such as knee arthroscopy or carpal tunnel release, the patient is placed in the supine position. For procedures involving the shoulder or elbow, a sitting or semisitting position is preferred. Surgery involving the hip joint requires that the patient be in a lateral position to allow efficient access.

Each position presents a challenge for the perioperative team. Complications from improper positioning can result in nerve compression, interference with venous return and cardiac output, compression of the eye or possibly corneal abrasions, accidental removal of the endotracheal tube, joint strain, and other position-specific sequelae. In a position where the operative site is higher than the right atrium (such as the sitting position for cervical laminectomy), the patient may be at risk for venous air embolism; an esophageal stethoscope, transthoracic Doppler device, and end-tidal carbon dioxide monitors will be required. A right atrial catheter may be inserted in high-risk patients to permit removal of air.

The RN first assistant in orthopedics must maintain a practical knowledge of the use of positioning aids and operative beds, including increasingly complex fracture tables with special attachments. These present special patient care considerations as well; ensuring safety for the unconscious and paralyzed patient during positioning maneuvers must be a joint effort of the anesthesiologist, surgeon, and perioperative nursing team.

Skin preparation and draping techniques also vary depending on the surgical intervention and patient characteristics. Many different products can be used in skin prep, including film-forming iodophor complexes, povidone-iodine in solutions or gels, and iodine soap suspensions. Agents containing iodine are bactericidal against gram-negative and gram-positive organisms. Alcohol in combination promotes the rapid action of the agent's bactericidal properties. The area to be prepped is always inspected for integrity. If the skin is broken, even slightly, an alcohol-based agent is not recommended for use.

Applying surgical drapes, observing aseptic techniques, and providing adequate surgical site exposure are important RN first assistant activities. Many orthopedic surgeries involve manipulation of an extremity or a joint at some point in the procedure. The drapes must be placed to allow this activity. Many facilities use disposable drapes, many of which are designed to meet the manipulation requirements as well as the surgical site exposure and barrier requirements. In general, whichever type of draping system is chosen, the drapes should be nonlinting, provide an effective bacterial barrier, provide maximum patient coverage, permit freedom for manipulation, transmit heat and water vapor, and be nonflammable or flame retardant. The basic principles for aseptic technique and the handling of sterile drapes are observed. When plastic incise drapes are used, those with an antiseptic incorporated into the adhesive may be selected.

To begin the surgical procedure, the surgeon makes the skin incision with a scalpel blade and dissects the fascia with the electrosurgical pen tip or scalpel. As the incision progresses, the surgeon uses the electrosurgical pen to transect blood vessels and muscle. The RN first assistant applies slight pressure with a lap sponge to the area already exposed to assist. The lap sponge can also be used to provide retraction of the skin edges, depending on the procedure.

Self-retaining retractors are used during the procedure, placed in the shallow area of the incision. The position of the self-retaining retractors may be changed frequently to provide exposure. Whenever a retractor is placed, care must be taken to observe all structures it is to retract. The nerves and blood vessels must be identified before retractor placement. As the procedure progresses, the type of retractor needed changes from one designed for tissue retraction to one designed to elevate or secure bone. Caution is needed when manipulating any type of retractor. Too much upward force can result in a fracture; too little will not provide the correct exposure. Also, the downward pressure exerted while using a retractor may place unwanted stress on the underlying structures, causing interruption in the blood flow and possible damage to the muscle.

A hand-held retractor such as a rake retractor is often used superficially, to retract the skin or superficial fascia. It may also be used at the beginning of the procedure, after the skin incision has been made, to assist in the discovery of blood vessels severed during the incision. Used to retract the skin, this instrument permits exposure so that hemostasis can occur. A rake can also be used to retract the fibrous tissue covering a bone or joint capsule and ensure that the tissue is not twisted onto the drill bit, preventing visual inspection during the drilling procedure and possibly obscuring the hole after drilling.

A power saw, drill, or reamer (nitrogen, electrical, or battery-driven) is frequently used to resect, perforate, or cannulate a bone. Care must be taken to protect the surrounding tissue from injury related to mechanical (pressure from the angle of use or wound entry) or physical (thermal effects from the friction between the metal and the bone) events. The Midas Rex equipment is frequently used in total hip revisions. This particular instrumentation is very effective in removing old cement. Pulsating irrigation systems are used with antibiotic irrigating solutions throughout many orthopedic procedures to remove bone or cement fragments.

Tourniquets are often useful in minimizing blood loss. The RN first assistant may either apply the tourniquet or assist with application. In general, the width of the tourniquet cuff should be more than half the limb diameter, and the cuff should be applied over smooth padding that is kept wrinkle-free and dry. During prepping, it may be necessary to protect the cuff with an impermeable plastic drape placed just distal to the cuff. A properly applied and monitored pneumatic tourniquet is reasonably safe. The RN first assistant should carefully implement the AORN's recommended practice for the use of the pneumatic tourniquet.[38]

Hemostasis is maintained during surgery by means of pressure, suctioning, irrigation, and electrosurgery. When using the electrosurgical pencil, care must be taken to touch only the hemostat holding the bleeding end of the blood vessel or the area of uncontrolled bleeding. Touching any other tissue can cause thermal damage and increase the risk of postoperative wound infection. Because blood loss can be significant in certain procedures, the RN first assistant must participate in measures to calculate blood loss by weighing sponges, measuring suction canister contents, estimating the amount of blood on the drapes, and tracking the amount of irrigation fluid. If chemical/topical hemostatic adjuncts are required, oxidized regenerated cellulose is less likely to promote infection than are gelatin sponges or microfibrillar collagen.[39] This may be especially important when other foreign bodies, such as a prosthesis, are also left in the wound.

Wound closure techniques and materials will vary depending on the location of the surgical incision. Generally, an interrupted technique is used for closure. Each stitch is placed separately so that if one stitch breaks or loosens, the remaining sutures will still maintain the integrity of the closure. Stress on the primary suture line is of particular concern in procedures involving a joint. For procedures involving a capsule (hip or shoulder), a nonabsorbable synthetic, multifilament, braided suture is used to secure the internal tissue approximations. Next to surgical steel, this type of suture is the strongest available, and it retains its tensile strength for a long time. The nonabsorbable suture remains embedded in the body tissues (unless it is surgically removed), becoming encapsulated in fibrous tissue during wound healing. A retention suture—interrupted nonabsorbable suture material placed through tissue on each side of the primary suture line—is often used to relieve tension.

For smaller incisions, incisions in areas of less stress (*e.g.*, the arm), or incisions in areas where sutures will not be removed, an absorbable, synthetic, multifilament braided suture is used. The suturing technique will be either continuous or interrupted, depending on the site and the surgeon's preference. This suture is usually absorbed within 60–90 days by a process of slow hydrolysis.

Skin closure commonly is achieved using skin staples. Drains are used to reduce the dead space and decrease the risk of infection. For major orthopedic procedures (*e.g.*, total hip replacement, total knee replacement, shoulder procedures), the drain is placed by means of a secondary stab wound made distal to the surgical wound. Depending on the location, this drain may be secured with a heavy silk suture or taped securely in place as part of a bulky dressing.

Postoperatively, the orthopedic patient requires stabilization of the extremity. This is achieved by means of a cast, a splint, a sling, or a restricting device (such as an abduction pillow for the postoperative total hip patient). The patient may remain under anesthesia while the orthopedic appliance is secured. Postoperatively, the extremity is elevated to minimize swelling and decrease discomfort. Before transfer from the operating room, a check of the patient's vascular status is performed. This includes assessment of the pulses in the operative extremity, tissue perfusion, and sensory/motor function. Postoperative application of an ice pack is indicated to reduce swelling and decrease pain. Application of antiembolic stockings is indicated if the patient's mobility is limited by the surgery performed.

CONCLUSION

Advances in orthopedic surgery have changed and will continue to change the types of patients and patient procedures with which RN first assistants are involved. As the population continues to age, there will be more age-related orthopedic problems amenable to surgical intervention. New materials from space-age technology will invite new applications for orthopedic patients. Lasers are being considered in future orthopedic procedures; for arthroscopic procedures, the CO2 laser has proven effective. Fortunately, for all patients who require orthopedic surgery, the surgeon and RN first assistant, along with biomechanical engineers, will continue to contribute innovation and the knowledge of experience to alleviate pain and improve patients' functional abilities.

REVIEW QUESTIONS

Answer questions 1–9 regarding the following scenario: Theresa Bollens is admitted to the hospital with nausea and abdominal pain following ingestion of a meal high in fat content. She is diagnosed with cholecystitis and scheduled for laparoscopic cholecystectomy.

1. In a preoperative interview, Ms. Bollens, while intrigued by the notion of minimally invasive surgery, asks the RN first assistant what the advantages are. An appropriate explanation would include
   a. fewer incisions
   b. less postoperative pain and discomfort
   c. a lengthened hospital stay but earlier return to work
   d. better visualization of the anatomy
2. An important question for the RN first assistant to ask Ms. Bollens during the preoperative assessment would be about
   a. any previous abdominal surgery
   b. her menstrual history and possibility of current pregnancy
   c. previous episodes of dyspepsia following carbohydrate ingestion
   d. frequency of eructation and sensation of fullness
3. Which of the following would be a contraindication to the laparoscopic approach for Ms. Bollens?
   a. the presence of severe pain
   b. massive obesity
   c. clay-colored, fatty stools
   d. the need for common duct exploration
4. During explanation of anticipated perioperative events, the RN first assistant would ordinarily *not* prepare Ms. Bollens to expect
   a. an intravenous line insertion
   b. an indwelling urinary catheter
   c. temporary abdominal distention
   d. a preoperative enema
5. Most likely, Ms. Bollens will be placed in the supine position with which of the following modifications?
   a. left side elevated
   b. slight Trendelenburg
   c. reverse Trendelenburg
   d. low lithotomy
6. Because Ms. Bollens has had previous abdominal surgery, the surgeon and RN first assistant anticipate abdominal wall adhesions. Therefore, they might decide to modify the insertion site of the veress needle and insert it
   a. infraumbilically
   b. umbilically
   c. in the right upper quadrant
   d. in the cul de sac

7. To prevent the risk of air embolism and diaphragmatic damage, the RN first assistant will ensure that the intraabdominal pressure monitor is set for an upper limit of
   a. 4–6 mm Hg
   b. 6–12 mm Hg
   c. 12–16 mm Hg
   d. 16–25 mm Hg
8. During the surgery, the pressure monitor sounds. The RN first assistant should
   a. discontinue insufflation
   b. reduce the flow rate
   c. close the trocar valve
   d. check for kinks in the insufflation tubing
9. In assisting with hemostasis, the RN first assistant has many options during endoscopic surgery. The knot is tied outside the abdomen and slid down the trocar before final securing in which technique?
   a. extracorporeal
   b. pretied endoligature
   c. ski needle technique
   d. suture introducing technique
10. While reviewing the laboratory data for a patient undergoing mitral valve replacement, the RN first assistant notices that the urinalysis shows WBCs in the urine. An appropriate action at this point in time would be to
    a. disregard the report; it has no direct bearing on cardiovascular status
    b. inform the anesthesiologist; a broad-spectrum antibiotic should be given perioperatively
    c. inform the surgeon; patients with remote, concurrent infections are at risk for prosthetic infection
    d. request a urology consult
11. Which of the following are *not* normal breath sounds?
    a. vesicular
    b. bronchovesicular
    c. bronchial
    d. crackles
12. On assessment of a 74-year-old patient, the RN first assistant observes that the patient has had bilateral vein strippings. Before notifying the surgeon, the RN first assistant should
    a. assess the lesser saphenous vein
    b. determine how the patient feels about a prosthetic conduit
    c. explain to the patient that a porcine graft will be required; determine if this presents religious or cultural problems
    d. explain to the patient that not all five coronary vessels will be able to be grafted

Answer questions 13–16 regarding the following scenario: Mrs. Smith, age 76, is scheduled for CABG.

13. Which of the following factors would be most significant for preventing additional postoperative discomfort for Mrs. Smith?
    a. type of sternal retractor used
    b. use of ESU and bonewax during sternal opening

c. position of the sternal retractor
d. amount of homologous blood given

14. Postoperatively, the RN first assistant checks Mrs. Smith's chest tube drainage system. Which of the following would be considered the most normal in the first 24 hours postoperatively?
    a. no fluctuation in the water-seal tube
    b. intermittent, slight bubbling from the water-seal tube
    c. bright-red, bloody drainage
    d. orders to maintain suction at 30 cm H_2O
15. Which action might the RN first assistant recommend to best facilitate effective coughing and deep breathing by Mrs. Smith postoperatively?
    a. encourage her to take one day at a time and do her best
    b. see that she receives a back rub to relax her before coughing and deep breathing
    c. suggest that she request her pain medication about 20 minutes before coughing and deep breathing
    d. position her for postural drainage with cupping and vibration 10–15 minutes before coughing and deep breathing
16. Mrs. Smith's vital signs have been stable and she has been alert and oriented. However, today she has several episodes of confusion. Arterial blood gases are drawn; the values are pH 7.5, $PaCO_2$ 33.5, PaO_2 71.8, and oxygen saturation 95.6%. Which value is within normal limits?
    a. Oxygen saturation
    b. $PaCO_2$
    c. PaO_2
    d. none
17. A 70-year-old patient is scheduled for a redo CABG. He has patent saphenous veins to the right coronary artery (RCA) and internal mammary to the left anterior descending artery (LAD). Angiography shows a diseased marginal vessel. The RN first assistant should anticipate that the surgical position of choice might be
    a. right lateral
    b. left lateral
    c. modified supine
    d. semisitting
18. The RN first assistant in orthopedics often is involved in trauma patient care. When a patient with a compound fracture of the shaft of the right femur is admitted, the RN first assistant is present with the trauma team. What is the first thing the nursing team should do?
    a. cover the patient's open wound
    b. obtain a blood pressure
    c. clean the fracture site
    d. assess respiratory status
19. To determine the presence of effusion in the knee, the RN first assistant will use
    a. McMurray's test
    b. Apley's test
    c. ballottement
    d. passive and active range of motion assessment

20. A common postoperative device which is patient-guided and provides passive exercise is
    a. PCA
    b. CPM
    c. TENS
    d. ROM

Answer questions 21–23 regarding the following scenario: John Carry is admitted for arthroscopic knee surgery.

21. During preoperative patient education, the RN first assistant should explain to Mr. Carry
    a. the importance of early weight-bearing
    b. the type of general anesthesia he will receive
    c. methods of crutch walking
    d. the type of immobilization device used postoperatively
22. In the postanesthesia care area, the RN first assistant will be alert to the nursing diagnosis of Altered Peripheral Tissue Perfusion. Accordingly, the RN first assistant will
    a. monitor neurovascular status of the operative leg
    b. encourage ROM to the affected knee to improve tissue perfusion
    c. check that perioperative antibiotics have been prescribed
    d. encourage Mr. Carry to increase ambulation as tolerated
23. A potential complication for Mr. Carry is compartment syndrome. If left untreated, this could cause
    a. gas gangrene
    b. necrosis with loss of extremity
    c. liver failure
    d. metabolic alkalosis
24. Following total hip arthroplasty, the RN first assistant would expect the patient's ESR to return to preoperative levels within
    a. 1–2 months
    b. 2–3 months
    c. 3–6 months
    d. 6–9 months
25. The antibiotic usually selected for prophylaxis for major orthopedic procedures is a
    a. cephalosporin
    b. second-generation tetracycline
    c. penicillin or penicillin derivative
    d. aminoglycoside

Answers

1. b	6. c	11. d	16. d	21. c
2. a	7. c	12. a	17. b	22. a
3. b	8. d	13. c	18. d	23. b
4. c	9. a	14. b	19. c	24. c
5. c	10. c	15. c	20. b	25. a

REFERENCES

1. Phillips JM: Laparoscopy, pp vii; 6–15. Baltimore, Williams & Wilkins, 1977
2. Semm K: Operative manual for endoscopic abdominal surgery, pp v–x; 1–16; 20–23. Chicago, Year Book Medical Publishers, 1987
3. Gotz F, Pier A, Bacher C: Modified laparoscopic appendectomy in surgery. Surg Endoscopy 4:6–9, 1990
4. Corbitt JD: Early experience with laparoscopic guided colectomy. Proceedings of the 39th Annual Association of Operating Room Nurses' Congress, March 15–20, 1992
5. Llorente J, McHenry WS: Laparoscopic cholecystectomy. Proceedings of the 39th Annual Association of Operating Room Nurses Congress, March 15–20, 1992.
6. Ibid
7. Zucker KA: Surgical Laparoscopy, pp 31–39. St Louis, Quality Medical Publishing, 1991
8. Ibid
9. Endoscopic Suturing and Knot Tying Manual. Somerville, NJ, ETHICON Inc, 1991
10. Raza ST, et al: Changing trends and risk factors in coronary artery bypass surgery. Abstract, American Heart Association Scientific Session 1171, November 1990.
11. Personal communication. Phil Thompson, Cardiovascular Registered Nurse First Assistant, St Francis Medical Center, Monroe, LA, 1991
12. Meeker MH, Rothrock JC: Alexander's Care of the Patient in Surgery, p 898. St Louis, Mosby–Year Book, 1991
13. Dodd H, Cockett FB: The Pathology and Surgery of the Veins of the Lower Limb, p 111. Edinburgh, Livingstone, 1976
14. Lajos TZ, Espersen C: Anatomical considerations in venous drainage of the lower extremities: Clinical implications. J Surg Res 34:1–6, 1983
15. Siclari F, Heublein B, Schaps D: Total arterial revascularization of the heart using both mammary arteries and the right gastroepiploic artery, J Card Surg 5:309–314, 1990
16. Rothrock JC: Preoperative psychoeducational interventions. In Perioperative Nursing Research: A Ten-Year Review, pp 1–14. Denver, Association of Operating Room Nurses, 1989
17. Devine EC, et al: Clinical and financial effects of psychoeducational care provided by staff nurses to adult surgical patients in the post-DRG environment. Am J Pub Health, 78:1293–1297, 1988
18. Cupples S: Effects of timing and reinforcement of preoperative education on knowledge and recovery of patients having coronary artery bypass graft surgery. Heart & Lung, 20:654–660, 1991
19. Carr JA, Powers MJ: Stressors associated with coronary bypass surgery. Nurs Res 35:243–246, 1986
20. Keller C: Seeking normalcy: the experience of coronary artery bypass surgery. Res in Nurs and Health, 14:173–178, 1991
21. King KB, Norsen LH, Robertson RK, Hicks GL: Patient management of pain medication after cardiac surgery. Nurs Res 36:145–150, 1987
22. Cardiac rehabilitation programs enhance recovery of heart surgery patients. In Research Activities, No 150. Agency for Health Care Policy and Research, 1992
23. Gortner SR, et al: Improving recovery following cardiac surgery: A randomized clinical trial. J Adv Nurs 13:649–661, 1988
24. Garding BS, Kerr JC, Bay K: Effectiveness of a program of information and support for myocardial infarction patients recovering at home. Heart & Lung, 17:355–362, 1988
25. Ruiz BA, Dibble SL, Gillis CL, Gortner SR: Predictors of general activity 8 weeks after cardiac surgery. Appl Nurs Res, 5(2):59–64, 1992
26. Reichert SLA, et al: Intraoperative transesophageal color-coded doppler echocardiography for evaluation of residual regurgitation after mitral valve repair. J Thor and Cardio Surg, 100:756–761, 1990
27. Docker CS, Muthusamy MB, Balasundaram SG, Duran CG: Intraoperative echocardiography: An essential tool in cardiac surgery. AORN J 55:167–176, 1992

28. Grosner G, et al: Left thoracotomy reoperation for coronary artery disease. J Card Surg, 5:304–308, 1990
29. Teoh KHT, et al: Optimal visualization of coronary artery anastomosis by gas jet. Ann Thor Surg, 52:564, 1991
30. David TE, Bos J, Rakowski H: Mitral valve repair by replacement of chordae tendineae with polytetrafluoroethylene sutures. J Thor and Cardio Surg, 101:495–501, 1991
31. Paschal S, Zardus M: Sports Medicine: Surgery of the Knee and Shoulder, pp 95–104. Proceedings of the 39th Annual Association of Operating Room Nurses Congress, March 1992.
32. Seidel HM, Ball JW, Dains JE, Benedict GW: Mosby's Guide to Physical Examination, pp 551–554. St Louis, CV Mosby, 1987
33. Epstein O, Perkin GD, deBono DP, Cookson J: Clinical Examination, pp 11.35–11.39. New York, Gower Medical Publishing, 1992
34. Tucker SM, Canobbio MM, Paquette EV, Wells MF: Patient Care Standards, pp 370–372. St Louis, Mosby–Year Book, 1992
35. Kelley H: Patient perceptions of pain and disability after joint arthroplasty. Ortho Nurs 10(6):43–50, 1991
36. Dougherty SH: Prosthetic Devices. In Care of the Surgical Patient, pp 2-1–2-22. New York, Scientific American Medicine, 1991
37. Cuckler JM, et al: Diagnosis and management of infected total joint arthroplasty. Ortho Clin N Am 22:523–530, 1991
38. Association of Operating Room Nurses: Recommended Practices for Use of Pneumatic Tourniquet, III, 13-1–13-4. Denver, Association of Operating Room Nurses, 1992
39. Dougherty, p 2-13

PREAMBLE

Perioperative nursing practice has historically included the role of the RN as assistant at surgery. As early as 1980, documents issued by the American College of Surgeons supported the appropriateness for qualified RNs to first assist.

AORN officially recognized this role as a component of perioperative nursing in 1983 and adopted the first Official Statement on RN First Assistants (RNFA) in 1984. Acceptance of this official statement by many state boards of nursing has supported that RNFA behaviors are recognized within the scope of nursing practice.

AORN's official statement delineates the definition, scope of practice, qualifications, educational requirements, and clinical privileges that must be met by the perioperative nurse who practices as an RNFA. AORN further recognizes the need for appropriate compensation/reimbursement to RNs who fulfill this role in providing perioperative patient care.

DEFINITION OF RN FIRST ASSISTANT

The RN first assistant at surgery collaborates with the surgeon in performing a safe operation with optimal outcomes for the patient. The RN first assistant practices perioperative nursing and must have acquired the necessary specific knowledge, skills, and judgment. The RN first assistant practices under the supervision of the surgeon during the intraoperative phase of the perioperative experience. The RN first assistant does not concurrently function as a scrub nurse.

SCOPE OF PRACTICE

The scope of practice of the nurse performing as first assistant is a part of perioperative nursing practice. Perioperative nursing is a specialized area of practice. The activities included in first assisting are further refinements of perioperative nursing practice which are executed within the context of the nursing process. The observable nursing behaviors are based on an extensive body of scientific knowledge. These intraoperative nursing behaviors may include

- ☐ handling tissue,
- ☐ providing exposure,
- ☐ using instruments,
- ☐ suturing, and
- ☐ providing hemostasis.

These behaviors may vary depending on patient populations, practice environments, services provided, accessibility of human and fiscal resources, institutional policy, and state nurse practice acts.

The decision by an RN to practice as a first assistant must be made voluntarily and deliberately, with an understanding of the professional accountability that the role entails.

QUALIFICATIONS OF THE RN FIRST ASSISTANT

Qualifications for RN first assistants should include, but not be limited to

- ☐ certification in perioperative nursing (CNOR);
- ☐ documentation of proficiency in perioperative nursing practice as both a scrub and circulating nurse;
- ☐ ability to apply principles of asepsis and infection control;
- ☐ knowledge of surgical anatomy, physiology, and operative technique related to the operative procedures in which the RN assists;
- ☐ ability to perform cardiopulmonary resuscitation;
- ☐ ability to perform effectively in stressful and emergency situations;
- ☐ ability to recognize safety hazards and initiate appropriate preventive and corrective action;
- ☐ ability to perform effectively and harmoniously as a member of the operative team;
- ☐ ability to demonstrate skill in behaviors unique to the RN first assistant (as defined); and
- ☐ meets requirements of statutes, regulations, and institutional policies relevant to RN first assistants.

PREPARATION FOR THE RN FIRST ASSISTANT

The AORN has stated, "The complexity of knowledge and skill required to effectively care for recipients of operating room nursing services compels nurses to be well educated and to continue their education beyond generic nursing programs."[1]

Perioperative nurses who wish to practice as RN first assistants must develop a set of cognitive, psychomotor, and affective behaviors that demonstrate accountability and responsibility for identifying and meeting the needs of the recipients of their nursing services.

Development of this set of behaviors begins with and builds upon the education program leading to licensure as an RN, which provides basic knowledge, skills, and attitudes essential to the practice of perioperative nursing. Further preparation for the RN first assistant includes perioperative nursing practice with diversified experience in scrubbing and circulating. This should culminate in the nurse achieving certification as a CNOR. Additional preparation is then acquired through completion of formal education programs including didactic instruction and supervised clinical learning activities.

These programs should consist of curricula that address all of the content areas of the modules in the *Core Curriculum for the RN First Assistant*, take place in institutions approved by The Association of Higher Education (or its equivalent), and award a degree or certificate upon successful program completion.

ESTABLISHMENT OF CLINICAL PRIVILEGES FOR THE RN FIRST ASSISTANT

To determine if an RN qualifies for clinical privileges as a first assistant, an approval process must be established by the institution in which the individual will practice.

The process of granting clinical privileges should include mechanisms for

- ☐ assessing individual qualifications for practice,
- ☐ assessing continuing proficiency,
- ☐ revaluating annual performance,
- ☐ assessing compliance with relevant institutional and departmental policies,
- ☐ defining lines of accountability,
- ☐ retrieving documentation of participation as first assistant, and
- ☐ establishing systems for peer review.

Each RN first assistant demonstrates behaviors that progress on a continuum from basic competency to excellence. Once having met the educational and experiential requirements, the RNFA is encouraged to attain a bachelor of science in nursing degree and to achieve and maintain certification (CRNFA) for this specific role.

NOTE

1. D L Davis, J A Kneedler, B J Manuel, *Surgical Experience: A Model for Professional Nursing Practice in the Operating Room* (Denver: Association of Operating Room Nurses, Inc, 1978).

SUGGESTED READING

Association of Operating Room Nurses, Inc. "Perioperative patient care quality." *Chapter Resource Manual.* Denver: Association of Operating Room Nurses, Inc, 1992.

"Standards of perioperative nursing." In *AORN Standards and Recommended Practices for Perioperative Nursing.* Denver: Association of Operating Room Nurses, Inc, 1992, II:2-1.

"Competency statements in perioperative nursing." In *AORN Standards and Recommended Practices for Perioperative Nursing.* Denver: Association of Operating Room Nurses, Inc, 1992, I:2-1.

Association of Operating Room Nurses, Inc. *Core Curriculum for the RN First Assistant.* Denver: Association of Operating Room Nurses, Inc, 1990.

Joint Commission on Accreditation of Healthcare Organizations. *AMH/92 Accreditation Manual for Hospitals.* Chicago: Joint Commission on Accreditation of Healthcare Organizations, 1991.

American College of Surgeons. "Statements on principles." *1991-1992 Socioeconomic Factbook.* Chicago: American College of Surgeons, 1989, 10.

"Medicare and Medicaid programs: Conditions of participation for hospitals," *Federal Register* 51 (June 17, 1986) 22048.

(Source: AORN official statement on RN first assistants, 1993. Reprinted with permission from AORN, Inc., Denver, CO.

APPENDIX: II
Diagnostic Studies and Their Meaning

Abbreviations

Conventional Units

kg = kilogram
g = gram
mg = milligram
μg = microgram
μμg = micromicrogram
ng = nanogram
pg = picogram
dl = 100 milliliters
ml = milliliter
mm^3 = cubic millimeter
fl = femtoliter
mM = millimole
nM = nanomole

mOsm = milliosmole
mm = millimeter
μm = micron or micrometer
mm Hg = millimeters of mercury
U = unit
mU = milliunit
μU = microunit
mEq = milliequivalent
IU = International Unit
mIU = milliInternational Unit

SI Units

g = gram
L = liter
d = day
hr = hour
mol = mole
mmol = millimole
μmol = micromole
nmol = nanomole
pmol = picomole

From Goodman D. Appendix I: Diagnostic Studies and Their Meaning. In The Lippincott Manual of Nursing Practice, 5th ed. Philadelphia, JB Lippincott, 1991.

*Reference Ranges—Hematology**

Determination	Reference Range: *Conventional Units*	Reference Range: *SI Units*	Clinical Significance
A_2 hemoglobin	1.5%–3.5% of total hemoglobin	Mass fraction: 0.015–0.035 of total hemoglobin	Increased in certain types of thalassemia
Bleeding time	2–8 min	2–8 min	Prolonged in thrombocytopenia, defective platelet function, and aspirin therapy
Factor V assay (proaccelerin factor)	60%–140%		
Factor VII assay (antihemophiliac factor)	50%–200%		Deficient in classical hemophilia
Factor IX assay (plasma thromboplastin component)	75%–125%		Deficient in Christmas disease (pseudohemophilia)
Factor X (Stuart factor)	60%–140%		Deficient in Stuart clotting defect
Fibrinogen	200–400 mg/dl	2–4 g/dl	Increased in pregnancy, infections accompanied by leukocytosis, nephrosis Decreased in severe liver disease, abruptio placentae
Fibrin split products	<10 mg/L	<10 mg/L	Increased in disseminated intravascular coagulopathy
Fibrinolysins (whole blood clot lysis time)	No lysis in 24 hr		Increased activity associated with massive hemorrhage, extensive surgery, transfusion reactions
Partial thromboplastin time (activated)	20–45 sec		Prolonged in deficiency of fibrinogen, factors II, V, VIII, IX, X, XI, and XII, and in heparin therapy
Prothrombin consumption	>20 sec		Impaired in deficiency of factors VIII, IX, and X
Prothrombin time	9.5–12 sec		Prolonged by deficiency of factors, I, II, V, VII, and X, fat malabsorption, severe liver disease, coumarin-anticoagulant therapy
Erythrocyte count	Males: 4,600,000–6,200,000/mm^3 Females 4,200,000–5,400,000/mm^3	$4.6–6.2 \times 10^{12}$/L $4.2–5.4 \times 10^{12}$/L	Increased in severe diarrhea and dehydration, polycythemia, acute poisoning, pulmonary fibrosis Decreased in all anemias, in leukemia, and after hemorrhage, when blood

Erythrocyte indices			
Mean corpuscular volume (MCV)	80–94 (μm^3)	80–94 fl	Increased in macrocytic anemias; decreased in microcytic anemia
Mean corpuscular hemoglobin (MCH)	27–32 $\mu\mu g$/cell	27–32 pg	Increased in macrocytic anemias; decreased in microcytic anemia
Mean corpuscular hemoglobin concentration (MCHC)	33%–38%	Concentration fraction: 0.33–0.38	Decreased in severe hypochromic anemia
Reticulocytes	0.5%–1.5% of red cells	Number fraction: 0.005–0.015	Increased with any condition stimulating increase in bone marrow activity (*i.e.*, infection, blood loss [acute and chronic]); after iron therapy in iron deficiency anemia, polycythemia rubra vera Decreased with any condition depressing bone marrow activity, acute leukemia, late stage of severe anemias
Erythrocyte sedimentation rate (ESR)—Westergren method	Males under 50 yr: <15 mm/hr	<15 mm/hr	Increased in tissue destruction, whether inflammatory or degenerative; during menstruation and pregnancy; and in acute febrile diseases
	Males over 50 yr: <20 mm/hr	<20 mm/hr	
	Females under 50 yr: <20 mm/hr	<20 mm/hr	
	Females over 50 yr: <30 mm/hr	<30 mm/hr	
Erythrocyte sedimentation ratio—Zeta centrifuge	41%–54% in both sexes	Fraction: 0.41–0.54	Significance similar to ESR
Hematocrit	Males: 42%–50%	Volume fraction: 0.42–0.5	Decreased in severe anemias, anemia of pregnancy, acute massive blood loss
	Females: 40%–48%	Volume fraction: 0.4–0.48	Increased in erythrocytosis of any cause, and in dehydration or hemoconcentration associated with shock
Hemoglobin	Males: 13–18 g/dl Females: 12–16 g/dl	2.02–2.79 mmol/L 1.86–2.48 mmol/L	Decreased in various anemias, pregnancy, severe or prolonged hemorrhage, and with excessive fluid intake

* Laboratory values vary according to the techniques used in different laboratories.

(continued)

Reference Ranges—Hematology* *(continued)*

Determination	Reference Range: Conventional Units	Reference Range: SI Units	Clinical Significance
			Increased in polycythemia, chronic obstructive pulmonary diseases, failure of oxygenation because of congestive heart failure, and normally in people living at high altitudes
Hemoglobin F	<2% of total hemoglobin	Mass fraction: <0.02	Increased in infants and children, and in thalassemia and many anemias
Leukocyte alkaline phosphatase	Score of 40–100		Increased in polycythemia vera, myelofibrosis, and infections Decreased in chronic granulocytic leukemia, paroxysmal nocturnal hemoglobinuria; hypoplastic marrow, and viral infections, particularly infectious mononucleosis
Leukocyte count	Total: 5,000–10,000/mm^3	5–10 × 10^9/L	Elevated in acute infectious diseases, predominantly in the neutrophilic fraction with bacterial diseases, and in the lymphocytic and monocytic fractions in viral diseases Elevated in acute leukemia, following menstruation, and following surgery or trauma Depressed in aplastic anemia, agranulocytosis, and by toxic agents such as chemotherapeutic agents used in treating malignancy Eosinophils elevated in collagen disease, allergy, intestinal parasitosis
Neutrophils	60%–70%	Number fraction: 0.6–0.7	
Eosinophils	1%–4%	Number fraction: 0.01–0.04	
Basophils	0%–0.5%	Number fraction: 0.00–0.05	
Lymphocytes	20%–30%	Number fraction: 0.2–0.3	
Monocytes	2%–6%	Number fraction: 0.02–0.06	
Osmotic fragility of red cells	Increased if hemolysis occurs in over 0.5% NaCl Decreased if hemolysis is incomplete in 0.3% NaCl		Increased in congenital spherocytosis, idiopathic acquired hemolytic anemia, isoimmune hemolytic disease, ABO hemolytic disease of newborn Decreased in sickle cell anemia, thalassemia

Platelet count	$100,000–400,000/mm^3$	$0.1–0.4 \times 10^{12}/L$	Increased in malignancy, myeloproliferative disease, rheumatoid arthritis, and postoperatively; about 50% of patients with unexpected increase of platelet count will be found to have a malignancy Decreased in thrombocytopenic purpura, acute leukemia, aplastic anemia, and during cancer chemotherapy, infections, and drug reactions

Reference Ranges—Serum, Plasma, and Whole Blood Chemistries

	Normal Adult Reference Range		Clinical Significance	
Determination	*Conventional Units*	*SI Units*	*Increased*	*Decreased*
Acetoacetate	0.2–1.0 mg/dl	19.6–98 μmol/L	Diabetic acidosis Fasting	
Acetone	0.3–2.0 mg/dl	51.6–344.0 μmol/L	Toxemia of pregnancy Carbohydrate-free diet High-fat diet	
Adrenocorticotropic hormone (ACTH) (plasma)—RIA*	Less than 50 pg/ml	Less than 50 mg/mL	Pituitary-dependent Cushing's syndrome Ectopic ACTH syndrome Primary adrenal atrophy	Adrenocortical tumor Adrenal insufficiency secondary to hypopituitarism
Aldolase	3–8 Sibley-Lehninger U/dl at 37°C	22–59 mU/L at 37°C	Hepatic necrosis Granulocytic leukemia Myocardial infarction Skeletal muscle disease	
Aldosterone (plasma)—RIA	Supine: 3–10 ng/dl Upright: 5–30 ng/dl Adrenal vein: 200–800 ng/dl	0.08–0.30 nmol/L 0.14–0.90 nmol/L 5.54–22.16 nmol/L	Primary aldosteronism (Conn's syndrome) Secondary aldosteronism	Addison's disease
Alpha-1-antitrypsin	200–400 mg/dl	2–4 g/L		Certain forms of chronic lung and liver disease in young adults

(continued)

Reference Ranges—Serum, Plasma, and Whole Blood Chemistries (continued)

	Normal Adult Reference Range		Clinical Significance	
Determination	*Conventional Units*	*SI Units*	*Increased*	*Decreased*
Alpha-1-fetoprotein	None detected		Hepatocarcinoma Metastatic carcinoma of liver Germinal cell carcinoma of the testis or ovary Fetal neural tube defects—elevation in maternal serum	
Alpha-hydroxybutyric dehydrogenase	Up to 140 U/ml	Up to 140 U/L	Myocardial infarction Granulocytic leukemia Hemolytic anemias Muscular dystrophy	
Ammonia (plasma)	40–80 μg/dl (enzymatic method); varies considerably with method	22.2–44.3 μmol/L	Severe liver disease Hepatic decompensation	
Amylase	60–160 Somogyi U/dl	111–296 U/L	Acute pancreatitis Mumps Duodenal ulcer Carcinoma of head of pancreas Prolonged elevation with pseudocyst of pancreas Increased by drugs that constrict pancreatic duct sphincters: morphine, codeine, cholinergics	Chronic pancreatitis Pancreatic fibrosis and atrophy Cirrhosis of liver Pregnancy (2nd and 3rd trimesters)
Arsenic	6–20 μg/dl; $\geq$ 50 μg/dl, suspect toxicity	0.78–2.6 μmol/L	Accidental or intentional poisoning Excessive occupational exposure	
Ascorbic acid (vitamin C)	0.4–1.5 mg/dl	23–85 μmol/L	Large doses of ascorbic acid as a prophylactic against the common cold	
Bilirubin	Total: 0.1–1.2 mg/dl Direct: 0.1–0.2 mg/dl	1.7–20.5 μmol/L 1.7–3.4 μmol/L	Hemolytic anemia (indirect) Biliary obstruction and disease	

	Indirect: 0.1–1 mg/dl	1.7–17.1 μmol/L	Hepatocellular damage (hepatitis) Pernicious anemia Hemolytic disease of newborn	
Blood gases				
Oxygen, arterial (whole blood)				
Partial pressure (PaO_2) Saturation (SaO_2)	95–100 mm Hg 94%–100%	12.64–13.30 kPa Volume fraction: 0.94–1	Polycythemia Anhydremia	Anemia Cardiac decompensation Chronic obstructive pulmonary disease
Carbon dioxide, arterial (whole blood): partial pressure ($PaCo_2$)	35–45 mm Hg	4.66–5.99 kPa	Respiratory acidosis Metabolic alkalosis	Respiratory alkalosis Metabolic acidosis
pH (whole blood arterial)	7.35–7.45	7.35–7.45	Vomiting Hyperpnea Fever Intestinal obstruction	Uremia Diabetic acidosis Hemorrhage Nephritis
Calcitonin	Basal: nondetectable 400 pg/ml	400 ng/L	Medullary carcinoma of the thyroid Some nonthyroid tumors Zollinger-Ellison syndrome	
Calcium	8.5–10.5 mg/dl	2.125–2.625 mmol/L	Tumor or hyperplasia of parathyroid Hypervitaminosis D Multiple myeloma Nephritis with uremia Malignant tumors Sarcoidosis Hyperthyroidism Skeletal immobilization Excess calcium intake: milk-alkali syndrome	Hypoparathyroidism Diarrhea Celiac disease Vitamin D deficiency Acute pancreatitis Nephrosis After parathyroidectomy
CO_2 venous	Adults: 24–32 mEq/L Infants: 18–24 mEq/L	24–32 mmol/L 18–24 mmol/L	Tetany Respiratory disease Intestinal obstruction Vomiting	Acidosis Nephritis Eclampsia Diarrhea Anesthesia

(continued)

Reference Ranges—Serum, Plasma, and Whole Blood Chemistries (continued)

	Normal Adult Reference Range		Clinical Significance	
Determination	*Conventional Units*	*SI Units*	*Increased*	*Decreased*
Carcinoembryonic antigen (CEA)–RIA	0–2.5 ng/ml	0–2.5 μg/L	The repeatedly high incidence of this antigen in cancers of the colon, rectum, pancreas, and stomach suggests that CEA levels may be useful in the therapeutic monitoring of these conditions.	
Catecholamines (plasma)–RIA	Epinephrine, random: up to 90 pg/ml Norepinephrine, random: 100–550 pg/ml Dopamine, random: up to 130 pg/ml	Up to 490 pmol/L 590–3240 pmol/L Up to 850 pmol/L	Pheochromocytoma	
Ceruloplasmin	30–80 mg/dl	300–800 mg/L		Wilson's disease (hepatolenticular degeneration)
Chloride	95–105 mEq/L	95–105 mmol/L	Nephrosis Nephritis Urinary obstruction Cardiac decompensation Anemia	Diabetes Diarrhea Vomiting Pneumonia Heavy metal poisoning Cushing's syndrome Burns Intestinal obstruction Febrile conditions
Cholesterol	150–200 mg/dl	3.9–5.2 mmol/L	Lipemia Obstructive jaundice Diabetes Hypothyroidism	Pernicious anemia Hemolytic anemia Hyperthyroidism Severe infection Terminal states of debilitating disease
Cholesterol esters	60%–70% of total	Fraction of total cholesterol 0.6–0.7		The esterified fraction decreases in liver diseases
Cholinesterase	Serum: 0.6–1.6 delta pH Red cells: 0.6–1 delta pH	0.6–1.6 U 0.6–1 U	Nephrosis Exercise	Nerve gas intoxication (greater effect on red cell activity) Insecticides, organic phosphates (greater effect on plasma activity)

Chorionic gonadotropin, beta subunit—RIA	0–5 IU/L	0–5 IU/L	Pregnancy Hydatidiform mole Choriocarcinoma	
Complement, human C_3	Males: 88–252 mg/dl Females: 88–206 mg/dl	880–2520 mg/L	Some inflammatory diseases	Acute glomerulonephritis Disseminated lupus erythematosus with renal involvement
Complement C_4	14–51 mg/dl	140–510 mg/L	Some inflammatory diseases	Often decreased in immunologic disease, especially with active systemic lupus erythematosus Hereditary angioneurotic edema
Complement, total (hemolytic)	90%–94% complement		Some inflammatory diseases	Acute glomerulonephritis Epidemic meningitis Subacute bacterial endocarditis
Copper	70–165 μg/dl	11–25.9 μmol/L	Cirrhosis of liver Pregnancy	Wilson's disease
Cortisol–RIA	8 AM: 7–25 μg/dl 4 PM: 2–9 μg/dl	193–690 nmol/L 55–248 nmol/L	Stress: infectious disease, surgery, burns, etc. Pregnancy Cushing's syndrome Pancreatitis Eclampsia	Addison's disease Anterior pituitary hypofunction
C peptide reactivity	1.5–10 ng/ml	1.5–10 μg/L	Insulinoma	Diabetes
Creatine	0.2–0.8 mg/ml	15.3–61 μmol/L	Pregnancy Skeletal muscle necrosis or atrophy Starvation Hyperthyroidism	
Creatine phosphokinase (CPK)	Males: 50–325 mU/ml Females: 50–250 mU/ml	 50–325 U/L 50–250 U/L	Myocardial infarction Skeletal muscle diseases Intramuscular injections Crush syndrome Hypothyroidism Alcohol withdrawal delirium Alcoholic myopathy Cerebrovascular disease	
Creatine phosphokinase isoenzymes	MM band present (skeletal muscle); MB band absent (heart muscle)		MB band increased in myocardial infarction, ischemia	

(continued)

Reference Ranges—Serum, Plasma, and Whole Blood Chemistries (continued)

	Normal Adult Reference Range		Clinical Significance	
Determination	*Conventional Units*	*SI Units*	*Increased*	*Decreased*
Creatinine	0.7–1.4 mg/dl	62–124 μmol/L	Nephritis Chronic renal disease	Kidney diseases
Creatinine clearance	100–150 ml of blood cleared of creatinine per min	1.67–2.5 ml/sec		
Cryoglobulins, qualitative	Negative		Multiple myeloma Chronic lymphocytic leukemia Lymphosarcoma Systemic lupus erythematosus Rheumatoid arthritis Infective subacute endocarditis Some malignancies Scleroderma	
11-Deoxycortisol	1 μg/dl	<0.029 μmol/L	Hypertensive form of virilizing adrenal hyperplasia due to an 11-β-hydroxylase defect	
Dibucaine number	Normal: 70%–85% inhibition Heterozygote: 50%–65% inhibition Homozygote: 16%–25% inhibition			Important in detecting carriers of abnormal cholinesterase activity who are susceptible to succinyldicholine anesthetic shock
Dihydrotestosterone	Males: 50–210 ng/dl Females: none detectable	1.72–7.22 nmol/L		Testicular feminization syndrome
Estradiol—RIA	Females: Follicular: 10–90 pg/ml Midcycle: 100–500 pg/ml Luteal: 50–240 pg/ml	 37–370 pmol/L 367–1835 pmol/L 184–881 pmol/L	Pregnancy	Depressed or failure to peak—ovarian failure

	Follicular phase: 2–20 ng/dl Midcycle: 12–40 ng/dl Luteal phase: 10–30 ng/dl Postmenopausal: 1–5 ng/dl Males: 0.5–5 ng/dl			
Estriol—RIA	Nonpregnant females: <0.5 ng/ml	<1.75 nmol/L	Pregnancy	Depressed or failure to peak—ovarian failure
	Pregnant females: 1st trimester: up to 1 ng/ml	Up to 3.5 nmol/L		
	2nd trimester: 0.8–7 ng/ml	2.8–24.3 nmol/L		
	3rd trimester: 5–25 ng/ml	17.4–86.8 nmol/L		
Estrogens, total—RIA	Females: cycle days:		Pregnancy Measured on a daily basis, can be used to evaluate response of hypogonadotrophic, hypoestrogenic women to human menopausal or pituitary gonadotropin	Fetal distress Ovarian failure
	Days 1–10: 61–394 pg/ml	61–394 ng/L		
	Days 11–20: 122–437 pg/ml	122–437 ng/L		
	Days 21–30: 156–350 pg/ml	156–350 ng/L		
	Males: 40–115 pg/ml	40–115 ng/L		
Estrone—RIA	Females:		Pregnancy	Depressed or failure to peak—ovarian failure
	Days 1–10: 4.3–18 ng/dl	15.9–66.6 pmol/L		
	Days 11–20: 7.5–19.6 ng/dl	27.8–72.5 pmol/L		
	Days 21–30: 13–20 ng/dl	48.1–74 pmol/L		
	Males: 2.5–7.5 ng/dl	9.3–27.8 pmol/L		
Ferritin—RIA	Males: 10–270 ng/ml	10–270 μg/L	Nephritis Hemochromatosis Certain neoplastic diseases Acute myelogenous leukemia Multiple myeloma	Iron deficiency
	Females: 5–100 ng/ml	5–100 μg/L		

(continued)

Reference Ranges—Serum, Plasma, and Whole Blood Chemistries *(continued)*

	Normal Adult Reference Range		Clinical Significance	
Determination	***Conventional Units***	***SI Units***	***Increased***	***Decreased***
Folic acid—RIA	4–16 ng/mi	9.1–36.3 nmol/L		Megaloblastic anemias of infancy and pregnancy Inadequate diet Liver disease Malabsorption syndrome Severe hemolytic anemia Pituitary failure
Follicle stimulating hormone (FSH)—RIA	Females: Follicular phase: 5–20 mIU/ml Peak of middle cycle: 12–30 mIU/ml Luteinic phase: 5–15 mIU/ml Menopausal females: 40–200 mIU/ml	 5–20 IU/L 12–30 IU/L 5–15 IU/L 40–200 IU/L	Menopause and primary ovarian failure	
Galactose	<5 mg/dl	<0.28 mmol/L		Galactosemia
Gamma glutamyl transpeptidase	Males: <45 IU/L Females: <30 IU/L	45 U/L 30 U/L	Hepatobiliary disease Anicteric alcoholics Drug therapy damage Myocardial infarction Renal infarction	
Gastrin—RIA	Fasting: 50–155 pg/ml Postprandial: 80–170 pg/ml Zollinger-Ellison syndrome: 200–over 2000 pg/ml Pernicious anemia: 130–2260 pg/ml (mean 912)	50–155 ng/L 80–170 ng/L 200–over 2000 ng/L 130–2260 ng/L (mean 912)	Zollinger-Ellison syndrome Peptic ulceration of the duodenum Pernicious anemia	
Glucose	Fasting: 60–110 mg/dl Postprandial (2 hr): 65–140 mg/dl	3.3–6.05 mmol/L 3.58–7.7 mmol/L	Diabetes Nephritis Hyperthyroidism Early hyperpituitarism Cerebral lesions Infections Pregnancy Uremia	Hyperinsulinism Hypothyroidism Late hyperpituitarism Pernicious vomiting Addison's disease Extensive hepatic damage

Glucose tolerance (oral)	Features of normal response: 1. Normal fasting between 60–110 mg/dl 2. No sugar in urine 3. Upper limits of normal: Fasting = 125 1 hour = 190 2 hours = 140 3 hours = 125	3.3–6.05 mmol/L 6.88 mmol/L 10.45 mmol/L 7.70 mmol/L 6.88 mmol/L	(Flat or inverted curve) Hyperinsulinism Adrenal cortical insufficiency (Addison's disease) Anterior pituitary hypofunction Hypothyroidism Sprue and celiac diseases	(High or prolonged curve) Diabetes Hyperthyroidism Primary adrenal cortical tumor or hyperplasia Severe anemia Certain central nervous system disorders
Glucose-6-phosphate dehydrogenase (red cells)	Screening: Decolorization in 20–100 min Quantitative: 1.86–2.5 IU/ml RBC	1860–2500 U/L		Drug-induced hemolytic anemia Hemolytic disease of newborn
Glycoprotein (alpha-1-acid)	40–110 mg/dl	400–1100 mg/L	Neoplasm Tuberculosis Diabetes complicated by degenerative vascular disease Pregnancy Rheumatoid arthritis Rheumatic fever Infectious liver disease Lupus erythematosus	
Growth hormone—RIA	<10 ng/ml	<10 mg/L	Acromegaly	Failure to stimulate with arginine or insulin—hypopituitarism
Haptoglobin	50–250 mg/dl	0.5–2.5 g/L	Pregnancy Estrogen therapy Chronic infections Various inflammatory conditions	Hemolytic anemia Hemolytic blood transfusion reaction
Hemoglobin (plasma)	0.5–5 mg/dl	5–50 mg/L	Transfusion reactions Paroxysmal nocturnal hemoglobinuria Intravascular hemolysis	
Hemoglobin A1 (glycohemoglobin)	Nondiabetics & diabetics whose control of glucose is: Good: 4.4%–8.2% Fair: 8.3%–9.2% Poor: >9.2%			

(continued)

Reference Ranges—Serum, Plasma, and Whole Blood Chemistries (continued)

Determination	Normal Adult Reference Range: Conventional Units	SI Units	Clinical Significance: Increased	Decreased
Hexosaminidase, total	Controls: 333–375 nM/ml/h Heterozygotes: 288–644 nM/ml/h Tay-Sachs disease: 284–1232 nM/ml/h Diabetics: 567–3560 nM/ml/h	333–375 μmol/L/h 288–644 μmol/L/h 284–1232 μmol/L/h 567–3560 μmol/L/h	Diabetes Tay-Sachs disease	
Hexosaminidase A	Controls: 49%–68% of total Heterozygotes: 26%–45% of total Tay-Sachs disease: 0%–4% of total Diabetics: 39%–59% of total	Fraction of total: 0.49–0.68 0.26–0.45 0–0.04 0.39–0.59		Tay-Sachs disease and heterozygotes
High-density lipoprotein cholesterol (HDL cholesterol)				HDL cholesterol is lower in patients with increased risk for coronary heart disease

Age (yr)	Males (mg/dl)	Females (mg/dl)	Males (mmol/L)	Females (mmol/L)
0–19	30–65	30–70	0.78–1.68	0.78–1.91
20–29	35–70	35–75	0.91–1.81	0.91–1.94
30–39	30–65	35–80	0.78–1.68	0.91–2.07
40–49	30–65	40–85	0.78–1.68	1.04–2.2
50–59	30–65	35–85	0.78–1.68	0.91–2.2
60–69	30–65	35–85	0.78–1.68	0.91–2.2

Determination	Conventional Units	SI Units	Increased	Decreased
17-Hydroxyprogesterone—RIA	Males: 0.4–4 ng/ml Females: 0.1–3.3 ng/ml Children: 0.1–0.5 ng/ml	1.2–12 nmol/L 0.3–10 nmol/L 0.3–1.5 nmol/L	Congenital adrenal hyperplasia Pregnancy Some cases of adrenal or ovarian adenomas	

Immunoglobulin A	Adults: 50–300 mg/dl (in children the normal values are lower and vary with age)	0.5–3 g/L	Gamma A myeloma Wiskott-Aldrich syndrome Autoimmune disease Hepatic cirrhosis	Ataxia telangiectasis Agammaglobulinemia Hypogammaglobulinemia, transient Dysgammaglobulinemia Protein-losing enteropathies
Immunoglobulin D	0–30 mg/dl	0–300 mg/L	IgD multiple myeloma Some patients with chronic infectious diseases	
Immunoglobulin E	20–740 ng/ml	20–740 μg/L	Allergic patients and those with parasitic infestations	
Immunoglobulin G	Adults: 635–1400 mg/dl	6.35–14 g/L	IgG myeloma Following hyperimmunization Autoimmune disease states Chronic infections	Congenital and acquired hypogammaglobulinemia IgA myelomas, Waldenstrom's (IgM) macroglobulinemia Some malabsorption syndromes Extensive protein loss
Immunoglobulin M	Adults: 40–280 mg/dl	0.4–2.8 g/L	Waldenstrom's macroglobulinemia Parasitic infections Hepatitis	Agammaglobulinemias Some IgG and IgA myelomas Chronic lymphatic leukemia
Insulin—RIA	5–25 μU/ml	0.2–1 μg/L	Insulinoma Acromegaly	Diabetes mellitus
Iron	65–170 μg/dl	11.6–30.4 μmol/L	Pernicious anemia Aplastic anemia Hemolytic anemia Hepatitis Hemochromatosis	Iron deficiency anemia
Iron-binding capacity	IBC: 150–235 μg/dl TIBC: 250–420 μg/dl % Saturation: 20–50	26.9–42.1 μmol/L 44.8–75.2 μmol/L Fraction of total ironbinding capacity: 0.2–0.5	Iron deficiency anemia Acute and chronic blood loss Hepatitis	Chronic infectious diseases Cirrhosis
Isocitric dehydrogenase	50–180 U	0.83–3 U/L	Hepatitis: cirrhosis Obstructive jaundice Metastatic carcinoma of the liver Megaloblastic anemia	
Lactic acid (whole blood)	Venous: 5–20 mg/dl Arterial: 3–7 mg/dl	0.6–2.2 mmol/L 0.3–0.8 mmol/L	Increased muscular activity Congestive heart failure Hemorrhage Shock	

(continued)

Reference Ranges—Serum, Plasma, and Whole Blood Chemistries *(continued)*

	Normal Adult Reference Range		Clinical Significance	
Determination	*Conventional Units*	*SI Units*	*Increased*	*Decreased*
			Some varieties of metabolic acidosis Some febrile infections May be increased in severe liver disease	
Lactic dehydrogenase (LDH)	100–225 mU/ml	100–225 U/L	Untreated pernicious anemia Myocardial infarction Pulmonary infarction Liver disease	
Lactic dehydrogenase isoenzymes				
Total lactic dehydrogenase	100–225 mU/ml	100–225 U/L Fraction of total LDH:	LDH-1 and LDH-2 are increased in myocardial infarction, megaloblastic anemia, and hemolytic anemia LDH-4 and LDH-5 are increased in pulmonary infarction, congestive heart failure, and liver disease	
LDH-1	20%–35%	0.2–0.35		
LDH-2	25%–40%	0.25–0.4		
LDH-3	20%–30%	0.2–0.3		
LDH-4	0–20%	0–0.2		
LDH-5	0–25%	0–0.25		
Lead (whole blood)	Up to 40 μg/dl	Up to 2 μmol/L	Lead poisoning	
Leucine aminopeptidase	80–200 U/ml	19.2–48 U/L	Liver or biliary tract diseases Pancreatic disease Metastatic carcinoma of liver and pancreas Biliary obstruction	
Lipase	0.2–1.5 U/ml	55–417 U/L	Acute and chronic pancreatitis Biliary obstruction Cirrhosis Hepatitis Peptic ulcer	
Lipids, total	400–1000 mg/dl	4–10 g/L	Hypothyroidism Diabetes Nephrosis Glomerulonephritis Hyperlipoproteinemias	Hyperthyroidism

Lipoprotein Phenotype: Summary of Findings in the Primary Hyperlipoproteinemias

Type	Frequency	Appearance	Triglyceride	Cholesterol	Lipoprotein Staining				Secondary Causes
					Beta	*Pre-Beta*	*Alpha*	*Chylomicrons*	
Normal		Clear	Normal	Normal	Moderate	Zero to moderate	Moderate	Weak	
I	Very rare	Creamy	Markedly increased	Normal to moderately increased	Weak	Weak	Weak	Markedly increased	Dysglobulinemia
II	Common	Clear	Normal to slightly increased	Slightly to markedly increased	Strong	Zero to strong	Moderate	Weak	Hypothyroidism, myeloma, hepatic syndrome, macroglobulinemia, and high dietary cholesterol
III	Uncommon	Clear, cloudy, or milky	Increased	Increased	Broad intense band	Extends into beta	Moderate	Weak	
IV	Very common	Clear, cloudy, or milky	Slightly to markedly increased	Normal to slightly increased	Weak to moderate	Moderate to strong	Weak to moderate	Weak	Hypothyroidism, diabetes mellitus, pancreatitis, glycogen storage diseases, nephrotic syndrome, myeloma, pregnancy, and oral contraceptives
V	Rare	Cloudy to creamy	Markedly increased	Increased	Weak	Moderate	Weak	Strong	Diabetes mellitus, pancreatitis, and alcoholism

Type I and II are fat induced; types III and IV are carbohydrate induced; type V is fat and carbohydrate induced.

Lithium	Usual maintenance level: 0.5–1 mEq/L	0.5–1 mmol/L	
Low-density lipoprotein cholesterol (LDL cholesterol)	Age (yr) mg/dl	mmol/L	LDL cholesterol is higher in patients with increased risk for coronary heart disease
	0–19 50–170	1.30–4.40	
	20–29 60–170	1.55–4.40	
	30–39 70–190	1.80–4.92	
	40–49 80–190	2.07–4.92	
	50–59 80–210	2.07–5.44	

(continued)

Reference Ranges—Serum, Plasma, and Whole Blood Chemistries (continued)

	Normal Adult Reference Range		Clinical Significance	
Determination	*Conventional Units*	*SI Units*	*Increased*	*Decreased*
Luteinizing hormone—RIA	Males: 6–30 mIU/ml	1.4–6.9 mg/L	Pituitary tumor Ovarian failure	Depressed or failure to peak—pituitary failure
	Females:			
	Follicular phase: 2–3 mIU/ml	0.5–6.9 mg/L		
	Ovulatory peak: 40–200 mIU/ml	9.2–46 mg/L		
	Luteal phase: 0–20 mIU/ml	0–5 mg/L		
	Postmenopausal: 35–120 mIU/ml	8–27.5 mg/L		
Lysozyme (muramidase)	2.8–8 μg/ml	2.8–8 mg	Certain types of leukemia (acute monocytic leukemia) Inflammatory states and infections	Acute lymphocytic leukemia
Magnesium	1.3–2.4 mEq/L	0.7–1.2 mmol/L	Excess ingestion of magnesium-containing antacids	Chronic alcoholism Severe renal disease Diarrhea Defective growth
Manganese	0.04–1.4 μg/dl	72.9–255 nmol/L		
Mercury	Up to 10 μg/dl	Up to 0.5 μmol/L	Mercury poisoning	
Myoglobin—RIA	Up to 85 ng/ml	Up to 85 μg/ml	Myocardial infarction Muscle necrosis	
5′ Nucleotidase	3.2–11.6 IU/L	3.2–11.6 U/L	Hepatobiliary disease	
Osmolality	280–300 mOsm/kg	280–300 mmol/L	Useful in the study of electrolyte and water balance	Inappropriate secretion of antidiuretic hormone
Parathyroid hormone	160–350 pg/ml	160–350 ng/L	Hyperparathyroidism	
Phenylalanine	1.2–3.5 mg/dl 1st week 0.7–3.5 mg/dl thereafter	0.07–0.21 mmol/L 0.04–0.21 mmol/L	Phenylketonuria	
Phosphatase, acid, total	0–11 UL	0–11 UL	Carcinoma of prostate Advanced Paget's disease Hyperparathyroidism Gaucher's disease	
Phosphatase, acid, prostatic—RIA	0–10 ng/ml Borderline: 2.5–3.3 IU/L	0–10 μg/L	Carcinoma of prostate	

Phosphatase, alkaline	Adults: 30–115 mU/ml	30–115 μ/L	Conditions reflecting increased osteoblastic activity of bone Rickets Hyperparathyroidism Liver disease	
Phosphatase, alkaline, thermostable fraction	Thermostable fraction >35%: hepatic disease and combined disease with predominant hepatic component Thermostable fraction between 25% and 35% combined hepatic and skeletal disease Thermostable fraction <25%: skeletal disease with increased osteoblastic activity		Hepatic disease	
Phosphohexose isomerase	20–90 IU/L	20–90 U/L	Malignancy Disease of heart, liver, and skeletal muscles	
Phospholipids	125–300 mg/dl	1.25–3 g/L	Diabetes Nephritis	
Phosphorus, inorganic	2.5–4.5 mg/dl	0.8–1.45 mmol/L	Chronic nephritis Hypoparathyroidism	Hyperparathyroidism Vitamin D deficiency
Potassium	3.8–5 mEq/L	3.8–5 mmol/L	Addison's disease Oliguria Anuria Tissue breakdown or hemolysis	Diabetic acidosis Diarrhea Vomiting
Progesterone—RIA	Follicular phase: up to 0.8 ng/ml Luteal phase: 10–20 ng/ml End of cycle: <1 ng/ml Pregnant: up to 50 ng/ml in 20th week	2.5 nmol/L 31.8–63.6 nmol/L <3 nmol/L Up to 160 nmol/L	Useful in evaluation of menstrual disorders and infertility and in the evaluation of placental function during pregnancies complicated by toxemia, diabetes mellitus, or threatened miscarriage	

(continued)

Reference Ranges—Serum, Plasma, and Whole Blood Chemistries *(continued)*

	Normal Adult Reference Range		Clinical Significance	
Determination	*Conventional Units*	*SI Units*	*Increased*	*Decreased*
Prolactin—RIA	6–24 ng/ml	6–24 μg/L	Pregnancy Functional or structural disorders of the hypothalamus Pituitary stalk section Pituitary tumors	
Protein, total	6–8 g/dl	60–80 g/L	Hemoconcentration	Malnutrition
Albumin	3.5–5 g/dl	35–50 g/L	Shock	Hemorrhage
Globulin	1.5–3 g/dl	15–30 g/L	Multiple myeloma (globulin fraction) Chronic infections (globulin fraction) Liver disease (globulin)	Loss of plasma from burns Proteinuria
Electrophoresis (cellulose acetate)				
Albumin	3.5–5 g/dl	35–50 g/L		
Alpha-1 globulin	0.2–0.4 g/dl	2–4 g/L		
Alpha-2 globulin	0.6–1 g/dl	6–10 g/L		
Beta globulin	0.6–1.2 g/dl	6–12 g/L		
Gamma globulin	0.7–1.5 g/dl	7–15 g/L		
Protoporphyrin erythrocyte (whole blood)	15–100 μg/dl	0.27–1.80 μmol/L	Lead toxicity Erythropoietic porphyria	
Pyridoxine	3.6–18 ng/ml			A wide spectrum of clinical conditions such as mental depression, peripheral neuropathy, anemia, neonatal seizures, and reactions to certain drug therapies
Pyruvic acid (whole blood)	0.3–0.7 mg/dl	34–80 μmol/L	Diabetes Severe thiamine deficiency Acute phase of some infections, possibly secondary to increased glycogenolysis and glycolysis	

Renin (plasma)—RIA	Normal diet: Supine: 0.3–1.9 ng/ml/hr Upright: 0.6–3.6 ng/ml/hr Low salt diet: Supine: 0.9–4.5 ng/ml/hr Upright: 4.1–9.1 ng/ml/hr	0.08–0.52 ng/L/sec 0.16–1.00 μg/L/sec 0.25–1.25 μg/L/sec 1.13–2.53 μg/L/sec	Renovascular hypertension Malignant hypertension Untreated Addison's disease Primary salt-losing nephropathy Low-salt diet Diuretic therapy Hemorrhage	Frank primary aldosteronism Increased salt intake Salt-retaining steroid therapy Antidiuretic hormone therapy Blood transfusion
Sodium	135–145 mEq/L	135–145 mmol/L	Hemoconcentration Nephritis Pyloric obstruction	Alkali deficit Addison's disease Myxedema
Sulfate (inorganic)	0.5–1.5 mg/dl	0.05–0.15 mmol/L	Nephritis Nitrogen retention	
Testosterone—RIA	Females: 25–100 ng/dl Males: 300–800 ng/dl	0.9–3.5 nmol/L 10.5–28 nmol/L	Females: Polycystic ovary Virilizing tumors	Males: Orchidectomy for neoplastic disease of the prostate or breast Estrogen therapy Klinefelter's syndrome Hypopituitarism Hypogonadism Hepatic cirrhosis
T_3 (triiodothyronine) uptake	25%–35%	Relative uptake fraction: 0.25–0.35	Hyperthyroidism TBG deficiency Androgens and anabolic steroids	Hypothyroidism Pregnancy TBG excess Estrogens and antiovulatory drugs
T_3, total circulating—RIA	75–200 ng/dl	1.15–3.1 nmol/L	Pregnancy Hyperthyroidism	Hypothyroidiam
T_4 (thyroxine)—RIA	4.5–11.5 μg/dl	58.5–150 nmol/L	Hyperthyroidism Thyroiditis Elevated thyroxine-binding proteins caused by oral contraceptives Pregnancy	Primary and pituitary hypothyroidism Idiopathic involvement Cases of diminished thyroxine-binding proteins caused by androgenic and anabolic steroids Hypoproteinemia Nephrotic syndrome
T_4, free	1–2.2 ng/dl	13–30 pmol/L	Euthyroid patients with normal free thyroxine levels may have abnormal T_3 and T_4 levels caused by drug preparations	

(continued)

Reference Ranges—Serum, Plasma, and Whole Blood Chemistries (continued)

Determination	Normal Adult Reference Range		Clinical Significance	
	Conventional Units	*SI Units*	*Increased*	*Decreased*
Thyroid-stimulating hormone (TSH)—RIA		0.3–5 m/IU/L	Hypothyroidism	Hyperthyroidism
Thyroid-binding globulin	10–26 μg/dl	100–260 μg/L	Hypothyroidism Pregnancy Estrogen therapy Oral contraceptives Genetic and idiopathic	Androgens and anabolic steroids Nephrotic syndrome Marked hypoproteinemia Hepatic disease
Transaminase, serum glutamic-oxaloacetate (SGOT, aspartate aminotransferase)	7–40 U/ml	4–20 U/L	Myocardial infarction Skeletal muscle disease Liver disease	
Transaminase, serum glutamic-pyruvic (SGPT, alanine aminotransferase)	10–40 U/ml	5–20 U/L	Same conditions as SGOT, but increase is more marked in liver disease than SGOT	
Transferrin	230–320 mg/dl	2.3–3.2 g/L	Pregnancy Iron-deficiency anemia due to hemorrhaging Acute hepatitis Polycythemia Oral contraceptives	Pernicious anemia in relapse Thalassemia and sickle cell anemia Chromatosis Neoplastic and hepatic diseases
Triglycerides	10–150 mg/dl	0.10–1.65 mmol/L	See lipoprotein phenotype table, pp. 1999–2000	
Tryptophan	1.4–3 mg/dl	68.6–147 nmol/L		Tryptophan-specific malabsorption syndrome
Tyrosine	0.5–4 mg/dl	27.6–220.8 mmol/L	Tyrosinosis	
Urea nitrogen (BUN)	10–20 mg/dl	3.6–7.2 mmol/L	Acute glomerulonephritis Obstructive uropathy Mercury poisoning Nephrotic syndrome	Severe hepatic failure Pregnancy
Uric acid	2.5–8 mg/dl	0.15–0.5 mmol/L	Gouty arthritis Acute leukemia Lymphomas treated by chemotherapy Toxemia of pregnancy	Xanthinuria Defective tubular reabsorption

Viscosity	1.4–1.8 relative to water at 37°C (98.6°F)		Patients with marked increases of the gamma globulins	
Vitamin A	50–220 μg/dl	1.75–7.7 μmol/L	Hypervitaminosis A	Vitamin A deficiency Celiac disease Sprue Obstructive jaundice Giardiasis Parenchymal hepatic disease
Vitamin B_1 (thiamine)	1.6–4 μg/dl	47.4–135.7 nmol/L		Anorexia Beriberi Polyneuropathy Cardiomyopathies
Vitamin B_6 (pyridoxal phosphate)	3.6–18 ng/ml	14.6–72.8 nmol/L		Chronic alcoholism Malnutrition Uremia Neonatal seizures Malabsorption, such as celiac syndrome
Vitamin B_{12}—RIA	130–785 pg/ml	100–580 pmol/L	Hepatic cell damage and in association with the myeloproliferative disorders (the highest levels are encountered in myeloid leukemia)	Strict vegetarianism Alcoholism Pernicious anemia Total or partial gastrectomy Ileal resection Sprue and celiac disease Fish tapeworm infestation
Vitamin E	0.5–2 mg/dl	11.6–46.4 μmol/L		Vitamin E deficiency
Xylose absorption test	2 hr, 30–50 mg/dl	2–3.35 mmol/L		Malabsorption syndrome
Zinc	55–150 μg/dl	7.65–22.95 μmol/L	Zinc is essential for the growth and propagation of cell cultures and the functioning of several enzymes	

Reference Ranges—Urine Chemistry

	Normal Adult Reference Range		Clinical Significance	
Determination	*Conventional Units*	*SI Units*	*Increased*	*Decreased*
Acetone and acetoacetate	Zero		Uncontrolled diabetes Starvation	

(continued)

Reference Ranges—Urine Chemistry *(continued)*

Determination	Normal Adult Reference Range		Clinical Significance	
	Conventional Units	*SI Units*	*Increased*	*Decreased*
Acid mucopolysaccharides	Negative		Hurler's syndrome Marfan's syndrome Morquio-Ulrich disease	
Aldosterone	Normal salt: Normal: 4–20 μg/24 hr Renovascular: 10–40 μg/24 hr Tumor: 20–100 μg/24 hr	11.1–55.5 nmol/24 hr 27.7–111 nmol/24 hr 55.4–227 nmol/24 hr	Primary aldosteronism (adrenocortical tumor) Secondary aldosteronism Salt depletion Potassium loading ACTH in large doses Cardiac failure Cirrhosis with ascites formation Nephrosis Pregnancy	
Alpha amino nitrogen	50–200 mg/24 hr	3.6–14.3 mmol/24 hr	Leukemia Diabetes Phenylketonuria Other metabolic diseases	
Amylase	35–260 units excreted per hr	6.5–48.1 U/hr	Acute pancreatitis	
Arylsulfatase A	>2.4 U/ml			Metachromatic leukodystrophy
Bence-Jones protein	None detected		Myeloma	
Calcium	<150 mg/24 hr	<3.75 mmol/24 hr	Hyperparathyroidism Vitamin D intoxication Fanconi syndrome	Hypoparathyroidism Vitamin D deficiency
Catecholamines	Total: 0–275 μg/24 hr Epinephrine: 10%–40% Norepinephrine: 60%–90%	0–275 μg/24 hr Fraction total: 0.10–8.4 Fraction total: 0.60–0.90	Pheochromocytoma Neuroblastoma	
Chorionic gonadotrophin, qualitative (pregnancy test)	Negative		Pregnancy Chorionepithelioma Hydatidiform mole	

Copper	20–70 μg/24 hr	0.32–1.12 μmol/ 24 hr	Wilson's disease Cirrhosis Nephrosis	
Coproporphyrin	50–300 μg/24 hr	0.075–0.45 μmol/ 24 hr	Poliomyelitis Lead poisoning Porphyria hepatica Porphyria erythropoietica Porphyria cutanea tarda	
Cortisol, free	20–90 μg/24 hr	55.2–248.4 nmol/day	Cushing's syndrome	
Creatine	0–200 mg/24 hr	0–1.52 mmol/24 hr	Muscular dystrophy Fever Carcinoma of liver Pregnancy Hyperthyroidism Myositis	
Creatinine	0.8–2 g/24 hr	7–17.6 mmol/24 hr	Typhoid fever Salmonella infections Tetanus	Muscular atrophy Anemia Advanced degeneration of kidneys Leukemia
Creatinine clearance	100–150 ml of blood cleared of creatinine per min	1.67–2.5 ml/sec		Measures glomerular filtration rate Renal diseases
Cystine and cysteine	10–100 mg/24 hr	0.08–0.83 mmol/ 24 hr	Cystinuria	
Delta aminolevulinic acid	0–0.54 mg/dl	0–40 μmol/L	Lead poisoning Porphyria hepatica Hepatitis Hepatic carcinoma	
11-Desoxycortisol	20–100 μg/24 hr	0.6–2.9 μmol/day	Hypertensive form of virilizing adrenal hyperplasia due to an 11-beta hydroxylase defect	

(continued)

Reference Ranges—Urine Chemistry (continued)

	Normal Adult Reference Range		Clinical Significance	
Determination	*Conventional Units*	*SI Units*	*Increased*	*Decreased*
Estriol (placental)	**Weeks of Pregnancy**	**µm/24 hr**	**nmol/24 hr**	Decreased values occur with fetal distress of many conditions, including preeclampsia, placental insufficiency, and poorly controlled diabetes mellitus
	12	<1	<3.5	
	16	2–7	7–24.5	
	20	4–9	14–32	
	24	6–13	21–45.5	
	28	8–22	28–77	
	32	12–43	42–150	
	36	14–45	49–159	
	40	19–46	66.5–160	
Estrogens, total (fluorometric)	Females:		Hyperestrogenism due to gonadal or adrenal neoplasm	Primary or secondary amenorrhea
	Onset of menstruation: 4–25 µg/24 hr	4–25 µg/24 hr		
	Ovulation peak: 28 µg/24 hr	28 µg/24 hr		
	Luteal peak: 22–105 µg/24 hr	22–105 µg/24 hr		
	Menopausal: 1.4–19.6 µg/24 hr	1.4–19.6 µg/24 hr		
	Males: 5–18 µg/24 hr	5–18 µg/24 hr		
Etiocholanolone	Males: 1.9–6 mg/24 hr	6.5–20.6 µmol/24 hr	Adrenogenital syndrome Idiopathic hirsutism	
	Females: 0.5–4 mg/24 hr	1.7–13.8 µmol/24 hr		
Follicle-stimulating hormone—RIA	Females:		Menopause and primary ovarian failure	Pituitary failure
	Follicular: 5–20 IU/24 hr	5–20 IU/day		
	Luteal: 5–15 IU/24 hr	5–15 IU/day		
	Midcycle: 15–60 IU/24 hr	15–60 IU/day		
	Menopausal: 50–100 IU/24 hr	50–100 IU/day		
	Males: 5–25 IU/24 hr	5–25 IU/day		

Glucose	Negative		Diabetes mellitus Pituitary disorders Intracranial pressure Lesion in floor of 4th ventricle	
Hemoglobin and myoglobin	Negative		Extensive burns Transfusion of incompatible blood Myoglobin increased in severe crushing injuries to muscles	
Homogentisic acid, qualitative	Negative		Alkaptonuria Ochronosis	
Homovanillic acid	Up to 15 mg/24 hr	Up to 82 μmol/day	Neuroblastoma	
17-hydroxycorticosteroids	2–10 mg/24 hr	5.5–27.5 μmol/day	Cushing's disease	Addison's disease Anterior pituitary hypofunction
5-Hydroxyindoleacetic acid, qualitative	Negative		Malignant carcinoid tumors	
Hydroxyproline	15–43 mg/24 hr	0.11–0.33 μmol/day	Paget's disease Fibrous dysplasia Osteomalacia Neoplastic bone disease Hyperparathyroidism	
17-Ketosteroids, total	Males: 10–22 mg/24 hr Females: 6–16 mg/24 hr	 35–76 μmol/day 21–55 μmol/day	Interstitial cell tumor of testes Simple hirsutism, occasionally Adrenal hyperplasia Cushing's syndrome Adrenal cancer, virilism Arrhenoblastoma	Thyrotoxicosis Female hypogonadism Diabetes mellitus Hypertension Debilitating disease of mild to moderate severity Eunuchoidism Addison's disease Panhypopituitarism Myxedema Nephrosis
Lead	Up to 150 μg/24 hr	Up to 60 μmol/24 hr	Lead poisoning	
Luteinizing hormone	Males: 5–18 IU/24 hr Females: Follicular phase: 2–25 IU/24 hr Ovulatory peak: 30–95 IU/24 h	 2–25 IU/day 30–95 IU/day	Pituitary tumor Ovarian failure	Depressed or failure to peak—pituitary failure

(continued)

Reference Ranges—Urine Chemistry (continued)

Determination	Normal Adult Reference Range		Clinical Significance	
	Conventional Units	*SI Units*	*Increased*	*Decreased*
	Luteal phase: 2–20 IU/24 hr Postmenopausal: 40–110 IU/24 hr	2–20 IU/day 40–100 IU/day		
Metanephrines, total	Less than 1.3 mg/24 hr	Less than 6.5 μmol/day	Pheochromocytoma; a few patients with pheochromocytoma may have elevated urinary metanephrines but normal catecholamines and VMA	
Osmolality	Males: 390–1090 mM/kg Females: 300–1090 mM/kg	390–1090 mmol/kg 300–1090 mmol/kg	Useful in the study of electrolyte and water balance	
Oxalate	Up to 40 mg/24 hr	Up to 456 μmol/day	Primary hyperoxaluria	
Phenylpyruvic acid qualitative	Negative		Phenylketonuria	
Phosphorus, inorganic	0.8–1.3 g/24 hr	26–42 mmol/24 hr	Hyperparathyroidism Vitamin D intoxication Paget's disease Metastatic neoplasm to bone	Hypoparathyroidism Vitamin D deficiency
Porphobilinogen, qualitative	Negative		Chronic lead poisoning Acute porphyria Liver disease	
Porphobilinogen, quantitative	0–1 mg/24 hr	0–4.4 μmol/24 hr	Acute porphyria Liver disease	
Porphyrins, qualitative	Negative		See porphyrins, quantiative	
Porphyrins, quantitative (coproporphyrin and uroporphyrin)	Coproporphyrin: 50–160 μg/24 hr Uroporphyrin: up to 50 μg/24 hr	0.075–0.24 μmol/24 hr Up to 0.06 μmol/24 hr	Porphyria hepatica Porphyria erythropoietica Porphyria cutanea tarda Lead poisoning (only coproporphyrin increased)	

Potassium	40–65 mEq/24 hr	40–65 mmol/24 hr	Hemolysis	
Pregnanediol	Females:		Corpus luteum cysts	Placental dysfunction
	Proliferative phase: 0.5–1.5 mg/24 hr	1.6–4.8 μmol/24 hr	When placental tissue remains in the uterus following parturition	Threatened abortion Intrauterine death
	Luteal phase: 2–7 mg/24 hr	6–22 μmol/24 hr	Some cases of adrenocortical tumors	
	Menopause: 0.2–1 mg/24 hr	0.6–3.1 μmol/24 hr		
	Pregnancy:			
	Weeks of Gestation	**mg/24 hr**	**μmol/24 hr**	
	10–12	5–15	15.6–47	
	12–18	5–25	15.6–78.0	
	18–24	15–33	47.0–103.0	
	24–28	20–42	62.4–131.0	
	28–32	27–47	84.2–146.6	
	Males: 0.1–2 mg/24 hr	0.3–6.2 μmol/24 hr		
Pregnanetriol	0.4–2.4 mg/24 hr	1.2–7.1 μmol/24 hr	Congenital adrenal androgenic hyperplasia	
Protein	Up to 100 mg/24 hr	Up to 100 mg/24 hr	Nephritis Cardiac failure Mercury poisoning Bence-Jones protein in multiple myeloma Febrile states Hematuria	
Sodium	130–200 mEq/24 hr	130–200 mmol/24 hr	Useful in detecting gross changes in water and salt balance	
Titratable acidity	20–40 mEq/24 hr	20–40 mmol/24 hr	Metabolic acidosis	Metabolic alkalosis
Urea nitrogen	9–16 gm/24 hr	0.32–0.57 mol/L	Excessive protein catabolism	Impaired kidney function
Uric acid	250–750 mg/24 hr	1.48–4.43 mmol/24 hr	Gout	Nephritis
Urobilinogen	Random urine: <0.25 mg/dl 24-hour urine: up to 4 mg/24 hr	<0.42 mol/24 hr Up to 6.76 μmol/24 hr	Liver and biliary tract disease Hemolytic anemias	Complete or nearly complete biliary obstruction Diarrhea Renal insufficiency
Uroporphyrins	Up to 50 μg/24 hr	Up to 0.06 μmol/24 hr	Porphyria	

(continued)

Reference Ranges—Urine Chemistry (continued)

Determination	Normal Adult Reference Range		Clinical Significance	
	Conventional Units	*SI Units*	*Increased*	*Decreased*
Vanillylmandelic acid (VMA)	0.7–6.8 mg/24 hr	3.5–34.3 μmol/24 hr	Pheochromocytoma Neuroblastoma Coffee, tea, aspirin, bananas, and several different drugs	
Xylose absorption test (5 hour)	16%–33% of ingested xylose	Fraction absorbed: 0.16–0.33		Malabsorption syndromes
Zinc	0.15–1.2 mg/24 hr	2.3–18.4 μmol/24 hr	Zinc is an essential nutritional element	

Reference Ranges—Cerebrospinal Fluid

Determination	Normal Adult Reference Range		Clinical Significance	
	Conventional Units	*SI Units*	*Increased*	*Decreased*
Albumin	15–30 mg/dl	150–300 mg/L	Certain neurologic disorders Lesion in the choroid plexus or blockage of the flow of CSF Damage to the blood–CNS barrier	
Cell count	0–5 mononuclear cells per mm^3	$0–5 \times 10^6$/L	Bacterial meningitis Neurosyphilis Anterior poliomyelitis Encephalitis lethargica	
Chloride	100–130 mEq/L	100–300 mmol/L	Uremia	Acute generalized meningitis Tuberculous meningitis
Glucose	50–75 mg/dl	2.75–4.13 mmol/L	Diabetes mellitus Diabetic coma Epidemic encephalitis Uremia	Acute meningitides Tuberculous meningitis Insulin shock
Glutamine	6–15 mg/dl	0.41–1 mmol/L	Hepatic encephalopathies, including Reye's syndrome Hepatic coma Cirrhosis	

IgG	0–6.6 mg/dl	0–66 mg/L	Damage to the blood–CNS barrier Multiple sclerosis Neurosyphilis Subacute sclerosing panencephalitis Chronic phases of CNS infections
Lactic acid	<24 mg/dl	<2.7 mmol/L	Bacterial meningitis Hypocapnia Hydrocephalus Brain abscesses Cerebral ischemia
Lactic dehydrogenase	1/10 that of serum	Activity fraction: 0.1 that of serum	CNS disease
Protein:			Acute meningitis
Lumbar	15–45 mg/dl	150–450 mg/L	Tubercular meningitis
Cisternal	15–25 mg/dl	150–250 mg/L	Neurosyphilis
Ventricular	5–15 mg/dl	50–150 mg/L	Poliomyelitis Guillain-Barré syndrome
Protein electrophoresis	% of total:	Fraction:	An increase in the level of albumin alone can be the result of a lesion in the choroid plexus or a blockage of the flow of CSF. An elevated gamma globulin value with a normal albumin level has been reported in multiple sclerosis, neurosyphilis, subacute sclerosing panencephalitis, and the chronic phase of CNS infections. If the blood–CNS barrier has been damaged severely during the course of these diseases, the CSF albumin level may also be elevated.
(cellulose acetate)	3–7	0.03–0.07	
Prealbumin	56–74	0.56–0.74	
Albumin	2–6.5	0.02–0.065	
$Alpha_1$ globulin	3–12	0.03–0.12	
$Alpha_2$ globulin	8–18.5	0.08–0.185	
Beta globulin	4–14	0.04–0.14	
Gamma globulin			

Gastric Analysis

	Normal Adult Reference Range		Clinical Significance	
Determination	*Conventional Units*	*SI Units*	*Increased*	*Decreased*
pH	<2	<2		Pernicious anemia
Basal acid output	0–6 mEq/hr	0–6 mmol/hr	Peptic ulcer	Gastric carcinoma
Maximum acid	5–50 mEq/hr	5–40 mmol/hr	Zollinger-Ellison syndrome	Chronic atrophic gastritis
				Decreased normally with age

Miscellaneous Values

		Clinical Significance	
Determinations	**Normal Value**	*Conventional Units*	*SI Units*
Acetaminophen	0	Therapeutic level: 10–20 μg/ml	10–20 mg/L
Aminophylline (theophylline)	0	Therapeutic level: 10–20 μg/ml	10–20 mg/L
Bromide	0	Therapeutic level: 5–50 mg/dl	50–500 mg/L
Carbon monoxide	0%–2%	Symptoms with >20% saturation	
Chlordiazepoxide	0	Therapeutic level: 1–3 μg/ml	1–3 mg/L
Diazepam	0	Therapeutic level: 0.5–2.5 μg/dl	5–25 μg/L
Digitoxin	0	Therapeutic level: 5–30 ng/ml	5–30 μg/L
Digoxin	0	Therapeutic level: 0.5–2 ng/ml	0.5–2 μg/L
Ethanol	0%–0.01%	Legal intoxication level: 0.10% or above 0.3%–0.4%: marked intoxication 0.4%–0.5%: alcoholic stupor	
Gentamicin	0	Therapeutic level: 4–10 μg/ml	4–10 mg/L
Methanol	0	May be fatal in concentration as low as 10 mg/dl	100 mg/L
Phenobarbital	0	Therapeutic level: 15–40 μg/ml	10–20 mg/L
Phenytoin	0	Therapeutic level: 10–20 μg/ml	10–20 mg/L
Primidone	0	Therapeutic level: 5–12 μg/ml	5–12 mg/L
Quinidine	0	Therapeutic level: 0.2–0.5 mg/dl	2–5 mg/L
Salicylate	0	Therapeutic level: 2–25 mg/dl	20–250 mg/L
		Toxic level: >30 mg/dl	300 mg/L
Sulfonamide	0	Therapeutic levels:	
		Sulfadiazine 8–15 mg/dl	80–150 mg/L
		Sulfaguanidine 3–5 mg/dl	30–50 mg/L
		Sulfamerazine 10–15 mg/dl	100–150 mg/L
		Sulfanilamide 10–15 mg/dl	100–150 mg/L

SUBJECT INDEX

ISBN 0-397-55014-6